MALPRACTICE RISK MANAGEMENT IN PSYCHIATRY

A Comprehensive Guide

MALPRACTICE RISK MANAGEMENT IN PSYCHIATRY

A Comprehensive Guide

Edited by
FREDERIC FLACH, M.D.

A HATHERLEIGH CME BOOK
HATHERLEIGH PRESS
New York

Hatherleigh Press
1114 First Avenue, Suite 500
New York, NY 10021
1-800-906-1234
www.hatherleigh.com

DISCLAIMER
This book does not give legal or medical advice.
Always consult your physician, attorney, and other professionals.
The names of people who contributed anecdotal material have been changed.

The ideas and suggestions contained in this book are not intended
as a substitute for consulting with a physician or attorney.
All matters regarding your health require medical supervision.

Library of Congress Cataloging-in-Publication Data

Malpractice risk management in psychiatry : a comprehensive guide / edited
by Frederic Flach.
p.   cm.
Includes bibliographical references and index.
ISBN 1-57826-013-2 (alk. paper)
1. Psychiatrists—Malpractice—United States. I. Flach, Frederic F.
[DNLM: WM 33 AA1 M259 1997]
KF2910.P753M354   1997
344.73'04121—dc21
DNLM/DLC
Library of Congress   97-3799
                                                                    CIP

All Hatherleigh Press titles are available for bulk purchase,
special promotions, and premiums. For more information, please contact
the manager of our Special sales department at 1-800-906-1234.

Designed by Dede Cummings Designs

10 9 8 7 6 5 4 3 2 1

Printed in Canada

CONTENTS

CONTRIBUTING AUTHORS

EDWARD E. BARTLETT, PHD.
Dr. Bartlett is Associate Adjunct Professor in the Department of Community and Family Medicine at Georgetown University, Washington, DC

KENNETH DUCKWORTH, M.D. AND
THOMAS G. GUTHEIL, M.D.
Dr. Duckworth is Instructor in Psychiatry at the Massachusetts Mental Health Center, Harvard Medical School, Department of Psychiatry, Boston, MA.

Dr. Gutheil is Professor of Psychiatry at the Massachusetts Mental Health Center, Harvard Medical School, Department of Psychiatry, Boston, MA.

MARK S. GOLD, M.D., FCP, FAPA
Dr. Gold is Professor, University of Florida Brain Institute, Departments of Neuroscience, Psychiatry, and Community Health & Family Medicine, Gainesville, FL.

OTTO KAUSCH, M.D. AND PHILIP J. RESNICK, M.D.
Dr. Kausch is Assistant Professor, Case Western Reserve University, and Attending Psychiatrist, VA Medical Center, Brecksville, OH.

Dr. Resnick is Professor of Psychiatry, Case Western Reserve University, and Director of Forensic Psychiatry, University Hospitals of Cleveland, OH.

LAWRENCE L. KERNS, M.D., AND
CAROL GERNER, J.D.
Dr. Kerns is in private practice with Kerns and Associates in Barrington, IL.

Ms. Gerner is an attorney with the Chicago office of Sedgwick, Detert, Moran, and Arnold, specializing in malpractice litigation and managed care liability problems.

KATHLEEN MERO MOGUL, M.D.
Dr. Mogul is Associate Professor of Psychiatry at Tufts University Medical School, Boston, MA.

DOUGLAS MOSSMAN, PHD.

Dr. Mossman is Associate Clinical Professor and Director, Division of Forensic Psychiatry, Wright State University School of Medicine, and adjunct faculty member, University of Dayton School of Law, Dayton, OH.

JEROME A. MOTTO, M.D.

Dr. Motto is Professor of Psychiatry at University of California School of Medicine, San Francisco.

SILVIA W. OLARTE, M.D.

Dr. Olarte is Clinical Professor of Psychiatry and faculty member of the Psychoanalytic Institute, Department of Psychiatry, New York Medical College, Valhalla, NY.

MICHAEL L. PERLIN, ESQ.

Mr. Perlin is the Professor of Law at the New York Law School, New York, NY.

JARRETT W. RICHARDSON, M.D.

Dr. Richardson is Consultant in Psychiatry, Mayo Clinic, Rochester, MN

JAMES E. ROSENBERG, M.D.

Dr. Rosenberg is Assistant Clinical Professor of Psychiatry, UCLA School of Medicine, and Chief, Psychiatric Intensive Care Units, West Los Angeles VA Medical Center, Los Angeles, CA.

ROBERT L. SADOFF, M.D.

Dr. Sadoff is Clinical Professor of Psychiatry and Director of the Center for Studies in Social-Legal Psychiatry, University of Pennsylvania, Philadelphia.

JOAN SALTMAN, ESQ.

Ms. Saltzman is a practicing attorney in Philadelphia whose practice is limited to medical malpractice law, mental health law, and appellate cases. She is a teacher at the National Institute for Trial Advocacy, Notre Dame Law School, South Bend, IN.

GEORGE S. SIGEL, M.D.

Dr. Sigel is Director of Admission Services at Bridgewater State Hospital, Bridgewater, MA.

ROBERT I. SIMON, M.D.

Dr. Simon is Clinical Professor of Psychiatry and Director of the Program in Psychiatry and Law at Georgetown University School of Medicine, Washington, DC.

INTRODUCTION

The number of psychiatric malpractice cases has grown significantly in the past two to three decades. Patients have become more litigious and plaintiffs' lawyers have become increasingly creative in finding reasons to blame psychiatrists for negative reactions, some of which may be totally unpredictable, unexpected, or unforeseen.

Furthermore, the practice of psychiatry has changed significantly over this time span. Laws affecting the mentally ill, restricting involuntary committment, and providing patients with rights when hospitalized have changed considerably. And then there's managed care. Managed care has added a new dimension to the malpractice issues psychiatrists must confront. When third party payers have the power to dictate the quality of psychiatric care irrespective of a psychiatrist's assessment of his patient's needs, the likelihood of substandard care increases, and so, therefore, does the risk of malpractice claims. Management of malpractice risk is primarily geared toward maintaining a high standard of professional practice, and avoiding malpractice lawsuits.

Perhaps the two most important areas that have led to malpractice claims are the use of various psychotropic agents in the treatment of psychiatric patients and the concept of dangerousness, to oneself or others, that has become the standard for involuntary committment of the mentally ill. The rise in the utilization of psychotropic agents for a number of psychiatric conditions has given rise to standards of care concerning the use of such medication. The prudent practitioner must be aware of side effects of individual medications, effects of combinations of medications, and contraindications for the use of other medications. Failure to follow these standards and guidelines may jeopardize the patient's health and become an ever more prevalent basis for malpractice action.

Psychiatrists are charged with protecting society from the violent and self-destructive behavior of the mentally ill. We are regarded as having the special ability to predict dangerousness and are held responsible when our patients, current and former, behave inappropriately, violently, or self-destructively.

Other causes of malpractice in psychiatry include mishandling transference or boundary violations in the doctor-patient relationship; breach of confidentiality; violation of *Tarasoff* or duty-to-protect guidelines; and intentional infliction of emotional harm on patients.

The anatomy of a psychiatric malpractice suit involves the four D's: the damage to the patient is a direct result of dereliction of the duty the psychiatrist owes to the patient. Unless all four elements are present and related, there should be no valid lawsuit.

Finally, coping with a malpractice suit has been a problem for many psychiatrists who have difficulty handling the emotional trauma accompanying such a suit. First, the psychiatrist usually has difficulty processing emotions evoked by the charge that he or she is guilty of the transgressions enumerated in the complaint. Secondly, the lawsuit may progress for several years, invading the psychiatrist's privacy, interfering with his or her life, both personal or professional. The best way to handle such trauma is to avoid or prevent a lawsuit by following the various standards of care without exception.

Malpractice risks in psychiatry must be recognized and minimized wherever they occur for the same reason that the welfare of the patient must always be the primary concern of the doctor. It is simply good medicine.

—*Robert L. Sadoff, M.D.*

PART I

Psychiatric Malpractice

1

The Basis of
Medical Malpractice[*]

MICHAEL L. PERLIN, ESQ.

Editor's Note

Malpractice implies negligence. Each negligence case has five basic elements: (1) something is done or not done by (2) someone legally obligated to conform to a code of conduct to protect others from unreasonable risk which (3) exposed someone to an unreasonable risk of harm; (4) the action or inaction must be the proximate cause of the injury, and (5) the plaintiff must prove he or she has actually suffered damage to warrant liability. Medical malpractice is defined as the negligent performance of duties by a physician perforce the assumed contractual relations entered into with a patient. It is distinguished from ordinary negligence by the application of a standard of care determined by other medical experts in the field. Because of the varied approaches advocated for the treatment of psychiatric patients, establishing such a standard of care is quite complex.

---

[*]This and the following three sections by Mr. Perlin are largely adapted from Chapter 12 of Perlin, *Mental Disability Law: Civil and Criminal* (©Kluwer Law Books, 1988).

A Rising Incidence of Psychiatric Malpractice Suits

For the psychiatrist few topics are more anxiety-provoking than the threat (or fear) of malpractice litigation. Although such suits are still remarkably rare, their potentiality remains significant to all practitioners.

Traditionally, there have been dramatically fewer malpractice claims against psychiatrists than against nonpsychiatric physicians.[1] Standard estimates had suggested that only about 1.5 such claims were filed per 100 psychiatrists annually, while other medical practitioners were sued at the annual rate of 25 per 100.[2] Although the incidence of bringing suits against psychiatrists is clearly growing[3]—by 1993, the frequency had risen to about 6%[4]—it is still substantially lower than that for other medical specialties. In Dr. Paul Slawson's words, psychiatrists thus "continue to enjoy more favorable loss experience."[5]

Listed below are the numerous reasons which have been offered to explain the relatively low incidence of malpractice suits against psychiatrists:[6] The general reluctance of tort law to provide money damages for emotional injuries;[7] the difficulty of proving in a court of law an applicable standard of care and a causal relationship between the breach of the standard of care and the alleged injury;[8] the fact that psychiatric medicine remains "somewhat of an enigma to most trial lawyers";[9] the stigma which patients fear might result from making public their psychiatric history;[10] a patient's reluctance to sue as a result of emotional ties to his/her psychiatrist[11] and/or the patient's belief that successful psychotherapy requires full cooperation with the psychiatrist;[12] many patients' inability to either formulate clear expectations or assess the "success" of their treatment;[13] the ability of trained psychiatrists to therapeutically deal with patient hostility and thus avert a suit;[14] and the frequency with which many patients see their psychiatrists.[15]

This "most favored nation" status[16] which psychiatry benefits from is changing for a combination of reasons. First, tort law has become generally more receptive to suits alleging emotional injuries.[17] Second, to some extent, individuals who have sought psychotherapeutic treatment have been more open about it, thus lessening, for *some* potential plaintiffs, the stigma of having to divulge the fact of their treatment.[18] Third, the "explosion"[19] in litigation on behalf of the institutionalized mentally disabled has made judges and lawyers far more familiar with cases involving psychiatric treatment than they were twenty years ago.[20] Fourth, as more is learned about the side effects of neuroleptic drugs (specifically, tardive dyskinesia), it is inevitable that new litigation will increase.[21] Fifth, as a few idiosyncratic verdicts are publicized,[22] aggrieved patients may begin to feel that, in spite of stigma and embarrassment, it may be sufficiently financially worthwhile to file suit.

The Definition of Negligence[23]

There are five basic elements in a negligence case:[24]

1. An act: The actor must do something (or not do something for which he is under an affirmative duty to do).[25]
2. Duty of care: There must be a legal obligation requiring the defendant to conform to a certain conduct code so as to insulate others from unreasonable risks.[26] The standard is an objective one, reflecting a "reasonable person of ordinary prudence";[27] although evidence of custom, folkways, or statutory compliance is admissible,[28] it is not conclusive.[29]

   Courts have been forever split on the issue of to whom the duty is owed.[30] In the majority of jurisdictions, a defendant owes a duty of care to anyone who might suffer injury as a proximate result of a breach of duty.[31] In the minority, the duty of care is only to those persons within the "zone of danger" in which a reasonable person would have foreseen a risk of harm to the plaintiff.[32]
3. Breach: If a duty of care is present, there must be some evidence that the defendant breached that duty (by doing or failing to do something) which exposed the plaintiff to an unreasonable risk of harm.[33]
4. Causation: The defendant's conduct must be the "proximate cause" of the plaintiff's injuries.[34] It need not be the last act prior to the injury, but may be the one which actually aided, as a "direct and existing cause," in producing the injury.[35] If there is a question of "intervening causation"—that is, if there is an injury to which a defendant substantially contributed but was brought about, at a later date, by another cause of origin independent of the defendant—the court will ask whether it was reasonably foresee-

able that the subsequently intervening force would be involved and that the final result would thus occur.[36]

5. Damages: The plaintiff must prove that he/she suffered some damage in order for the defendant to be liable.[37] In any negligence case, there must be proof of actual damages.[38]

Medical Malpractice

Medical malpractice has been defined as the negligent performance of duties which are devolved upon a physician because of the implied contractual relations entered into with the patient.[39] It is distinguished from the ordinary negligence by the application of a standard of care determined by other medical experts in the field.[40] A specialist, such as a psychotherapist, is expected to adhere to the standard of care of a reasonably prudent and careful specialist in that specific area of practice.[41]

Thus, in the lead case of *Stone v. Proctor*,[42] which involved electroshock administration, the North Carolina Supreme Court determined that a psychiatrist must:

(1) possess the degree of professional learning, skill and ability which others similarly situated ordinarily possess; (2) exercise reasonable care and diligence in the application of his knowledge and skill to the patient's case; and (3) use his best judgment in the treatment and care of his patient.[43]

This, however, does not require that the specialist insure adequate results,[44] nor does it mean that the professional exercise "extraordinary skill and care or even the highest degree of skill and care possible."[45] A doctor is not liable for a "mere error of judgment, provided he does what he thinks is best after careful examination."[46] Reasonableness, not extraordinary ability, is the requirement.

Standards of Care for Mental Health Professionals

Generally, the law does not express a preference for one form of treatment over another. Practitioners are judged against the standards created by their own school of treatment,[47] as long as the method is supported "by a respectable minority of [practitioners, and] as long as the [defendant] has adhered to the acceptable procedures of administering the treatment as espoused by the minority."[48]

Because of the remarkable diversity of psychotherapeutic treatments (nearly 200 different approaches have been catalogued),[49] the problems of defining an appropriate standard are increased.[50] Since "respected minorities" are legion in psychotherapy,[51] in certain circumstances, courts have shifted the burden to the practitioner for justifying the use of unorthodox methods.[52] As the law has been traditionally concerned with "prevent[ing] quackery from insulating itself from outside scrutiny," a school—to be considered reputable—"must be grounded in sound scientific principles attested to by professional expert witnesses."[53]

Difficulties are further exacerbated because of the wide range of professional backgrounds of individuals characterized as mental health professionals—psychiatrists, psychologists, social workers, and others.[54] While there are clear differences in education, orientation, modalities of treatment employed, and organization, and in the degree to which such practitioners are regulated by state statute or by self-certification, unlicensed practitioners are generally held to the same standard of care as a qualified, licensed practitioner,[55] with court decisions often resting on the case made by the nonprofessional as to his or her qualifications.[56]

References

1. Klein & Glover, "Psychiatric Malpractice," 6 *Int'l J. L. & Psych*. 131 (1983). As of 1975, it was estimated that psychiatrists faced one malpractice action for every 50–100 years of practice. Trent & Muhl, "Professional Liability Insurance and the American Psychiatrist," 132 *Am. J. Psych*. 1312 (1975).

2. Klein & Glover, *supra* note I, at 131–132; see also, *e.g.,* Slawson, "Psychiatric Malpractice: A Regional Incidence Study," 126 *Am. J. Psych*. 1302 (1970) (Slawson I).

3. See Taub, "Psychiatric Malpractice in the 1980's: A Look at Some Areas of Concern," 11 *L., Med. & Health Care* 97 (1983) (Taub 1).

4. Slawson, "Psychiatric Malpractice: The Low-Frequency of Risk," 12 *Med Law* 673 (1993).

6. On malpractice issues affecting other mental health professionals, see generally, Cohen, "The Professional Liability of Behavioral Scientists: An Overview," I *Behav. Sci. & L.* 9 (1983).

7. Klein & Glover, *supra* note 2, at 132. There is some evidence that this doctrine has begun to erode, at least where the emotional injuries result in physical injuries. See, *e.g., Crivellaro v. Pennsylvania Power & Light Co.,* 341 Pa. Super. 173, 491 A. 2d 207, 209 (Super.Ct. 1985) (noting Pennsylvania's adoption of *Restatement (Second) Torts,* §§436 and 436A).

8. See Taub I, *supra* note 3; Nieland, "Malpractice Liability of Psychiatric Professionals," I *Am J. Forens. Psych.* 22, 26–27 (1979).

9. "More Patients Suing Their Psychiatrists," 68 *A.B.A.J.* 1353 (1982) (quoting Allen Wilkinson, a California trial lawyer).

10. Fishalow, "The Tort Liability of the Psychiatrist," 4 *Bull. Am. Acad. Psych. & L.* 191 (1975).

11. *Id.* at 191–192.

12. Taub 1, *supra* note 3; Shapiro & Zimmerly, "Current Medicolegal Issues in Psychiatry," in Wecht, ed., *Legal Medicine Annual* 1977, 327 (1979).

13. *Id.*

14. Fishalow, *supra* note 10.

15. At least one commentator has noted "an inverse correlation between the contact a physician has with his patients and the incidence of malpractice action." Note, "The Liability of Psychiatrists for Malpractice," 36 *U. Pitt. L. Rev.* 108, 130 (1974).

16. See generally, Perlin, "Institutionalization and the Law," in Amer. Hosp. Ass'n. eds., *Psychiatric Services in Institutional Settings* 75 (1978).

17. See generally, Ingber, "Rethinking Intangible Injuries: A Focus on Remedy," 73 *Calif. L. Rev.* 772 773 (1985): In the last twenty-five years, there has been a significant movement toward recognizing "intangible" interests by more fully protecting against the infliction of "emotional distress."

18. This may have been partially spurred on by a series of "confessional pieces" by well-known celebrities discussing their experiences with psychiatric treatment. See, e.g., Ashley "A Short Time Out," *New York* (August 14, 1978), at 37.

19. La Fond, "An Examination of the Purposes of Involuntary Civil Commitment," 30 *Buff. L. Rev.* 499 (1981).

20. See, *e.g.,* Perlin, "Ten Years After: Evolving Mental Health Advocacy and Judicial Trends," 15 *Ford. Urb. L.J.* 335 (1986–87).

21. See generally, Perlin, "Can Mental Health Professionals Predict Judicial Decision-making: Constitutional and Tort Liability Aspects of the Right of the Institutionalized Mentally Disabled to Refuse Treatment: At the Cutting Edge," 3 *Touro L. Rev.* 13 (1986) ("Cutting Edge"); Taub, "Tardive Dyskinesia: Medical Facts and Legal Fictions," 30 *St. Louis U. L.J.* 833 (1986) (Taub II); Furrow, *Malpractice in Psychotherapy* 60–63 (1980): Wettstein & Appelbaum, "Legal Liability for Tardive Dyskinesia," 35 *Hosp. & Commun. Psych.* 992 (1984).

22. See 68 A.B.A.J., *supra* note 9, at 1354 (discussing $4.6 million jury verdict in case where male psychiatrist induced female patient to have sex with him).

23. See generally, Perlin, "Torts," in Sidley, ed., *Law and Ethics: A Guide for the Mental Health Professional* 149 (1985).

24. In addition, there are important tort defenses to consider, including, but not limited to, statutory privileges, statutes of limitation, contributory negligence, assumption of risk, and constitutional tort immunity. These topics are all discussed at length in Chapter 12 of Perlin, *Mental Disability Law: Civil and Criminal* (Kluwer Law Books, 1988).

25. See, *e.g.*, *Fortugno Realty Co. v. Bonomo*, 39 N.J. 382, 189 A. 2d 7 (Sup. Ct. 1963).

26. See, *e.g.*, *Wytupek v. City of Camden*, 25 N.J. 450, 136 A. 2d 887 (Sup. Ct. 1958).

27. See, *e.g.*, *Rappaport v. Nichols*, 31 N.J. 188, 156 A. 2d 1 (Sup. Ct. 1960).

28. See, *e.g.*, *Levine v. Wiss & Co.*, 97 N.J. 242, 478 A. 2d 397 (Sup. Ct. 1984).

29. Se, *e.g.*, *Nesbitt v. Community Health of South Dade*, 467 So. 2d 711. 714–715 (Fla. Dist. Ct. Appl. 1985), quoting *Texas & Pacific Ry. Co. v. Behymer*, 189 U.S. 468, 470 (1903) ("What usually is done may be evidence of what ought to be done, but what ought to be done is fixed by a standard of reasonable prudence, whether it usually is complied with or not").

30. The classic case is *Palsgraf v. Long Island R. Co.*, 248 N.Y 339. 162 N.E. 99 (Ct. App. 1928).

31. See, *e.g.*, *Hartford Accident & Indemnity Co. v. Abdullah*, 94 Cal. App. 3d 81, 156 Cal. Rptr. 254 (Ct. App. 1979).

32. See, *e.g.*, *Kileen v. State, 104 App. Div. 2d 586, 479 N.Y.S. 2d 371, 373 (App. Div. 1984)* (citing *Palsgraf* in case duty of care owed by State to mentally retarded patient in outpatient program), rev'd 66 N.Y. 2d 850, 498 N.Y.S. 2d 358 (Ct. App. 1985).

33. *Rossell v. Volkswagen of America*, 147, Ariz. 160, 709 P. 2d 517 (Sup. Ct. 1985).

34. See, *e.g.*, *Doe v. Kaiser Foundation*, 12 Cal. App. 3d 488, 90 Cal. Rptr. 747, 751 (Ct. App. 1970) (plaintiff must prove "causal nexus" between negligence and the resultant injuries).

35. *C & H Const. & Paving Co., Inc., v. Citizens Bank*, 93 N.M. 150. 597 P. 2d 1190 (Sup. Ct. 1979).

36. See, *e.g.*, *Pullman Palace Car v. Bluhm*, 109 Ill. 20 (Sup. Ct. 1884).

37. See, *e.g.*, *Kirby v. Carlisle*, 178 Pa. Super. 389, 116 A. 2d 220 (Super. Ct. 1955).

38. See, *e.g.*, *Hall v. Cornett*, 193 Or. 634. 240 P. 2d 231 (Sup. Ct. 1952). Punitive damages are generally limited to cases where the defendant's actions were "intentionally fraudulent, malicious, willful or wanton." *Aladdin Mfg. Co. v. Mantle Lamp of America*, 116 F. 2d 708, 716–717 (7 Cir. 1941), citing *Scott v. Donald*. 165 U.S. 58 (1896). For an example of such a case in the medical malpractice setting, see *Brooke v. Clarke*, 57 Tex. 105, 114 (1882), discussed in Weigel, "Punitive Damages in Medical Malpractice Litigation," 28 *So. Tex. L. Rev.* 19, 129 (1987).

39. See Shea, "Legal Standard of Care for Psychiatrists and Psychologists," 6 *Western St. U. L. Rev.* 71, 73 (1979).

40. Furrow, *supra* note 21, at 23. On the role of expert testimony, see, *e.g.*, *Tucker v. Metro. Gov't of Nashville & Davidson County*, 686 S.W. 2d 87, 92–94 (Tenn. Ct. App. 1984).

41. *Id.* See, *e.g.*, *Christy v. Saliterman*, 288 Minn. 144, 179 N.W. 2d 288, 302 n.1 (Sup. Ct. 1970).

42. 256 N.C. 633. 131 S.E. 2d 297 (Sup. Ct. 1963).

43. *Stone*, 131 S.E. 2d at 299. For a classic institutional case finding liability where lack of psychiatric care was the "primary reason for the inordinate length of

[plaintiff's] incarceration, with the concomitant side effects of physical injury, moral degradation, and mental anguish," see *Whitree v. State,* 56 Misc. 2d 693, 290 N.Y.S. 2d 486, 495 (Ct. Cl. 1968).

44. See *Nicholson v. Han,* 12 Mich. App. 35, 162 N.W. 2d 313, 316 (Ct. App. 1968).

45. Shea, *supra* note 39, at 75; see generally, *Carroll v. Richardson,* 201 Va. 157, 100 S.E. 2d 193 (Sup. Ct. 1959).

46. *Pike v. Honsinger,* 155 N.Y. 201, 49 N.E. 760, 762 (Ct. App. 1898), quoted in *Hirschberg v. State,* 91 Misc. 2d 590, 398 N.Y.S. 2d 470, 472 (Ct. Cl. 1977).

47. See generally, Cohen & Mariano, *Legal Guide Book in Mental Health 98–100 (1982).* The general rule is stated in *Nelson v. Dahl,* 174 Minn. 574 219 N.W. 2d 941, 942 (Sup. Ct. 1928).

48. *Hood v. Phillips,* 537 S.W. 2d 291, 294 (Tex. Civ. Ct. App. 1976).

49. Cohen & Mariano, *supra* note 47, at 99.

50. On the statutory regulation of psychotherapists in general, see Freiberg, "The Song is Ended but the Malady Lingers On: Legal Regulation of Psychotherapy," 22 *St. Louis U.L.J.* 519, 530–533.

51. See Note, "Tort Liability of the Psychotherapist," 8 *U. San. Fran. L. Rev.* 405, 419 (1973) ("San Francisco Note").

52. See, *e.g.,* Note, "Standard of Care in Administering Non-Traditional Psychotherapy," 7 *U.S. Davis L. Rev.* 56 (1974).

53. Furrow, *supra* note 21, at 23.

54. See, *e.g.,* "San Francisco Note," *supra* note 51, at 406–408. The author notes the proliferation of non-professional practitioners, and suggests that while some are "sincere and competent, others are cynical exploitationists." *Id.* at 408.

55. See Cohen & Mariano, *supra* note 47, at 448 450.

56. See, *e.g., Bogust v. Iverson,* 10 Wisc. 2d 129, 102 N.W. 2d 228 (Sup. Ct. 1960).

2

Risk Issues in Psychiatric Malpractice

MICHAEL L. PERLIN, ESQ.

Editor's Note

The more obvious issues that can give rise to malpractice complaints include:

- *Failure to make an accurate diagnosis.*
- *The often-overlooked obligation to be sure a patient presenting with an emotional problem does not suffer with a contributing or coexistent physical illness.*
- *Failure to obtain informed consent, particularly with regard to biological treatment.*
- *Failure to provide adequate biological treatment, particularly among professionals biased against, lacking proficiency in, or reluctant to obtain consultation for such treatment.*
- *Complications of electroconvulsive therapy.*
- *Complications of psychopharmacologic treatments, such as tardive dyskinesia.*
- *Sexual misconduct.*
- *Failure to protect the patient from self-harm.*

Interestingly, psychotherapeutic issues have not yet emerged as a common basis for malpractice suits.

Misdiagnosis

Courts have been fairly lenient in cases involving psychiatric misdiagnosis, because of the inherently inexact nature of such diagnosis,[1] and because the accuracy of the diagnosis depends to a significant extent on the adequacy of the information communicated to the physician by the patient.[2] In such court cases a patient must prove not only that a diagnosis was incorrect, but that it was arrived at negligently.[3] In other words, he or she must show "an unreasonable departure by the physician from accepted procedures."[4]

A mistake in physician judgment will generally be a defense if the defendant can show: (1) the existence of reasonable doubt as to the nature of the condition involved, (2) a split in opinion among the medical authorities as to the diagnostic procedure to be followed, and that one of the conflicting procedures was, in fact, used or (3) the diagnosis was made after a conscientious effort by the physician to inform himself about the patient's condition.[5]

An Appropriate Physical Examination[6]

As there is a "growing awareness of the high percentage of undetected physical illness in psychiatric patients":[7]—because such patients are likely to be in poorer physical condition, receive poorer medical care, and have a higher death rate than the public at large[8]—it is inevitable that there will be an increase in litigation on the question of whether or not it is a breach of duty for a psychiatrist to fail to perform such an examination.

Although it has been suggested that it is the physician's duty to conduct such an examination as a necessary predicate to an accurate diagnosis,[9] arguments have also been advanced as to why psychiatrists should *not* perform physicals: The doctor's potential incompetence resulting from lack of consistent use of the necessary skills,[10] lack of time,[11] and the possibility of unmanageable transference.[12] Perhaps as a result of this conflict, while there is no customary practice regarding the personal performance of such examinations,[13] it has become customary for psychiatrists to rely on medical examinations performed by other medical professionals, when such an examination is considered at all.[14]

Predictably, there have been fewer than a handful of cases litigated on the issues in question. In two New York public hospital cases, liability for failure to initiate a complete physical examination was found (1) where staff psychiatrists failed to adequately examine for (and diagnose) salicylate poisoning[15] and (2) where doctors failed to discover that a patient, diagnosed as an epileptic, suffered from severe barbiturate addiction.[16] Both cases reflect the courts' concern "with the quality of the examination performed, and whether one was performed at all in circumstances under which even a layman would have suspected a physical problem."[17]

Electroconvulsive Therapy

Suits premised on the use of nonverbal therapy—including electroconvulsive therapy (ECT) and other organic interventions—have generally involved claims (1) that the psychiatrist failed to warn a patient of a hazard inherent to the treatment, (2) that he failed to respond to the patient's complaints during therapy and (3) that he (or his agents) were negligent during the administration of the therapy.[18]

Until recently, the administration of ECT created the highest risk of liability for the therapist,[19] to such an extent that, as of the early 1950s, malpractice carriers were reluctant to insure doctors and hospitals using this form of treatment.[20] At this time, however, such claims amount to less than 1% of the total malpractice claims filed against psychiatrists.[21] This significant decrease is probably attributable to a combination of factors: (1) a significant decline in the use of ECT as a therapy,[22] (2) technological advances which have reduced considerably the possibility of secondary fractures and other injuries,[23] and (3) the use of muscle relaxants and other sedative and paralyzing agents which minimize muscular contractions during the convulsive phase of the treatment.[24]

On the other hand, other side effects from ECT (including both retrograde and anterograde memory loss, characterized as a "prominent side effect . . . unrelated to therapeutic efficacy,"[25] spontaneous seizures and temporary organic psychosis,[26] depression of respiratory and cardiovascular functions,[27] and, in the rare case, "permanent brain damage and death"[28]) have not disappeared, and there has thus been some significant recent litigation dealing with the therapist's liability in the use of this treatment.[29]

Thus, after the Seventh Circuit Court initially held that a Veterans' Administration psychiatrist was not immune from a suit brought by a patient alleging the imposition of nonconsensual ECT[30] in a case where the action alleged a battery under applicable state law[31] and a federal constitutional due process violation,[32] it subsequently ruled that the treating psychiatrist was entitled to qualified immunity from suit stemming from the theory that the constitutional right to refuse treatment had not yet been "clearly established" by the courts at the time of the psychiatrist's actions.[33]

In addition, ECT has become subject to increasingly greater statutory regulations.[34] By 1983, 26 states had enacted some sort of state law regulating the use of ECT in institutional settings, and another eight had promulgated analogous regulations.[35] Although it does not appear that malpractice issues were a major precipitant in the passage of such statutes, it is reasonable to predict that the fact of such legislative recognition of the possible peril of the use of ECT in an institutional setting may have a "spillover" effect in potential future litigation in nonhospital settings.

Improper Administration of Medication
General Considerations:

The improper administration of medication is a potential minefield for the psychiatrist who regularly uses this modality of treatment. In addition to the specific problems posed by neurological side effects such as tardive dyskinesia, the psychiatrist risks liability for negligent injuries in a variety of other areas:

> [A]bsence of an adequate history, physical examination, and laboratory evaluation prior to treatment [including failing to obtain a history of allergies and failing to inquire about other medications the patient is taking which might interact with the prescribed drug], prescription of a drug where it is not indicated, prescription of the wrong dosage, prescription of medication for inappropriately short or long time periods, failure to recognize, monitor or treat side effects or toxicity, failure to abate the possibility of drug reactions or interactions, and failure to consult with the necessary experts.[36]

While there are still relatively few decisions in this area,[37] such suits are becoming more common.[38] At the very least, dosage guidelines set forth in the *Physician's Desk Reference* will be given considerable weight by reviewing courts.[39] In one case where such guidelines were not held to establish a standard of care, they were considered evidential on the question of whether a defendant physician had notice of a drug's contraindications;[40] in another, deviation from the guidelines was considered prima facie evidence of negligence.[41]

Tardive Dyskinesia:[42]

In *Clites v. State,*[43] the first major case that has considered the impact of a constitutional right to refuse treatment on tort liability, the Iowa Court of Appeals affirmed a jury's negligence verdict of over $750,000 which it had awarded to a long-term resident of a state facility for the mentally retarded.[44] The plaintiff had been institutionalized since age eleven. Seven years later, hospital doctors began to prescribe antipsychotic drugs to "curb [his] aggressive behavior."[45] After receiving such drugs for five years, the plaintiff was diagnosed as suffering from tardive dyskinesia.[46]

The plaintiff sued in state court, arguing that the defendants failed to provide him with "reasonable medical treatment," and that his condition was proximately caused by their negligence.[47] The jury awarded him $385,000 for further medical expenses, and $375,000 for past and future pain and suffering. The defendants appealed this verdict,[48] but it was upheld.

In affirming this verdict, the Court of Appeals found that the defendants' actions were to be assessed by the standard of "such reasonable care and skill as is exercised by the ordinary physician of good standing under like circumstances,"[49] i.e., the traditional test for negligence.[50] It found, on the record before it, that there was "substantial support" for a series of fact-findings that the trial court had made regarding the appropriate "industry standards of care."[51]

Thus, while it was standard for patients receiving major tranquilizers to be closely monitored via tests, physical exams, and regular examinations by physicians, the plaintiff had not been visited by a physician for a three-year period.[52] The hospital staff's failure to react to the plaintiff's symptoms and alter his treatment program similarly fell short of industry standards, as did the hospital's failure to provide interim consultations with specialists, especially in light of the plaintiff's attending doctor's conceded unfamiliarity with tardive dyskinesia.[53]

Given the plaintiff's status and the type of drugs involved, the court noted that the practice of polypharmacy was not warranted by industry standards.[54] Finally, the major tranquilizers which the plaintiff received were "designed as a convenience or expediency program rather than a therapeutic program," constituting "substandard medical conduct."[55]

Further, under Iowa state law, defendants were obliged to "make a reasonable disclosure to [a] patient [or his guardians] of the nature and probable consequences of the suggested or recommended treatment."[56] This was not done in the *Clites* case. The court noted, "The concept of a therapeutic alliance between doctor and patient presumes a communication of information as to the pros and cons of a particular treatment program."[57]

Although the obtaining of informed written consent was a "recognized industry standard,"[58] the plaintiff's parents were "never informed of the potential side effects of the use, and prolonged use, of major tranquilizers, nor was consent to their use obtained."[59] On the issue of damages, the court again found "substantial evidence" to support the jury's verdict:[60]

Before Timothy was administered the major tranquilizers, he exhibited little aggressive or self-abusive behavior. Timothy could adequately communicate his needs to others, could dress himself, comb his hair, brush his teeth and make his bed. After the major tranquilizer treatment began, a marked change occurred. Timothy became aggressive and self-abusive. He began uncontrolled movements of his arms and legs. There is evidence of deterioration in the results of Timothy's psychological summaries and IQ testing. His hygiene habits worsened. In the words of the trial court, Timothy was, after the effects of tardive dyskinesia manifested themselves, "only a fraction of his former self."[61]

It had been predicted balefully that *Clites* would lead to "increased litigation for psychiatrists,"[62] and there were reports of increased filings in the case's aftermath.[63] However, the expected "flood" has not yet materialized. Although *Clites* was characterized as "disquieting" by Drs. Paul Appelbaum and Robert Wettstein,[64] those authors also suggested that it was "premature" to use the case as a standard by which to assess the general direction of caselaw developments in this area.[65] They suggested that the development of "appropriate written policies and procedures for the systematic monitoring of patients being treated with antipsychotic medication, whether or not tardive dyskinesia . . . [is] present"[66] would be the first step in limiting the future litigation risk of mental health professionals in the field.

Psychotherapy

Malpractice cases involving psychotherapeutic treatment[67] are especially problematic and difficult to sustain. In fact, according to Tancredi, "[t]hroughout the history of psychiatric malpractice cases there has not been a reported decision of an American appellate court that has established psychiatric malpractice based on improper conduct of psychotherapy alone."[68]

In addition to the general explanations for the paucity of malpractice suits in general[69] (and their low success rates[70]), there are particular difficulties in cases dealing solely with nonphysical interventions. First, the word "intervention" is probably an overstatement, since the therapist's "action" typically consists of "mere suggestion, or, at most, a prescription of behavior that the patient must follow."[71] Because there is no true "direct intervention,"[72] the defendant will usually be able to avoid liability.[73]

Second, the court is generally reluctant to take a patient's word over a therapist's,[74] especially in cases where there is no physical touching[75] (either through standard treatments such as chemical or pharmacologic intervention or other organic therapies or unacceptable "treatments" such as sexual contact).

Third, it may be especially difficult to establish a "nexus or connection between what was done in psychotherapy and an untoward outcome."[76]

Fourth, the generally ambiguous criteria for establishing psychiatric malpractice and the great diversity of psychotherapeutic techniques and goals are even less precise and more diffuse in the case of purely verbal therapy unaccompanied by an "overt act."[77]

Sexual Misconduct

Few aspects of psychiatric practice have engendered the controversy[78] and near-blanket[79] condemnation[80] that the issue of sexual relations between psychotherapist and patient has.[81] Although a few therapists have suggested that such contacts are not inherently improper,[82] and while it is not clear how many therapists have engaged in sexual relations with their patients,[83] such behavior has been rejected unequivocally by the American Psychiatric Association as "always unethical."[84] According to Klein and Glover, as of 1982, "every reported case involving a psychiatrist who was shown to have had sex with a patient has resulted in a verdict against the therapist."[85]

Three infamous cases have been well publicized in the legal, medical, and popular literatures.[86] In *Roy v. Hartogs,*[87] the court upheld a damage award to a patient whose psychiatrist had engaged in sexual intercourse with her. The court specifically rejected the defendant's claim that it was a legitimate part of therapy. Importantly, the court relied strongly on the public policy argument demanding the protection of patients from the "deliberate and malicious abuse of power and breach of trust" by a therapist.[88] In the "particularly outrageous circumstances"[89] of *Zipkin v. Freeman,*[90] where the therapist persuaded his patient—characterized as "a very frightened person"[91]—to increase her social contacts with him (including participation in nude swimming parties), leave her husband, invest her money in business ventures and have sexual relations with him,[92] the court found these actions to deviate from acceptable psychiatric standards.[93] There seems to be no basis upon which to contradict Professor Furrow's conclusion that this "litany of acts . . . leaves little doubt of the abuse of the psychiatric role."[94]

The English case of *Landau v. Werner*[95]—characterized by Furrow as "the most suggestive case as to liability for mishandling . . . transference"[96]—posed a slightly different set of facts. An "intelligent, middle-aged woman" told her therapist (who had treated her for anxiety for five months) that she was in love with him. After he explained the transference phenomenon to her, they began to date, and discussed the possibility of taking a vacation together, although, apparently, they never engaged in sexual relations.[97] The patient's condition worsened, and formal treatment was resumed, but was unsuccessful. In affirming a damages award, the Queen's Bench found the doctor's deviation from standard practice unjustified, and that his decision to see the plaintiff socially "led to the grave deterioration in the plaintiff's health."[98]

An important collateral issue[99] to be considered is the question of whether or not the defense of suits premised on sexual contact between therapist and patient will be covered by standard malpractice insurance policies.[100] Thus, in an intermediate appellate decision from Wisconsin, the court rejected the insurer's claim that the actions giving rise to the suit—the performance of sexual acts with the plaintiff—were not professional services covered by the policy, reasoning that the claim was for damages based on services "rendered or which should have been rendered."[101] On the other hand, in an action arising out of *Roy v. Hartogs,* the court held that coverage was properly denied where the psychiatrist knew the actions were for his own personal satisfaction, and were not for treatment;[102] to rule otherwise would "indemnify immorality and pay the expenses of prurience."[103]

Protection of Patient from Self*

In addition to those cases dealing squarely with suicide and attempted suicide, a group of other opinions has dealt with the liability of psychiatrists and hospitals in cases where patients were injured by a passing vehicle after having wandered off the hospital grounds, were injured in escape attempts,[104] or were injured on the hospital premises, allegedly because of inadequate supervision. In these cases, "there exists a duty on the part of a psychiatrist and/or psychiatric facility to use reasonable care to prevent a patient, who a defendant knows or ought to know may injure himself or herself, from doing so."[105]

Thus, when a seriously mentally disturbed patient jumped into a vat of boiling soap in the hospital laundry, the court had little difficulty in finding that the hospital failed to exercise reasonable care for the patient's supervision,[106] because the state was aware of his suicidal tendencies but permitted him to remain unattended when he should have been closely supervised, and had left unguarded the vat where the incident occurred. In another case where there was no evidence that hospital personnel had improperly or negligently applied restraints, the

---

*Although the thrust of this section deals with inhospital incidents, it should be pointed out that there are a significant number of cases outside the hospital as well.

court found there was no negligence when a patient nonetheless extricated himself from restraints and fell from the ledge of the hospital's second floor.[107]

In a suit brought against a nursing home for allowing an elderly, mentally ill patient to dart out onto a highway (where she was hit by a passing motorcyclist), the Texas Court of Appeals held that the nursing home was under an obligation to take the patient's known tendency to wander into account in protecting and providing for her.[108] In a similar action against a private hospital, the Connecticut Appellate Court treated the case as one of ordinary negligence, rather than as medical malpractice, subject to proof of the standard of care owed by a reasonably prudent person under the particular facts and circumstances.[109]

Somewhat paradoxically, these cases[110]—especially those that call into question the so-called "open door" policy[111]—appear to conflict with the body of constitutional and statutory law which has developed in the past fifteen years suggesting that involuntarily committed mental patients have a right either to treatment in the least restrictive alternative setting[112] or to a "reasonably nonrestrictive" treatment setting.[113]

Although psychiatric hospitals had traditionally stressed confinement and supervision in closed settings, more recently many psychiatrists have rejected the notion of a predominantly "locked ward" hospital, reasoning that the earlier a patient is able to be exposed to society as a part of treatment, the earlier he or she will be able to return to society, and the better adjusted the individual will be upon such return.[114] Because such policies are not always without risks,[115] courts have determined that hospitals and doctors must balance the potential benefit to the patient with the possible likelihood and severity of risks to the patient or the general public. If, however, the patient's conduct indicates that he or she cannot safely be released unsupervised into society "for whatever length of time," the use of the policy might be inappropriate."[117]

References

1. See generally, *O'Connor v. Donaldson,* 422 U.S. 563, 575 (1975) (Burger, C.J., concurring), on the unreliability of psychiatric diagnosis.
2. Note, "Medical Malpractice: The Liability of Psychiatrists," 48 *Notre Dame L.* 693, 698 (1973) ("Notre Dame Note"); Note, "An Evaluation of Changes in

the Medical Standard of Care," 23 *Vand. L. Rev.* 729, 748 (1970) ("Vanderbilt Note"). But see, *O'Neil v. New York,* 66 Misc. 2d 936, 323 N.Y.S. 2d 56 (Ct. Cl. 1971), discussed *infra* note 16.

3. See, *e.g., Ries v. Reinhard,* 47 Cal. App. 2d 116, 117 P. 2d 386 (Dist. Ct. App. 1941); *Welsch v. Frisbee Memorial Hospital,* 90 N.H. 337, 9 A. 2d 761 (Sup. Ct. 1939).

4. "Notre Dame Note," *supra* note 2, at 698.

5. "Vanderbilt Note," *supra* note 2, at 749.

6. The aspects of liability discussed in this and the preceding chapter are not, of course, the only important tort theories relevant to this aspect of the law. In other cases, mentally disabled individuals and/or their guardians have filed suit in cases involving, *inter alia,* improper use of seclusion and restraint; improper use of unconventional and nontraditional psychotherapy; improper involuntary commitment; abandonment; assault and battery; breach of confidentiality; defamation and libel; and false imprisonment. In addition, there are important tort *defenses* to consider, including, but not limited to, statutory privileges, statutes of limitation, contributory negligence, assumption of risk, and constitutional tort immunity. These topics are all discussed at length in Chapter 12 of Perlin, *Mental Disability Law: Civil and Criminal* (©Kluwer Law Books 1988).

7. Busch & Cavanaugh, "Physical Examination of Psychiatric Outpatients: Medical and Legal Issues," 36 *Hosp. & Commun. Psych.* 958, 959 (1985).

8. See, *e.g.,* Hall *et al.,* "Unrecognized Physical Illness Prompting Psychiatric Admission: A Prospective Study," 138 *Am. J. Psych.* 629 (1981); Busch & Cavanaugh, *supra* note 2, at 961 nn.7–12.

9. Ficarra, *Surgical and Allied Malpractice* 698 (1968). It should be noted, however, that certain psychoanalysts specifically oppose the practice of conducting physical examinations of psychiatric outpatients. See Busch & Cavanaugh, *supra* note 2 at 959.

10. See, *e.g.,* Anderson, "The Physical Examination in Office Practice," 137 *Am. J. Psych.* 1188–1189 (1980) (listing objections).

11. Id.

12. Busch & Cavanaugh, *supra* note 2, at 959. For one of the few cases discussing transference and countertransference, see *Mazza v. Huffaker,* 61 N.C. App. 170, 300 S.E. 2d 833, 840 (Ct. App. 1983).

13. Busch & Cavanaugh, *supra* note 2. at 961.

14. *Id.* at 959; see Patterson, "Psychiatrists and Physical Examinations: A Survey," 135 *Am. J. Psych.* 967 (1978).

15. *Hirschberg v. New York,* 91 Misc. 2d 590, 398 N.Y.S. 2d 470 (Ct. Cl. 1977). In that case, the admitting doctor—licensed to practice only in Yugoslavia—did not conduct a physical examination because the patient arrived at the hospital after the normal time for such a procedure. *Id.* at 472.

16. *O'Neil* 323 N.Y.S. 2d at 61: The State's witness testified that no one informed him of defendant's drug addiction and that if he knew he would not have admitted her to [the state hospital]. This is incredulous. Patients desirous of obtaining medical attention are not responsible for diagnosing their own ailments.

17. Busch & Cavanaugh *supra* note 2 at 960.

18. Horan & Milligan, "Recent Developments in Psychiatric Malpractice," 1 *Behav. Sci. & L.* 23, 28 (1983).

19. Weiner, "Provider-Patient Relations: Confidentiality and Liability." in Brakel, Parry & Weiner, *Mental Disability and the Law* 559, 580 (3d rev. ed. 1985) (Weiner).

20. Rebein, "Liability for Injury Caused by ∞Shock∞ Treatment," 2 *Kan. L. Rev.* 393 (1954).

21. Slawson, "The Clinical Dimension of Psychiatric Malpractice," 14 *Psych. Annals* 358, 363 (1984).

22. Scovern & Kilmann, "Status of Electroconvulsive Therapy: Review of the Outcome Literature," 87 *Psycholog. Bull.* 260 (1980), as cited in Weiner, *supra* note 19, at 580 n.232.

23. Tancredi, "Psychiatric Malpractice," in 3 Cavenar, ed., *Psychiatry,* ch. 29 (1986 rev. ed.). at 1, 10.

24. *Id.* See also, Furrow, *Malpractice in Psychotherapy* 59 (1980), citing Amer. Psych. Ass'n Task Force Report No. 14, *Electroconvulsive Therapy* 117 (1978) (*ECT Report*), discussing the additional use of oxygen supplementation.

25. Furrow, *supra* note 24, at 57, citing *ECT Report, supra* note 24, at 57.

26. *Id.* at 74–75.

27. Beresford, "Professional Liability of Psychiatrists," 21 *Defense L. J.* 123, 130 (1972).

28. ECT Report, *supra* note 24, at 80.

29. See generally, Winslade *et al.,* "Medical, Judicial, and Statutory Regulation of ECT in the United States," 141 *Am. J. Psych.* 1347 (1984) .

30. On the specific empirical issues involved in consenting to ECT, see Kaufmann *et al.,* "Informed Consent and Patient Decision Making." 4 *Int'l J. L. & Psych.* 345 (1981), concluding, see *id.* at 359, that "the values of psychiatrists and lawyers may cause them to disagree about the evaluation of patient decision-making to refuse or consent to [such] treatment."

31. *Loduk v. Quandt,* 706 F. 2d 1456, 1463–1464 (7 Cir. 1983).

32. *Id.* at 1465–1468.

33. *Loduk v. Johnson,* 770 F. 2d 619, 631 (7 Cir. 1985). See also *Price v. Sheppard,* 239 N.W. 2d 905 (Minn. Sup. Ct. 1976), affirming—in an institutional case—a trial court's grant of summary judgment for defendant in suit alleging civil rights violations and assault and battery for the administration of an ECT series, but, see *id.* at 913, ordering state to adopt adversary procedures requiring the obtaining of consent prior to the administration of "intrusive" treatments such as ECT.

34. See generally, Weiner, *supra* note 19, at 357–365 (Table 6.2).

35. Winslade *et al., supra* note 29, at 1348.

36. Wettstein, "Tardive Dyskinesia and Malpractice," 1 *Behav. Sci. & L.* 85, 89 (1983).

37. Klein & Glover, "Psychiatric Malpractice," 6 *Int'l J. L. & Psych.* 131, 135 (1983).

38. *Id.* See, *e.g., Gowan, Conservator for Gowan v. United States,* 601 F. Supp. 1297 (D. Ore. 1985) (dosage of prescribed drug and subsequent decision to discontinue not psychiatric malpractice).

39. *Speer v. United States,* 512 F. Supp. 670, 676–678 (N.D. Tex. 1981).
40. *Meier v. Ross General Hospital,* 69 Cal. 2d 420, 71 Cal. Rptr. 903, 913, 445 P. 2d 519 (Sup. Ct. 1968).
41. *Ohligschlager v. Proctor Community Hospital,* 55 Ill. 2d 411. 303 N.E. 2d 392 (Sup. Ct. 1973).
42. This section of this article is substantially adapted from Perlin, "Can Mental Health Professionals Predict Judicial Decision-making? Constitutional and Tort Liability Aspects of the Right of the Institutionalized Mentally Disabled to Refuse Treatment: At the Cutting Edge," 3 *Touro L. Rev.* 13 (1986).
43. 322 N.W. 2d 917 (Iowa Ct. App. 1982).
44. *Id.* at 919.
45. *Id.* at 918.
46. *Id.*
47. *Id.* at 919.
48. *Id.*
49. *Id.,* citing *Speed v. State,* 240 N.W. 2d 901.908 (Iowa 1976).
50. See, *e.g., Scherempf v. State of New York,* 66 N.Y. 2d 289 (Ct. App. 1985); *Bell v. N.Y.C. Health & Hospital Corp.,* 90 App. Div. 270.456 N.Y.S. 2d 787 (App. Div. 1982), and cases cited in *id.,* 456 N.Y.S. 2d at 793–7 98.
51. *Clites,* 322 N.W. 2d at 920–921.
52. *Id.*
53. *Id.*
54. *Id.*
55. *Clites,* 322 N.W. 2d at 920–921.
56. *Id.* at 922. quoting *Grosjean v. Spencer,* 258 Iowa 685, 693, 140 N.W. 2d 139. 144 (1960).
57. *Clites,* 322 N.W. 2d at 922. quoting *Rogers v. Okin,* 478 F. Supp. 1342, 1347 (D. Mass. 1979). The *Rogers* litigation—see generally, *Mills v. Rogers,* 457 U.S. 291 (1982)—is discussed extensively in Perlin *supra* note 6, at Chapter 5.
58. *Clites,* 322 N.W. 2d at 922.
59. *Id.* The court here relied on *Rogers,* 478 F. Supp. at 1366, 1377, for the proposition that the decision to accept or refuse such medication is a "basic right of privacy and [that] the physician–patient relationship presumes the communication of the pros and cons of any particular treatment."
60. *Id.* at 923.
61. *Id.*
62. Klein and Glover, *supra* note 37, at 137.
63. See Baker, "Expect a Flood of Tardive Dyskinesia Malpractice Suits," *Clin. Psych. News* (Jan. 1984), at 3.
64. Wettstein and Appelbaum, "Legal Liability for Tardive Dyskinesia." 35 *Hosp. & Commun. Psych.* 992, 993 (1984).
65. *Id.*
66. *Id.* (emphasis added). Suggested the authors: Such policies could be included under existing guidelines with regard to the appropriate use and dosage of antipsychotic and antiparkinsonian medications, but would also address the need

for periodic evaluation for tardive dyskinesia; the use of standardized dyskine-sia-assessment instruments; the role of consulting neurologists in screening, diagnosis and treatment of tardive dyskinesia; the availability of costly neuro-logical diagnostic procedures ([EEG] or computerized tomography, for exam-ple); and the method of securing and periodically reviewing a meaningful informed consent from the patient or his or her guardian both on the use of an-tipsychotic medication and the management of tardive dyskinesia. The formu-lation of such a policy demands a consensus among clinical (psychiatric and neurologic), administrative, legal, financial, and ethical agendas.

67. See generally, Freiberg, "The Song is Ended But the Malady Lingers On: Le-gal Regulation of Psychotherapy," 22 *St. Louis U. L. J.* 519, 520–523 (1978), for a helpful overview.

68. Tancredi, *supra* note 23, at 13. See also, Weiner, *supra* note 19, at 581.

69. See generally, Chapter 1, *supra* (this volume).

70. See Slawson *supra* note 21.

71. Note, "Malpractice in Psychotherapy: Is There a Relevant Standard of Care?" 35 *Case West. Res. L. Rev.* 251, 260 (1984).

72. *Id.*

73. See Watkins & Watkins, "Malpractice in Clinical Social Work: A Perspective on Civil Liability in the 1980's," 1 *Behav. Sci. & L.* 55, 69 (1983).

74. See. *e.g.,* Heller, "Some Comments to Lawyers on the Practice of Psychiatry," 30 *Temp. U. L.Q.* 401 (1957).

75. See Freiberg, *supra* note 67, at 527.

76. Tancredi, *supra* note 23, at 12: Just because suicide was a topic of conversation during a psychotherapeutic hour does not mean that the discussion was in any way responsible for the patient's subsequent suicidal behavior.

77. Tancredi, *supra* note 23, at 12–13.

78. For a historical overview, see Davidson, "Psychiatry's Problem With No Name: Therapist-Patient Sex," 37 *Am. J. Psychoanal.* 43 (1977).

79. But see, Shepard, *The Love Treatment: Sexual Intimacy Between Patients and Psy-chotherapists* (1971); McCartney, "Overt Transference," 2 *J. Sex. Research* 227 (1966).

80. See, *e.g.,* American Psych. Ass'n, *Opinions of the Ethics Committee on the Principles of Medical Ethics* 13 (1983); Stone, "The Legal Implications of Sexual Activity Be-tween Psychiatrists and Patient," 133 *Am. J. Psych.* 1138 (1976); Klein & Glover, *supra* note 37, at 138–139. Cohen has asked, somewhat rhetorically, "[H]ow ob-jective can a therapist be with his pants down?" Cohen, *Malpractice* 92 (1979).

81. See, for a listing of pertinent articles, Cohen & Mariano, *Legal Guide Book in Mental Health* 470–471 (1982).

82. See Taylor & Wagner, "Sex Between Therapists and Clients: A Review and Analysis," 7 *Professional Psychol.* 593, 594 (1976) (survey indicated therapeutic results were positive for over one-fifth of patients sexually involved with their therapists). But see, Marmor, "Some Psychodynamic Aspects of the Seduction of Patients in Psychotherapy," 36 *Am. J. Psychoanal.* 319, 320–321 (1976) (most erotic breaches occur with physically attractive women, "almost never

with the aged, the infirm or the ugly, thus giving the lie to the oftheard rationalization on the part of such therapists that they were acting in the interests of the patient!").

83. Furrow interpolates the data to show that up to ten percent of all private practice psychiatrists and psychologists have engaged in such sexual contacts. Furrow, *Malpractice in Psychotherapy* 34 (1980). On the other hand, 25% of a sample of medical students surveyed indicated that they felt sexual relations with patients "might be beneficial <under the right circumstances.>" Freiberg, *supra* note 67, at 525 n.32, quoting Crinklaw, "Seduction and Women in Psychotherapy," St. Louis Post-Dispatch (Feb. 20, 1977), §G, at 3, 36.

84. Klein & Glover *supra* note 37, at 138. Klein, general counsel to the American Psychiatric Association, has recently characterized doctor-patient sex as "the biggest single problem affecting therapists' liability and the one that's most difficult to address." "The Professional Liability Crisis: An Interview with Joel Klein," 37 *Hosp. & Commun. Psych.* 1012 (1986).

85. Klein & Glover, *supra* note 37, at 138.

86. See, *e.g.,* Freeman & Roy, *Betrayal* (1976).

87. 81 Misc. 2d 350, 366 N.Y.S. 2d 297 (Civ. Ct. 1975), mod. 85 Misc. 2d 891.381 N.Y.S. 2d 587 (Sup. Ct. 1976).

88. *Id.* at 354. See also, on the issue of breach of trust in such situations, *Omer v. Edgren,* 38 Wash. App. 376, 685 P. 2d 635, 636–38 (Ct. App. 1984).

89. Klein & Glover, *supra* note 37, at 139.

90. 436 S.W. 2d 753 (Mo. Sup. Ct. 1968).

91. *Id.* at 759.

92. *Id.* at 755.

93. *Id.*

94. Furrow, *supra* note 83, at 35.

95. 105 Sol. J . 1008 (C.A. 1961).

96. Furrow, *supra* note 83, at 35.

97. *Landau,* 105 Sol. J. at 1008.

98. *Id.*

99. See, on the collateral question of whether intentional acts of a psychotherapist who engaged in sexual acts with patients were within the scope of *respondeat superior, Marston v. Minneapolis Clinic of Psychiatry & Neurology, Inc.,* 329 N.W. 2d 306 (Minn. Sup. Ct. 1983).

100. See Klein & Glover, *supra* note 37, at 138.

101. *L.L. v. Medical Protective Company,* 362 N.W. 2d 174 (Wis. Ct. App. 1984). See also *e.g.,* Zipkin, 436 S.W. 2d at 761; *St. Paul Fire & Marine Ins. Co. v. Mitchell,* 164 Ga. App. 215, 296 S.E. 2d 126 (Ct. App. 1982); *Aetna Life & Cas. Co. v. McCabe,* 556 F. Supp. 1342 (E.D. Pa. 1983); *Mazza v. Medical Mutual Ins. Co. of North Carolina,* 311 N.C. 621, 319 S.E. 2d 217 (Sup. Ct. 1984).

102. *Hartogs v. Employers Mutual Liability Ins. Co.,* 89 Misc. 2d 468, 391 N.Y.S. 2d 962, 965 (Sup. Ct. 1977).

103. *Id.* at 965. The malpractice insurance carrier of the American Psychological Association will not pay damages assessed against an insured psychologist based

upon sexual contact with a patient, but will pay the costs of legal defense, if the therapist denies the allegations. Riskin, "Sexual Relations Between Psychotherapists and Their Patients," *67 Calif. L. Rev.* 1000, 1013 n.70 (1979).

104. See generally, Annotation, "Hospital's Liability for Patient's Injury or Death Resulting from Escape or Attempted Escape," 37 *A.L.R.* 4th 200 (1985); see generally, *Weber v. City of New York,* 101 App. Div. 2d 757, 475 N.Y.S. 2d 401 (App. Div. 1984). aff'd 63 N.Y. 2d 866, 483 N.Y.S. 2d 200, 472 N.E. 2d 1028 (App. Div. 1985).

105. 3 Pegalis & Wachsman, *American Law of Medical Malpractice* (1982), §18:3 at 380. Cases are collected at id. at 380–384, and *id.* at 43–45 (1985 Supp.)

106. *Daley v. State,* 273 App. Div. 552 78 N.Y.S. 2d 584 (App. Div. 1948). aff'd 798 N.Y. 880, 84 N.E. 2d 801 (Ct. App. 1948). See also, Wilson v. State, 14 A.D. 2d 976, 221 N.Y.S. 2d 354 (App. Div. 1961) (patient jumped through unlocked laundry chute door, falling to basement); *Gunnarson v. New York,* 95 App. Div. 2d 797, 463 N.Y.S. 2d 853 (App. Div. 1983) (allowing heavily medicated patient access to a cigarette lighter).

107. *Coltraine v. Pitt County Memorial Hospital,* 35 N.C. App. 755, 242 S.E. 2d 538 (Ct. App. 1978).

108. *Golden Villa Nursing Home, Inc. v. Smith,* 674 S.W. 2d 343, 348–350 (Tex. Ct. App. 1984).

109. *Badrigian v. Elmcrest Psychiatric Institute,* 6 Conn. App. 383, 505 A. 2d 741, 743–744 (App. Ct. 1986).

110. See generally, Annotation, "Hospital's Liability for Mentally Deranged Patient's Self-Inflicted Injuries," 36 *A.L.R.* 4th 117 (1985); cases cited in 1 Louisell & Williams, *Medical Malpractice* (1986), ¶3.22, at 3–78 to –79 n.8.

111. For a relatively early overview of this policy, see Note, "Liability of Mental Hospitals for Acts of Their Patients Under the Open Door Policy," 57 *Va. L. Rev.* 156 (1971).

112. See, *e.g.,* Perlin, *supra* note 6, at Chapter 3; Perlin, "Civil Rights of Hospitalized Mental Patients," *Directions in Psychiatry,* Vol. 4, Lesson 29 (1984).

113. See *Youngberg v. Romeo,* 457 U.S. 307 (1982).

114. See 2 Louisell & Williams, *supra* note 110, at §17A.II, at 17A–31 to –32.

115. See, *e.g., M. W. v. Jewish Hospital Ass'n of St. Louis,* 637 S.W. 2d 74, 76 (Mo. Ct. App. 1982) (discussing "calculated risk" of "open door policy").

116. See, *e.g., White v. United States,* 244 F. Supp. 127 (E.D. Va. 1965), aff'd *p.c.* 359 F. 2d 989 (4 Cir. 1966); *Eanes v. United States,* 407 F. 2d 823, 824 (4 Cir. 1969) (while court refuses to "condemn, *per se,* the ∞open door∞ policy," it suggests that "great care and caution should be taken to provide reasonable assurances that the risks involved will not ultimately prove to have been underestimated or miscalculated").

117. 2 Louisell & Williams, *supra* note 110, at §17A–34.

3

Record Keeping in Psychiatric Practice

ROBERT L. SADOFF, M.D.

Editor's Note

One key to professional survival in the face of the malpractice crisis is the keeping of careful and accurate records.

Documentation.

The purpose of such records is apparent: as a reference source for the treating physician, to communicate information to other professionals as required, for research purposes, for public health and administrative reasons, and, if and when the spectre of a malpractice suit appears, to be able to show that standards of ordinary professional care were indeed met adequately.

Records should include basic data relevant to diagnosis and treatment. Assessments of risk of suicide or potential violence to others should be noted. If a medication is given, it should be charted, along with notes about monitoring the regimen. Evidence of informed consent is essential. If a patient refuses to comply with a particular recommendation, that, too, requires notation. In short, the records should be kept not only to inform, but to sustain and, if necessary, defend the observations and decisions the therapist has made throughout his contact with the patient.

Certain data, such as detailed accounts of sexuality, interpersonal conflicts, and the like that might later embarrass the patient or make him more vulnerable, can be excluded. However, once an official request or subpoena for records is issued, the law demands that nothing that exists may be destroyed.

Records should be kept for a minimum of five to seven years, and probably in some form more or less indefinitely.

Definition of Medical Records

Medical records include all notes, reports, hospital charts, laboratory tests, letters—all written information about a patient that is kept by the physician or that is kept in the hospital chart. Records may also include any movies, photographs, slides, audio or video tape recordings of the patient, and all consultation reports. For legal purposes, the medical record is not confined to the physician's or psychiatrist's notes.

At present there is no legal standing to a "primary" and "secondary" record. The dual record system has not been legally approved or accepted at this time, although suggestions have been made to consider such a system in which one set of medical records would be available for subpoena or for disclosure under certain conditions. The other set would be available only to the treatment team and would not be disclosed to outside sources such as insurance companies or courts. This consideration is especially relevant to teaching hospitals, where residents and medical students prepare elaborate reports for supervision purposes. Teaching notes by residents or medical students that are excessively detailed for teaching purposes should not in most cases be placed in the chart. A summary by the student is more appropriate. Teaching notes may be utilized for training purposes for a limited time and then discarded. Psychoanalysts' jottings should also be kept separate, and a summary of material is more appropriate for the records. However, no teaching material or memory joggers or psychoanalytic notes should ever be discarded or destroyed after official request or subpoena for the records is issued. All records must be available when a subpoena arrives. Destruction or alteration of records that are subpoenaed for legal purposes may be considered destruction of evidence, which is a felony in most states.

The Purpose of Medical Records

Records are kept on patients for several reasons:

1. Primarily the record serves as a continuing and permanent record of a patient's medical care and treatment at a particular time. It

serves the therapist in his or her ongoing treatment requirements.

2. The record also serves as an available source of information to others if the therapist is not available and information is required by subsequent treaters or by others needing information about a particular patient.

3. Medical records are also used for research purposes in detailing the specifics of a particular illness, comparing with others who have the same illness, observing the natural course of the illness, and observing treatment modalities.

4. Finally, medical records are used in data collection for administrative and public health reasons to determine incidence and prevalence of disease types.

Content of Psychiatric Records

There has been a running controversy among psychiatrists about how much material the medical record ought to contain. Some have advocated the barest minimum to satisfy the Internal Revenue Service regarding fee payments, but no other information. Others have included basic skeletal information such as diagnosis, prognosis, treatment method, and results of treatment attempts. Still others have elaborated on an ongoing and continuing record of patient responses on a regular basis. Finally, there are those who advocate a complete and detailed record with all data necessary for research, administrative, or legal purposes especially in the event of a malpractice suit, when such information will be necessary to defend the doctor's position.

Perhaps the best approach is one that includes the basic data about the patient necessary for statistical and identification purposes as well as other information that would aid subsequent psychiatrists in the treatment of the patient. The other data would include specific responses to various treatments attempted, side effects of various medications, and responses by the patient to various external and environmental stresses. What is perhaps not appropriate in most medical records is a detailed account of sexuality, interpersonal conflicts, or other data that would tend to embarrass the patient if disclosed. However, for some patients, a detailed account of prior arrests or previous violent behavior and even a detailed account of sexual development and behavior would be important, appropriate, and necessary. Such elaborations would be determined on an individual, case-by-case basis.

For hospitalized patients, regulatory committees require other information which is used for prognostic purposes and for determination of length of stay in the hospital. Occasionally hospital records will require a regular comment by the psychiatrist about the condition of the patient and his improvement with the particular treatment received.

Alteration of Medical Records

If an error is made in a medical record, alterations may be made in the following way:

1. Never erase in the medical record.
2. Never destroy a page of medical records and replace it with a subsequent page that has been rewritten at a later stage of treatment.
3. The most acceptable method is to draw a single line through the erroneous material, whether the error is one letter, one word, a sentence, or even a paragraph.
4. Date and initial the correction so that other readers of the record will know exactly when the correction was made and by whom.
5. It is important to write clearly and legibly in the medical record both for original entries and for corrections. Use only acceptable abbreviations and proper identifying information.

Security and Confidentiality of Medical Records

All medical records must be kept in a secure place either in the hospital or in the doctor's office. Diligent efforts must be made to maintain security so that records are not available indiscriminately to unauthorized individuals. Improper disclosure of medical records may include the negligent care of security measures such that patient information is leaked by careless handling of the medical record.

A more important consideration is the intentional distribution of medical records. To whom do the records belong? And who has appropriate and authorized access to these records? The medical record belongs to the doctor or to the hospital. The information contained in the record belongs to the patient. Thus, under the Freedom of Information Act of 1972, patients in federal hospitals or federally funded institutions have a right to read their medical records. But the right is not absolute and without discretion. Hospitals have developed guidelines for patients who wish to review their charts. Application must be made and an appointment for such review is considered regarding the potential harm such review can have on the patient. It may be deemed necessary to have the psychiatrist who prepared the record available for interpretation and discussion when the patient reads his or her records. Indiscriminate review of records by patients has led to emotional damage that could have been avoided by more careful handling of the right to see the records. The law and the regulation are clear, but the interpretation and management of the actual disclosure are a matter of professional judgment.

In discussing the disclosure of medical records, consideration of the concept of confidentiality, privileged communications, patient's right to privacy, and informed consent must be briefly discussed.

Confidentiality is an ethical concept that prohibits the physician from discussing his patient with anyone except under compelling legal circumstances. In the event of emergency, e.g., the patient is imminently suicidal or homicidal, the therapist must breach confidentiality in order to save his patient's life or the life of an intended victim.

Privilege, on the other hand, is a legal concept developed through legislation, belonging to the patient that prohibits the therapist from testifying in court about the patient without the patient's consent, unless the patient has waived his privilege in certain legal situations. These situations include the patient being involved in a criminal charge where his mental state is relevant to the adjudication or the patient being involved in a civil case where he or she raises his or her mental state as an issue before the court. Some states outline in their mental health legislation the prohibition against disclosure of medical information.

The patient's right to privacy has been developed very clearly in the past two decades. Courts have expressed the patient's right to maintain his or her privacy in prohibiting the disclosure of medical information even when a court orders such disclosure (e.g., see *In Re B Pennsylvania*, 1980).

Informed consent is the keystone around which all of these concepts are built. The patient must give consent to disclosure, but the consent must be based on proper information given to the patient by the physician about the effects of such disclosure. The patient may consent to the disclosure of medical records in a number of ways:

1. He may give consent in writing—perhaps the most important method, since a record exists of his consent. Such consent must be specific to the information, dated, and time-limited.
2. He may give consent by telephone after the information has been read to him and a note is placed in his record that such communication occurred.
3. The physician may send a copy of the information to be disclosed to the patient for the patient to distribute to the persons requesting information. This applies occasionally in cases of third-party payment by insurance companies or when the patient is applying for insurance and requires a statement by his former therapist. In this way the patient has had the opportunity to read the material and makes the decision to send the material to the third party requesting the information.

Does the patient have a right to refuse to have his medical records disclosed even to third-party payers? The answer is that the patient who is voluntary and competent to make decisions about his treatment may refuse to have his medical records sent to anyone. If he refuses to have the records sent to third-party payers, he may forfeit his right or privilege to have his medical treatment paid for by the insurance company. If he refuses to have his medical records sent to a subsequent therapist, that therapist may refuse to treat the patient without access to his prior records. In the case of involuntary patients, however, the medical records may be sent without the patient's consent to the hospital to which the patient has been involuntarily committed.

The concept of competency to give permission or consent to disclose records is also important. A patient may receive specific information from the physician with respect to his medical records but may not be competent to understand the impact of that information on his decision to disclose or to withhold the information. Thus, informed consent implies that the patient is competent to give such consent.

How much information is disclosed depends upon the needs and requirements of the individual requesting the information. Generally, insurance companies have developed a standard form which requests basic information that is necessary but does not go beyond what is required. Occasionally an insurance company will request an elaboration of the information given in order to make a determination about paying a claim. It is the medical judgment of the physician from whom the information is requested that determines how much information he should disclose. He may consult with his patient with respect to this decision.

In some cases, records are subpoenaed for court use through a record copy service. Usually these services are authorized by the court and are utilized by attorneys requiring the medical records in the pursuit of litigation in civil cases. The record copy services are used as a convenience for obtaining the records, which is usually appropriate but may be challenged by the physician who does not agree. The attorney will often obtain a court order for the medical records if they are not sent through the record copy service.

Medical records must be safeguarded in the doctor's offices and diligence must be taken in order to preserve the security of the records. However, under the case of *Zurcher v. Stanford Daily*, upheld by the United States Supreme Court, police are authorized on the basis of a search warrant to enter a doctor's office to take his records if it is suspected that the psychiatrist is treating a person who is a known criminal or a known suspect in a criminal case and if information may be available in the medical record that would help prosecute the individual. At the time of this writing, there are no known cases where this has occurred, but legal counsel to the American Psychiatric Association has alerted all psychiatrists that this is a possibility under the *Zurcher* Doctrine.

How Long Should Medical Records Be Kept?

There is no one good answer to this question.

For statistical and financial purposes, medical records should be kept for five to seven years. This would take into account all tax liability problems as well as contractual agreements and fee-paying problems. However, medical records probably ought to be kept indefinitely, since patients do return for treatment even as long as fifteen or twenty years later. It is most helpful to have an accurate record of previous treatment when a patient does return. It is not necessary to keep the records that long, however, especially when storage space becomes a problem. In sum, the minimum time for keeping records should be five to seven years. Beyond that, the physician is the best judge of his own needs for keeping such medical records. It is also possible to maintain a skeletal record on a patient without extraneous material that may have been sent for purposes that are no longer required. Stripping the chart to keep the essentials after seven years would help alleviate storage problems. Some hospitals or practitioners may transfer the medical records to microfilm or microfiche. Neither of these procedures is necessary for the average practitioner and may be quite expensive.

Summary

In summary, the medical record is an important part of the ongoing treatment of psychiatric patients. The information contained therein must be carefully and legibly prepared and diligently guarded against undue disclosure. The records not only serve as a continuing guide to the medical care and treatment of a particular patient, but also may have significant legal import, potentially affecting the therapist as well as the patient.

Selected Reading

1.   American Psychiatric Association Position Statement on the Confidentiality of Medical Research Records, *American Journal of Psychiatry,* 130:6. June 1973, p. 739.

2.   American Psychiatric Association Position Statement on Confidentiality and Privilege with Special Reference to Psychiatric Patients, *American Journal of Psychiatry,* 124:7, January 1968, p. 1015.

3.   Britton. A. H., "Rights to Privacy in Medical Records," *The Journal of Legal Medicine, July–August,* 1975, p. 24–31.

4.   *Doe v. Roe and Poe,* 400 New York Supplement, 2d series, November 21, 1977.

5.   Goldsmith. L. C.. "The Myth About Informed Consent," *The Journal of Legal Medicine,* September 1975, p. 17.

6.   Group for the Advancement of Psychiatry Report No. 45, "Confidentiality and Privileged Communication in the Practice of Psychiatry," May 1966.

7.   Halleck. S. L., *Law in the Practice of Psychiatry,* Plenum Medical Book Company, New York, 1980.

8.   *In Re B.* Appeal of Dr. Loren Roth, Pa., 394 A 2d 419.

9.   Meisel, A. & Roth, L. H., "What We Do and Do Not Know About Informed Consent," *Journal of the American Medical Association,* 246:21, November 27, 1981, p. 2473.

10. Noll, J. O., "The Therapist and Informed Consent," *American Journal of Psychiatry,* 133: 12, December 1976, p. 1451.

11. Rada. R. T., "Informed Consent in the Care of Psychiatric Patients," *National Association of Private Psychiatric Hospitals Journal,* 8:2, 1979, p.9.

12. Romano, J., "Reflections on Informed Consent," *Archives General Psychiatry,* 30:1, January 1974, p. 129.
13. Sadoff, R. L., "Informed Consent, Confidentiality and Privilege in Psychiatry: Practical Applications," *Bulletin, AAPL,* 2, 1974, pp. 101–106.
14. Sadoff, R. L., "Medical Legal Aspects of the Doctor-Patient Relationship," *Pa. Medicine,* 81, March 1978, pp. 24–27.
15. Sadoff. R. L., "The Importance of Informed Consent," *Journal of Legal Medicine,* May-June 1973, pp. 25–26.
16. Slovenko. R., *Psychotherapy, Confidentiality and Privileged Communications,* Charles C. Thomas, Springfield, Illinois, 1966.

4

Reducing the Risk of Psychiatric Malpractice

ROBERT L. SADOFF, M.D.

Editor's Note

Dr. Sadoff gives psychiatrists some clear guidelines to follow to reduce the risk of malpractice claims and to protect us in the event that a complaint should be lodged against us. Follow specific accepted standards of care. Be sure in making a diagnosis that the usual steps involved are carefully carried out and documented. Use reasonable precautions to prevent suicide. Be sure you have clearly communicated with patients and, when indicated, their families. Assess patients' potential for violence judiciously and take any steps that are necessary to protect others. When using medications, use standard dosages and, if deviating from those dosages and regimens, document the reasons. Always obtain informed consent. Inform patients of alternative methods of treatment when choices must be made. Observe patients' rights and balance them carefully against medical indications when considering involuntary hospitalization. Avoid sexual involvements with patients; some psychiatrists advocate the avoidance of sexual and love liaisons after treatment has been terminated as well. Remember, patients can justify

CME questions for this chapter begin on page 348.

malpractice only when damages have ensued due to a physician's presumed failure to observe standard measures of practice and conduct. Remember also that, even when all proper medical practices and expectations have been observed, a patient and his or her lawyer may still launch a suit for which one should also be prepared.

Introduction

Malpractice in psychiatry may occur in any of several different areas:

1. Improper diagnosis of the patient
2. Improper treatment of the patient
3. Patient suicide
4. Violent behavior of the patient toward third parties
5. Sexual exploitation of the patient by the therapist
6. Regulatory improprieties, e.g., improper informed consent, intruding on the rights of patients, improper commitment procedures, or breach of confidentiality

This chapter is not about the medicolegal aspects of malpractice, as that will be found in other publications. However, the purpose of this chapter is to review for the practitioner various practical situations that may result in malpractice claims. How can the practitioner avoid behavior that may result in a malpractice claim? How can the practitioner reduce the risk of being sued by his or her patient?

The first dictum in psychiatric or any medical treatment is "primum non nocere"—first, do not harm. The second is more specific: the practitioner must follow specific accepted standards of care for patients. The standard of care is defined in most jurisdictions as practicing medicine according to the standards of the average practitioner in the community. More specifically, the standards involve a reasonableness that is accepted by most practitioners. For example, it would be considered unreasonable by most psychiatrists to allow a highly suicidal patient to have access to the means of committing suicide while hospitalized. The standard of care also requires monitoring patients who are on medications that may cause side effects, and it demands the psychiatrist not abandon the patient. The list is endless, but its items are applicable to particular cases in specific situations.

Improper Diagnosis and Treatment

In the case of diagnosis, the psychiatrist may make an improper one but may believe it to be accurate, based on his or her assessment of the patient. The issue is not whether the diagnosis is correct but rather the methods by which the psychiatrist arrives at the diagnosis. If that method is acceptable and employed by most psychiatrists, no undue risk of malpractice should exist. If, however, the assessment is wanting or deficient in thoroughness or use of standardized methods, the psychiatrist may increase the risk of lawsuit *in the event of damage to the patient.*

It is conceded by most psychiatrists that some patients are confusing in their presentation of symptoms, and an accurate diagnosis may not be available at first blush. It is also accepted by most psychiatrists that some symptoms may indicate various diagnoses that require further studies to establish the precise diagnosis. For example, some extremely psychotic bipolar individuals may appear at first to be schizophrenic. The method of treatment, of course, will depend upon the diagnosis that is made. Giving lithium (Eskalith, Lithane) to a person who is schizophrenic will not be very helpful, nor will an antipsychotic be effective for a depressed bipolar individual. However, proper management can avoid the undue risk associated with medicating.

It should be noted that malpractice consists of four elements, sometimes referred to as the four "D's." First, the psychiatrist has a *duty* to assess, evaluate, or diagnose the patient accurately and to treat the patient according to standards developed by the profession. Second, if the psychiatrist is guilty of *dereliction* of duty that *directly* leads to *damage* to the patient, the four elements are present for a successful malpractice suit. Dereliction of duty is often described in the law as negligence. Negligence does not necessarily mean that the psychiatrist ignored the patient but rather deviated from the standard of care in the treatment of the patient. If that deviation is a direct cause (or proximate cause) of damage to the patient, there may be grounds for malpractice action. Direct cause does not necessarily mean, logically, that one action or omission caused the other but may be interpreted as being necessary for the damage to have occurred. Absent the negligence, damage may not have resulted. The damage may be a physical, emotional, or financial loss as a result of the doctor's deviation from the standard of care.

Sometimes the psychiatrist may deviate from the standard of care, but no damage befalls the patient. On other occasions, damage to the patient may not have been caused by the negligence of the doctor. Those are cases of unfortunate outcome but cannot be faulted to malpractice. All four elements must be provided by the plaintiff in order for the malpractice action to be successful.

Patient Suicide

Perhaps one of the most tragic situations in psychiatry is the suicide of a patient, either in the hospital or as an outpatient. It is fairly standard for incidents of inpatient suicide to precipitate malpractice claims. In such cases, the family feels they have placed their trust and the life of their family member in the hands of the hospital and the treating physician, and they do not anticipate the death of the loved one in such a setting. There is no absolute guarantee that suicidal patients will not succeed in killing themselves if they are hospitalized: it is possible through no fault of the staff or the treating physician. However, adequate measures must be taken to ensure that patients do not commit suicide when they are hospitalized and recognized as high suicide risks.

In discussing malpractice risks, it is tempting to be overly conservative in recommending safeguards to prevent malpractice. Especially in cases where a patient's life may be at stake, it is increasingly important to act in a manner that preserves the life of the patient, even when patients may resist appropriate treatment in that direction. Sometimes the psychiatrist must restrict the freedom of the patient and abridge his or her rights in order to save the patient's life. As patients' rights have emerged over the past several decades to be important considerations in legal matters and in the treatment of psychiatric patients, the law has become a partner in treatment. Psychiatrists may not involuntarily hospitalize a patient without the court's approval or order. Merely being mentally ill is no longer sufficient for involuntary commitment; the patient must also represent, as a result of mental illness, a clear and present danger of harm to self or others. The law interprets the "dangerous potential" of the patient in determining the need for involuntary confinement. With respect to discharging patients, psychiatrists have assumed the risk of the patient's behavior following discharge. If the patient has been committed as mentally ill and poses a clear and present danger to self, the psychiatrist must properly assess the patient's suicide risk in the community before discharging the patient. If the psychiatrist decides to discharge the patient to his or her family, requirements must be met in terms of communication to the family regarding the proper care of the patient at home and in the community. The family must be apprised of the suicide risk and the need for continued medication and proper safeguards within the home. Guns must be locked away and medications must not be readily available for overdose ingestion.

Violence Directed at a Third Party

If the patient is committed by the court because of being mentally ill and posing a clear and present danger to others, the psychiatrist, prior to discharging the patient, must assess the patient's potential for violent behavior to others in the community. It may be a general potential for harming unnamed or unidentified persons or a specific assessment of the potential for harming specific individuals whom the patient has threatened. If the patient is discharged and within a reasonable period of time harms a third party, the psychiatrist ordering the discharge may be held liable for the damage inflicted by his or her patient. Therefore, it behooves the psychiatrist to make and duly record a valid, accurate, and careful assessment of the patient, not only for mental illness but also for the potential for violent behavior when discharged.

In order to reduce the risk of lawsuit to the psychiatrist taking the responsibility for such discharge, it is recommended that if the psychiatrist is not certain of the patient's potential for violence or for self-destructive behavior, a court should make the final determination for discharge. If, after a proper hearing, the judge orders the patient to be discharged from the hospital, the psychiatrist must comply with the court's order. If the patient then harms self or another within a short period of time, the psychiatrist is protected by the judge's order. The psychiatrist had no choice but to discharge the patient according to the order of the court. Refusal to follow the court's order makes the psychiatrist liable for contempt of court by improperly incarcerating the patient.

The psychiatrist, however, must take proper care in the method of discharge and alert people in the community to the potential dangers that exist for the patient or by the patient. Just because the psychiatrist follows the order of the court in discharging the patient, it does not relieve the duty to discharge in a careful, proper manner with appropriate communication of safeguards for the patient and others in the community.

Use of Medications

In using medication for treatment of patients, the psychiatrist should use standard medications and standard dosages whenever possible. If the psychiatrist decides to deviate from the recommended dosage range or chooses to use combinations of medications that may pose a risk of harm to the patient, the psychiatrist must justify such deviation in the patient's record. In the case of a medication-resistant patient, it is possible to prescribe larger doses or various combinations that are not standard and to do so with safety by properly monitoring the patient. The reasons for the method of treatment selected should be indicated in the record. One should, of course, always get the informed consent of the patient to use those various treatment modalities whenever possible.

A word about informed consent is important, because it is a confusing issue for most therapists. Some consider it to be a legal maneuver to harm therapists or entrap them in legal malpractice. In fact, the concept of informed consent is a very humane matter that gives autonomy to the patient when competent to make decisions on his or her own behalf. The concept is a long-standing one in the law and is supported by a number of precedent cases. The theory is that people have a right to decide what will happen to their bodies and their minds, and the physician may not intrude on the privacy of the patient without the patient's consent. The consent must be competent and valid; and it may be given only after proper information about the treatment is provided to the patient. Judgments have gone against the psychiatrist when the information given was not sufficient.

Psychiatrists should tell the patient what medication they intend to use, what effect the medication will have on the patient's illness, and what side effects may occur as a result of using that medication. The patient should also be told what would happen if the medication were not used and how much longer the patient would remain ill or remain hospitalized without the treatment recommended by the psychiatrist.

In addition, the physician must inform the patient of alternative methods of treatment that are available but that the physician chooses not to use at that time. For example, if a patient is suffering from depression and the psychiatrist chooses intensive psychotherapy rather than medication, the physician must not only explain the rationale for the decision but also inform the patient that other psychiatrists may choose antidepressant medication for treatment of his or her depression—and that medication may be successful in alleviating the depression in a relatively short time. It is not sufficient for the physician to offer only the selected treatment modality and ignore alternatives.

Sexual Exploitation of the Patient

One of the increasing problems in psychotherapy has become the sexual exploitation of the patient. Usually involved are a middle-age male therapist and a young, histrionic or borderline female patient. Psychiatrists try to defend the claim by such a patient that sexual activities have occurred by stating: (a) they have fallen in love with the patient; (b) the patient was unduly seductive and the psychiatrist could not or did not withstand the patient's charms; or (c) that the sexual behavior was a part of the treatment for the patient. Finally, the psychiatrist may acknowledge that sexual behavior occurred, but only after the termination of therapy.

It must be stated clearly that sexual involvement of a patient with a therapist is to be prohibited and is condemned by all major therapeutic psychotherapy organizations. The sexual exploitation of patients is harmful to the patient and should never be condoned or accepted. However, several issues need to be discussed. The first is the matter of timing. Is it ever appropriate for a psychiatrist to have sexual relations with a former patient, and if so, how long after therapy has terminated? There is no standard response to this question, but most analysts currently recommend no social or sexual involvement with patients or former patients, because the transference phenomenon continues after the termination of therapy. It is unwise and improper for a psychiatrist to take advantage of the relationship that had developed during therapy for the purpose of sexual involvement after therapy has ended. It is certainly unethical and inappropriate for the psychiatrist to be involved sexually with a patient during the course of therapy, even if outside the therapeutic hour.

An offshoot of this problem arises when a therapist encounters a patient who claims to have been sexually exploited by a previous psychiatrist. What is the obligation of the second therapist to report the inappropriate behavior of the first? The answer lies in the evidence that may be gleaned during the course of therapy to substantiate the behavior, rather than an immediate knee-jerk response to report a colleague purely on the word of a disgruntled former patient. The second therapist does not know the veracity of such a claim and may be inappropriately harming a colleague on insufficient data. It is wise not to jump into the fray until evidence is clear. A much better (and safer) strategy for the second therapist would be to encourage the patient to report the inappropriate behavior as part of the therapy. If the second therapist improperly reports his colleague and the reputation of the first therapist is damaged, even though the claim is not substantiated by a thorough investigation, the second therapist may be liable.

Regulatory Improprieties

Some malpractice cases involve commitment proceedings. Most jurisdictions have immunity clauses that protect the psychiatrist who either commits a patient to a hospital or decides the patient is not committable at that time. Again, as in diagnostic proceedings, the final judgment is not the major issue. What is important is the method by which the psychiatrist arrived at a decision either to commit or to withhold involuntary hospitalization. If the patient is clearly psychotic, destructive, and out of control, as reported by the people with whom the patient lives, the assessing psychiatrist may see no clear-cut evidence of uncontrollable behavior by the time the patient is brought to the emergency room. However, the psychiatrist may not ignore the behavior as reported by the family and must consider history as well as examination. If the psychiatrist refuses to hospitalize and the patient kills the person who requested commitment, the psychiatrist will invariably be sued for negligence in not considering all the available information when making the assessment and recommendation.

On the other hand, if a psychiatrist chooses to hospitalize a person on insufficient data, thereby depriving the patient of liberty, the psychiatrist may be sued for false arrest or improperly confining the patient. Again, judgment is not the issue in question. Instead, it is the means by which the judgment is reached. If other psychiatrists were exposed to the same information or data, would the average psychiatrist commit or withhold commitment? In some cases the answer is not clear and, since the burden of proof is on the plaintiff, the psychiatrist may not lose the lawsuit but still must feel the emotional pain of going through such an experience.

Governing Principles of Psychiatry

It is important for all psychiatrists to be aware of the principles that govern our practice and that will help reduce the risk of psychiatric malpractice.

Do not neglect the patient. If a patient indicates emotional or mental difficulties and requires assessment, do not avoid a personal examination of the patient. As an alternative, refer the patient to a respected and competent colleague or to the emergency room of the hospital.

Conduct all necessary tests and evaluations of the patient in order to make a proper, thorough, and complete assessment. Only then should treatment begin.

Use standard and acceptable modes and forms of treatment rather than experimental ones. The only exception to that rule would come from informed consent to experimental or unusual treatment modalities. Such consent should be recorded in the patient's chart along with the reasons for the use of such methods.

In the case of suicidal patients, always place the patient on an appropriate level of suicide observation. Careful assessment of suicide risk is required by asking the proper questions, which should be documented in the patient's chart. When changes in the patient's status are noted, such changes must also be recorded. At discharge of a suicidal patient, it is insufficient to give "patient is not homicidal or suicidal" as a final statement. It is much better to indicate the basis of such a conclusion, specifically the questions and answers used to arrive at that conclusion.

Always adhere to hospital guidelines and regulations with respect to seclusion and restraint of patients. Careful coordination with nursing personnel is required in many cases where suicide or violent behavior is prevalent.

Carefully document all communications, questions, and advice to the patient and family in the patient's record. Courts and lawyers will later argue that if the matter was not recorded, it was never communicated or accomplished. Although that may not be true, it will be more difficult for the psychiatrist to prove what he did if it is not contemporaneously recorded.

Avoid vague concepts in communicating with patients or in putting on record words that are not properly defined, such as "dangerousness." They may later be used to accuse the psychiatrist of negligent behavior. It is always better to use words of act or behavior, such as "self-destructive behavior," which can be documented, or "violent behavior," which can also be noted. Dangerousness is not well defined and is a vague term that has caused great difficulty for psychiatrists.

Never become emotionally or physically involved with a patient, either during or following therapy. Sexual or physical exploitation of the patient is always improper and harmful to patients and is condemned by all professional organizations.

Closely advise the families of psychotic patients, especially if the patient is to return home under the care of the family. Within the confines of confidentiality, share with the family (with the consent of the patient) the important information necessary for continued proper care of the discharged patient. (It should be noted that families assume responsibilities for care of patients only if they are properly instructed by the physician. A family may choose not to follow the recommendations of the physician, but then it must accept the responsibility and not blame the psychiatrist for failure to protect the patient.) It is essential that the psychiatrist relieve himself or herself of the liability by properly communicating to the family and recording the communication in the patient's chart. It is often the guilty family that will attempt to assuage its guilt by projecting it onto the psychiatrist after an untoward event.

Adhere to specific guidelines of national organizations, courts, and regulations regarding the rights of patients, especially the right to refuse treatment. Carefully record the patient's responses to information about treatment modalities or medication when considering informed consent or emergency situations in which treatment is given without consent.

Consult attorneys, especially the hospital attorney, if questions arise about the legality of any contemplated procedure.

Finally, it is best to be reasonable in the treatment of patients. Who defines reasonableness? The court ultimately will provide a definition;

however, the reasonable approach may be found by the psychiatrist by consulting his or her own reason and experience and by consulting respected colleagues in cases that appear confusing or novel. If the psychiatrist wishes to take a risk with a patient, that risk must be carefully documented and agreed to by the patient whenever possible. If the patient is incompetent, then the family, guardian, or court must be consulted in order to give consent that is not available directly from the patient.

Summary

Malpractice cases will occur even when the psychiatrist exercises good judgment and reason in the treatment of patients. However, the risk of a malpractice suit can be reduced by following the guidelines noted above. Even if a lawsuit occurs, the reasonable psychiatrist that follows such governing principles may emerge victorious. The psychiatrist who wins a lawsuit is still scarred by the process, so it is far better for all concerned if a malpractice suit can be avoided in the first place.

Reading List

Robertson JD. *Psychiatric Malpractice: Liability of Mental Health Professionals.* New York: John Wiley & Sons; 1988.

Sadoff RL. *Forensic Psychiatry: A Practical Guide for Lawyers and Psychiatrists.* 2nd Ed. Springfield, Ill.: Thomas and Co.; 1988.

Simon RI. *Clinical Psychiatry and the Law.* Washington, D.C.: American Psychiatric Press; 1987.

Simon RI. *Concise Guide to Clinical Psychiatry and Law.* Washington, D.C.: American Psychiatric Press; 1988.

5

Vulnerability of Psychiatrists in Assessment of Risk for Malpractice

ROBERT L. SADOFF, M.D.

Editor's Note

Malpractice is a civil tort in which a care giver is accused of (a) deviating from a standard of care or (b) being derelict in their duty to their patients, that (c) causes damage to the patient (d) or others. In this lesson, the author alerts us to areas of special vulnerability that can increase the risk of malpractice claims and offers guidelines to reduce that risk.

The areas covered here include the matter of hospitalizing patients (voluntary versus involuntary), how to deal with the concept of "dangerousness," every patient's right to adequate treatment and his or her right to refuse treatment, release or discharge to the community, the Tarasoff "duty to protect," confidentiality, informed consent, and boundary violations.

Introduction

The practice of psychiatry has become increasingly complex over the last two or three decades. Changes have occurred in the treatment of patients, and especially in the civil rights arena, that affirm various

CME questions for this chapter begin on page 350.

rights of patients, including the right to treatment and the right to refuse treatment. Commitment laws have changed to include the concept of "dangerousness." Managed care and other third party payers have invaded the scene, often limiting length of stay in various hospitals, obtaining release of particular information for recording purposes, and occasionally limiting the types of treatment available to the patient. Ethical considerations have become more prominent in the practice of psychiatry, including issues of confidentiality and of reporting incidents of inappropriate doctor-patient relationships and boundary violations. Treatment techniques and modalities have changed with the advent of newer and more efficient and effective psychotropic medications. Confusion has reigned over such concepts as least restrictive alternative and Tarasoff considerations of duty to warn and duty to protect.

Those issues by no means constitute a complete list of changes that lead to areas of vulnerability for practicing psychiatrists. However, they represent a significant number of issues that need to be explored and discussed in order to decrease the risk of malpractice claims against psychiatrists. This presentation is designed to alert the practicing psychiatrist to these areas of vulnerability that can increase the risk of malpractice claims and offer guidelines that will reduce (if not eliminate) the risk of lawsuit against the psychiatrist for inappropriate behavior or for practice that deviates from the standards of care.

Malpractice

Malpractice is defined as a civil tort in which care givers are accused of deviating from a standard of care or being derelict in their duty to their patients. It is the *dereliction* of *duty* that *directly* leads to *damage* that encompass the four elements necessary for a successful malpractice lawsuit, commonly known as the four D's. Thus, psychiatrists have a duty to their patients not to harm them, a duty not to breach confidentiality unless it is appropriate or mandated, and a duty to follow various standards of care that have been established by peers through previous experience and practice. Malpractice claims against psychiatrists have increased in the past two decades, primarily because of the general increase in lawsuits against physicians, but also because changes in the practice of psychiatry have not always been adhered to by all psychiatrists.

Voluntary and Involuntary Hospitalization of Psychiatric Patients

Traditionally, psychiatric patients were found to be treated more effectively as voluntary rather than involuntary patients. Every effort was made to encourage the patient to sign himself or herself into the hospital as a voluntary patient for treatment. Sometimes issues of competency were neglected in an effort to have the patient admitted voluntarily. Even very seriously mentally ill patients who were psychotic—even delirious or hallucinating—were voluntarily admitted if they agreed to come into the hospital for treatment. Following the case of *Zinermon v. Burch*,[1] such practices are now prohibited. Incompetent patients (i.e., patients who do not know the nature and consequences of their legal situation) cannot legally sign themselves into the hospital. They may need to be involuntarily committed if they meet the criteria for the jurisdiction involved. In the rare event that such patients are not committable under the statute of that jurisdiction, other means must be found to hospitalize the patient. Such means may include having next of kin sign the patient in temporarily until competency proceedings may be held with an appointed guardian who would then legally sign the patient in the hospital. Some provision for emergency competency hearing and assumption of temporary guardianship by the court to effect the commitment or admission may also be considered.

The difficulty comes more often in the involuntarily committed patient. Most states have immunity clauses in their commitment statutes[2] that allow physicians to involuntarily commit patients without risk of being sued unless, for example, they act in an unprofessional manner, using gross negligence or willful misconduct. Merely making an error in judgment regarding the patient's condition would not suffice to uphold a lawsuit for improper commitment to the hospital. However, physicians in the emergency room must be thorough and careful in their assessment in order to document all means by which the decision to commit was determined. Cases have occurred in which doctors have been sued for improper commitment because they found evidence for "dangerousness," but no evidence for a bona fide mental illness linked to the "dangerousness." Occasionally, an individual will come into the emergency room intoxicated and appear to be threatening and violent and unable to cooperate with the examining physician. Formerly, these individuals were sent to the drunk tank of the local jail to dry out and be re-evaluated in the morning. However, drunk tanks apparently have been replaced by mental health institutions to treat the effects of acute intoxication when violence or self-destructive behavior is threatened. It may be preferable to hold the patient in the emergency room until the effects of the intoxication wear off and a proper assessment of committability may be determined.

Physicians frequently assess the committability of an individual in an emergency situation, determine the patient is not committable, and allow the patient to go home. Should there be an episode of violent, self-destructive, or suicidal behavior, the physician is often sued for improper assessment of the patient for committability. Other aspects of such negligence may occur when the patient is not evaluated when brought to the emergency room and is allowed to elope, or escape, from the emergency room and commit suicide or kill someone.

When assessing an individual for mental illness, the psychiatrist (or the physician in the emergency room acting in lieu of the psychiatrist) assumes a responsibility for proper diagnosis and medical evaluation. Sometimes the more difficult assessment occurs with reference to the issue of "dangerousness." Perhaps it is best to redefine this elusive concept in clinical terms such as potential violence to others under various clinical conditions, or potential self-destructive or suicidal behavior under various clinical conditions. In this way, the assessing physician has the opportunity and obligation to determine under what clinical conditions the individual may be violent or self-destructive. For example, is this a person who has a diagnosis of paranoid schizophrenia, and who is noncompliant with taking medication? Does the violence occur when the patient does not take the medication for several days and begins to hallucinate, acting out psychotic thoughts against others? Or is this patient one who becomes extremely depressed and suicidal when faced with rejection and anticipated loss? What factors in this person's life may be consistent with such clinical conditions that they may warrant hospitalization because he or she clearly poses a threat of harm to himself or herself. With the advent of the concept of "dangerousness" built into all commitment laws, psychiatrists are under pressure not only to determine whether the patient is psychiatrically ill and in need of hospitalization (as was the old criteria) but also whether the patient poses a threat of harm to self or others.

If the assessing physician or psychiatrist is uncertain about committability, in most states, he or she has the opportunity and obligation to call the representative of the local court system to determine whether commitment would be acceptable within the legal structure of the community. Should the mental health review officer decide that the patient is not committable under the circumstances, the assessing physician, who wishes to have the patient committed, should clearly document any communications to the mental health review officer in the patient's record and indicate that the court system, through the representative of the mental health review officer (referee, magistrate), refused to accept the physician's recommendation. Should the patient then go on to do harm to self or someone else in the immediate future, the physician may have decreased the risk of lawsuit because the matter has been referred for community legal decision rather than making the decision alone.

An alternative method is to consult with a respected colleague, who examines the patient independently and comes to an independent conclusion about committability. If both physicians are of the same mind to commit, some states will allow that to occur without consulting the mental health review officer. However, in decreasing risk of potential malpractice suits, it is always wise to consult with the legal system that controls or regulates commitment and/or discharge from the hospital.

Dangerousness

A word about dangerousness. This concept has been poorly defined, if at all, in legislation and/or cases brought against psychiatrists. Nevertheless, many cases have determined that a psychiatrist can, and should be able to, predict when a patient is going to become "dangerous" and has a duty to protect the community from the violent behavior of the patient. Since the advent of this concept into psychiatric practice, it has been suggested that psychiatrists communicate to the courts their findings in terms of clinical decisions such as violent behavior or self-destructive or suicidal behavior under certain clinical conditions, rather than the general term of "dangerousness." By this means, a physician has maintained a professional determination within the guidelines of psychiatric expertise and has not deviated beyond that expertise into the realm of legal conceptualization. If the psychiatrist has an ability to predict future violent or self-destructive behavior, he or she can do so within clinical guidelines or as imminent behavior, rather than in the generic terms of future dangerousness. In this way, the standards of care will be determined by the psychiatrists rather than by the law, in terms of abilities of psychiatrists rather than expectations of what psychiatrists can or cannot do by those outside the profession. Many of the standards of care in malpractice lawsuits are actually legal standards set by the legal profession rather than medical standards set by the psychiatric profession.

Treatment Modalities–Use of Psychotropic Medication

The past two decades have brought a clarification of the rights of patients who have been involuntarily committed to psychiatric hospitals. These rights include the right to adequate treatment[4] and the right to refuse treatment.[1] In cases involving the right to refuse treatment, the courts have narrowed the treatment that may be refused by competent patients who are not emergencies to the neuroleptic medications that may have long-term harmful side effects (e.g., tardive dyskinesia). The courts have found that negligent use of such medications may be harmful to patients when monitoring systems for assessment of side effects are not properly employed. Merely having a side effect that is an expected consequence of many such medications is not malpractice. However, improper monitoring of the patient may lead to a malpractice suit. Thus, it is important when treating a patient with various medications to adequately monitor the patient's response. Also, the use of various combinations of medications may have unexpected side effects and may damage the patient and trigger a subsequent lawsuit.

The other important consideration in the use of any treatment modality is that of informed consent. The patient must be given proper information about the medication to be used, including its effects and side effects. Alternative treatment modalities, whether less or more complicated, must be offered to the patient for autonomous choice when a choice exists. The physician may recommend a particular treatment but may not be coercive in that treatment choice to a competent patient who is involuntarily committed. The information must be given in the patient's language in order that he or she understands the information and can incorporate the information into his or her thought processes and voluntarily consent to the treatment.[5]

Should there be any question about the patient's ability to understand—whether the patient is competent to refuse or whether the patient poses an emergency so that involuntary medication may be administered over the short term (never using the long-acting neuroleptics in such situations)—a respected colleague should be consulted for an independent examination and assessment to determine whether involuntary medication may be administered. If both agree that the patient either is incompetent to refuse or poses an emergency that needs to be handled as an emergency, then the medication may be given involuntarily until such time the patient either agrees to take the medication or a court can hear the case with respect to the patient's competency to refuse or his or her state of emergency.

Release or Discharge of a Patient to the Community

When a decision is made to discharge a patient to the community, various determinations must be made and procedures followed in order to decrease the risk of a lawsuit in the event the patient is "prematurely" released and then goes on to do harm to self or others. Many cases of "premature release" have been filed when patients leave the hospital and commit suicide or homicide. The treating physician is the one who makes the final determination about release. This determination must be made on the basis of clinical findings and not economic determination. Cases have been brought with respect to private psychiatric hospitals that discharge patients at the end of their insurance coverage. This is not appropriate if the patient is not ready for discharge. The patient may be transferred to another hospital to avoid large monetary deficits on the part of the hospital or the family, which may have to pay after the insurance coverage expires. However, the determination for discharge must be a clinical one.

If the treating psychiatrist is uncertain about the likelihood of self-destructive or violent behavior when released, he or she should either consult the court that committed the patient for treatment or petition for commitment of the patient. Many psychiatrists have criticized this view, indicating that the determination for discharge remains a medical decision, not a legal one. Traditionally, that has been true, and psychiatrists have been able to safely discharge patients to the community following admission or commitment. However, with the advent of the concept of dangerousness, courts have held psychiatrists and hospitals responsible for the damage incurred by patients who had been prematurely released, even for as long as 6 months after discharge.[6] Thus, it is important in reducing the risk of malpractice suits for the psychiatrist to consult the legal system (in many cases, it was the legal system or the judge that originally committed the patient to the hospital, depriving him or her of liberty) to determine whether the patient's liberty interests should be restored and the patient be discharged from the hospital. Lawyers have indicated that liberty interests are important for determination only when they are abridged and not when they are restored. However, the psychiatrist has been singled out, in creative lawsuits, charging that persons who became violent or suicidal following discharge did so because of the negligence of psychiatrists.

If the psychiatrist consults with the legal system by bringing the case before the committing judge or before the sitting judge in that jurisdiction, the judge may decide, after hearing all testimony, that the patient should be discharged to the community. If the judge so decides and orders the patient to be discharged from the hospital, then it seems the doctor would not be responsible for the violent behavior of the patient who has been so judicially discharged. The doctor will be following the order of the court (indeed, would be in contempt of the court if he or she did not follow it) and thus should be spared the consequences of a subsequent lawsuit in the event violent behavior ensued.

Tarasoff-*like Cases: Duty to Warn or Protect*

Many cases arise with respect to the issue of the psychiatrist's duty to warn the intended victim of the patient's violent threats or the psychiatrist's duty to protect the community from the violent behavior of psychiatric patients. The original *Tarasoff* case enunciated the duty of the treating psychiatrist to warn the victim identified by the patient who, in the course of therapy, made a specific threat to that person.[7] However, 2 years later, the court restated a new *Tarasoff* duty for psychiatrists: the duty to protect.[8] That duty allowed the psychiatrist to take other steps in protecting the identifiable victim of the patient's specific threats by either hospitalizing the patient, calling in the family to help control the patient, or utilizing the appropriate police department to help prevent violent behavior. Only as a last resort would the identifiable victim be called and warned.

This duty to protect, which appears to be more appropriate than a limited duty to warn, also has affected psychiatrists in other jurisdictions where no specific threat is required and no identifiable victim was necessary in order for a lawsuit to be brought against the treating psychiatrist. These jurisdictions have enunciated a general duty to protect the community from the violent behavior of the psychiatric patient.[9] Thus, psychiatrists have been put on notice that they will be sued if their patients commit violent behavior while in the course of therapy, irrespective of whether specific threats are made or identifiable victims are known. This puts a great burden on the treating psychiatrist to be very cautious in treating persons who may act out internal conflicts through violent behavior toward others. Despite the rule of "least restrictive alternative," psychiatrists must use the court system and commitment procedures when they are faced with persons who are likely to become violent. In some jurisdictions, no specific threat and no identifiable victims are necessary. The psychiatrist will be sued if the patient hurts another person. Thus, the psychiatrist should interpret the "least restrictive alternative" concept in its true meaning: the least restrictive alternative of treatment for the patient's medical needs at that particular time.

Tarasoff cases require the psychiatrist to breach the duty of confidentiality in order to save the life or health of another. Psychiatrists breach that duty in order to save the patient's life in a suicidal case; thus, breaching it to save a third party's life is not inappropriate. Rather, it is sanctioned and approved by the ethical code of the AMA as applied to psychiatrists.[10]

Ethical Considerations and Boundary Violations

There are ethical standards of medical practice for physicians as applied to psychiatry. There are ethical interpretations of those standards with respect to various questions that arise in the practice of psychiatry. There is the standard of doing no harm to patients and the concept of maintaining confidentiality. One may breach confidentiality when it is appropriate and when subpoenaed or court ordered for records or for testimony about a patient who has waived his or her privilege of silence when entering into a civil or criminal legal matter.

Also, the question of confidentiality arises when discharging a patient from the hospital. Families, who become the new caregivers following discharge, need to know several specifics in order to care for the patient properly. The family should know what medication the patient is taking, what side effects may occur from that medication, what effects may occur if the patient does not take the medication, and what symptoms or signs are to be observed for deterioration or regression in the patient's condition. Other issues that may need to be discussed with families concern the security of the person and/or the community. For example, in some cases it may be appropriate to tell families to lock away dangerous weapons, such as guns, large knives, and/or caustic or poisonous substances. Families have become very active in the care and treatment of mental patients discharged to their care. They have formed the Alliance for the Mentally Ill and have chapters throughout the country. They wish to be informed, and need to be informed, about various issues that affect their family members without breaching confidentiality. Such issues as medication, compliance, side effects, and dangerous objects in the home should be discussed with the family, in front of the patient, during a discharge planning session.[11]

Boundary violations are another major ethical issue that may lead to a malpractice lawsuit. Clearly, sexual behavior between psychiatrist and patient is prohibited. Sexual behavior between psychiatrist and former patient is "almost always" unethical. But, some boundary violations in and of themselves are destructive to the patient and may lead to malpractice suits, even when sexual behavior does not occur. Many occur with patients who have borderline personality disorders and who demand breaching of boundaries as part of their illness and their attempt to relate to the psychotherapist. Psychiatrists must be very clearly aware of transference and countertransference phenomena that may affect the treatment of patients. Breaching boundaries is a serious matter that can harm the patient and lead to a malpractice lawsuit. Such boundaries may include excessive informality with the patient, hugging the patient at each session, inappropriate touching of the patient, inviting the patient for lunch or dinner, seeing the patient outside the therapy situation, and having a dual-agency relationship with the patient involving matters other than treatment.[12]

Other Considerations that Increase Risk of Lawsuit

The foregoing are the major issues to be considered with respect to vulnerable areas for psychiatric practice. However, others that are emerging need to be briefly discussed, as they may lead to an increased risk of malpractice suits in the future. These include the treatment of HIV-positive or AIDS patients. Laws regulating confidentiality information regarding AIDS patients are fairly well documented by various professional guidelines.[13] However, the issues regarding AIDS patients remain unclear and no precedents have been clearly established for regulating such treatment. Psychiatrists treating HIV-positive or AIDS patients, whether inpatient or outpatient, should be alerted to the uncertainties in this area and conduct themselves accordingly.

The recent phenomenon of false memory syndrome may also affect psychotherapists. Without entering into a lengthy discussion of this most controversial area of practice, it should be noted that a number of young women who have eating disorders or other disorders common during early adulthood later claim they have been sexually abused as youngsters, primarily by members of their families. No memory of such incestuous behavior had occurred until the person became involved in treatment. Often the treatment encouraged or suggested that such behavior must have occurred for the patient to have such symptoms. Hypnosis or other relaxation techniques may help bring out these memories, especially under encouragement and suggestions. Sometimes lawsuits are filed against the family for such inappropriate behavior. If the concept of false memory syndrome is upheld in a particular case in which the family is sued and the patient loses the lawsuit, the therapist may be countersued by the family for iatrogenically causing such problems with the patient. Therapists must be cautious to avoid excessive suggestion or encouragement of such memories, especially if they are distorted or false and lead to inappropriate legal action.

References

1. *Zinermon v. Burch*, 110 Sct. 975 (1990).
2. *Pennsylvania Mental Health and Mental Retardation Procedures Act*, 1976.

3. *Wyatt v. Stickney*, 325F Supp. 781 (MD Ala. 1971).

4. *Rogers v. Okin*, 478F Supp. 1342 (D Mass. 1979) and *Rennie v. Klein*, 462F Supp. 1131 (D NJ 1978).

5. Roth LH, Meisel A, Lidz CW. Tests of competency to consent to treatment. *Am J Psychiatry*. 1977;134:279–284.

6. *Naidu v. Laird*, 539A 2d, 1064 (Del. 1988).

7. *Tarasoff v. Regents of the University of California*, 188 Cal. Rptr. 129,529P 2d 553 (1974).

8. *Tarasoff v. Regents of the University of California*, 188 Cal. Rptr. 14,551P 2d 334 (1976).

9. *Schuster v. Altenberg*, 144 Wis 2d 223,424 NW 2d 159 (1988).

10. Official actions, APA, principles of medical ethics as applied to psychiatrists. *Am J Psychiatry*. 1973;130(9):1061–1064.

11. Petrila JP, Sadoff RL. Confidentiality and the family as caregiver. *Hosp Commun Psychiatry*. 1992;43(2):136—139.

12. Simon RI. Treatment boundary violations: clinical, ethical, and legal considerations. *Bull Am Acad Psychiatry Law*. 1992;20(3):269–288.

13. *AIDS–Confidentiality of HIV-Related Information Act, PA Legis. Service Act*, 148, 1990.

6

Practical Legal Considerations for the Psychiatrist Being Sued for Malpractice

JOAN SALTMAN, ESQ.

Editor's Note

This lesson deals with being as prepared as possible for malpractice suits. Some of the guidelines are simple and obvious. Carry adequate malpractice insurance. Report to your insurance company as soon as the first threat appears. Be honest at all times with the lawyer who will represent you. Don't try to play lawyer yourself.

Some of the guidelines address more subtle, but no less critical, issues. Don't be thrown off because you haven't received a subpoena yet, mistakenly speaking with a former patient's attorney who says he's just "gathering some information." Refer him to your lawyer. Be sure your records are straight. Respond to any initial suit papers at once by

CME questions for this chapter begin on page 351.

notifying your attorney. Know what is involved in the "discovery process," which may involve written interrogations or oral explorations posed at depositions. These stages in the process have a great influence on what may happen later on in the courtroom . . . provided the case is not settled. And what should you do if you are not satisfied with the attorney assigned to you by your insurance carrier?

Introduction

When psychiatrists are defendants in malpractice cases, they often find themselves adrift in a sea of legal terminology and forensic gamesmanship. The law can be demystified, however. Psychiatrists can understand how to respond at each stage of a malpractice case by comprehending those stages and the appropriate reaction at each stage. Often the sage response is to ask a lawyer's help. Psychiatrists can also learn how to make lawyers more responsive to their needs. No psychiatrist should stride into the fray of a psychiatric malpractice case without the advice of an attorney who is knowledgeable in professional negligence.

Psychiatrists should ask for legal help (probably more than they think they should) in determining how to shield themselves from malpractice judgments, in deciding when to release medical records, in responding to suit papers and discovery, in determining whether to settle a case, and in learning how to conduct themselves at trial. When in doubt about issues that arise in the legal arena, the psychiatrist should ask a lawyer. While that precept may seem like an advertisement for the legal profession and self-serving, it is also a good way to avoid the serious trouble occasioned by attempting to go it alone in a legal conflict.

This chapter will discuss the question of malpractice coverage; the pre-trial, trial, and post-trial process; and the psychiatrist's best responses at each stage, including when to ask for legal help and how to make effective use of that legal aid.

Malpractice Insurance

No matter how carefully a clinician practices psychiatry, he or she may be the target of a malpractice suit for one of two reasons: the doctor's care falls below the appropriate medical standard or the lawyer evaluating a potential lawsuit against the physician errs. Every physician should carry adequate malpractice insurance to protect against the financial hardship that would result from the staggering costs of defending against and satisfying malpractice judgments. What is considered to be adequate insurance differs from state to state and from person to person. Some statutes provide that all physicians buy minimum coverage and then contribute to another fund, often called a catastrophe loss fund, that pays any amount above that of minimum coverage. Other states do not regulate malpractice insurance so closely. Obviously, all physicians will not require the same amount of insurance. Coverage should be large enough so none of the physician's personal assets would be jeopardized as a result of a malpractice judgment. A psychiatrist who is unsure as to the kind of malpractice insurance to invest in and how much insurance to buy should consult with an attorney, preferably one familiar with both malpractice and insurance issues. Insurance coverage should be reviewed and updated periodically.

The psychiatrist should carefully read the malpractice insurance policy after purchase because failure to follow the mandates of a professional liability insurance policy could result in denial of coverage. In some circumstances, insurance companies will refuse to guarantee coverage because physicians have ignored the provisions of policies that require prompt claims reporting. If understanding the language of the policy is a problem (and there is no shame in admitting that the legal terminology used in many policies is hard to understand), the psychiatrist should seek legal advice to explain the terms of the policy.

Reporting the Claim

Although language varies between policies, the psychiatrist is usually required under the terms of the malpractice insurance policy to report any "threatened" claim, with full information about treatment rendered. When the physician reports the claim, he or she should be completely honest, and the insurance company should be supplied with all records relevant to the patient. If the alleged malpractice took place in a hospital, the claim should also be reported to the hospital administrator, because the hospital will very likely become a defendant in the suit. The physician should ask his or her insurance company to report the claim to the hospital administrator so that the doctor is not in the position of discussing the case with a potential adversary at trial.

The Investigation by the Patient's Lawyer

Many psychiatrists believe a lawsuit is not serious until the papers initiating the suit, whether a complaint or a summons, actually arrive. Important aspects of a lawsuit begin well before the sheriff delivers a complaint or summons (the usual means of lawsuit initiation) to a psychiatrist's door. Often a patient's lawyer will investigate a potential malpractice case for more than one year before formal papers are filed in court. The machinations of the precomplaint by a plaintiff's lawyer are important to understand so the psychiatrist can respond intelligently to the attorney's investigation and requests for information.

The plaintiff's lawyer will interview the patient, patient's guardian, or, if the patient has died, a member of the patient's family. The interview often takes place soon after the suspect action. Most lawyers require much more than simply the word of the client before bringing suit, and ethical considerations preclude attorneys from bringing meritless lawsuits.[1] Some states permit countersuits against both the attorney and the plaintiff for initiating groundless actions,[2] and a Federal rule of civil procedure permits sanctions for the initiation of a baseless claim.[3] After the interview, the plaintiff's lawyer proceeds with an investigation of the potential claim.

On rare occasions, an attorney may call the potential defendant-psychiatrist, identify himself or herself as a lawyer consulted by a patient or a patient's family, and ask to "just clear a few things up" or "to get some information so that I don't have to bring a lawsuit." The legal ethics of such an approach are questionable at best, since a lawyer is precluded from directly contacting a potential defendant who is represented by counsel.[4] An unsuspecting psychiatrist might respond to the lawyer's queries, but any response to such questions on the telephone would be a mistake for two reasons. First, unless a signed authorization has been provided, any response would obviously be a breach of confidentiality. Second, a lawyer who has been consulted for the purpose of bringing a malpractice action is usually seeking information that will be detrimental to the psychiatrist's interests. No matter how much the lawyer professes to be on the psychiatrist's side, what the psychiatrist sees as an innocuous phone conversation before the suit is filed may be the physician's undoing at the deposition or trial.

Should a lawyer phone a psychiatrist with seemingly innocent inquiries, the lawyer should be advised that the psychiatrist is insured and/or represented by counsel. The psychiatrist should call the insurance company or personal lawyer to report the phone contact. The insurance company or lawyer will then act as the intermediary between the psychiatrist and the patient's lawyer. Lawyers generally know what to say and what not to say to protect a psychiatrist's rights in the context of a threatened malpractice case. What the insurance company's lawyer or the psychiatrist's own lawyer says cannot be used directly against the physician in court. On the other hand, what the psychiatrist says may constitute an admission and might be used against the doctor at trial.

Most lawyers, after conducting an interview and before bringing a malpractice lawsuit, will request psychiatric records and will often have an independent expert review those records to determine the viability of a claim. If the patient's psychiatric records are requested by a lawyer who says he or she is investigating a potential malpractice claim (the usual initial contact between a psychiatrist and a patient's lawyer), the psychiatrist should enlist the aid of the malpractice insurer or, if uninsured, a lawyer schooled in malpractice issues. The insurer or lawyer can work with both the psychiatrist and the patient's lawyer or offer advice on what records to provide as a result of the lawyer's request. Many physicians err by deciding on their own which records to provide and which to withhold. A decision early in the case to reveal less than the complete record may be disastrous if a document originally held back is later produced at trial. The inference by the judge or jury that the psychiatrist concealed the record because it contained something detrimental will be inescapable.

Some psychiatrists keep two sets of records—one that documents sessions and treatment and another "personal" set that includes highly confidential material that could prove embarrassing to the patient if revealed, as well as the psychiatrist's thoughts and impressions. Should a psychiatrist reveal only the records documenting treatment and withhold the "personal" ones, he or she should be aware that the "personal" records may surface. That would leave the physician in the unenviable position of explaining to a judge or jury why the concealed "personal" records contain information adverse to his or her case and why two sets of records are kept. A lawyer should be consulted to determine whether, under applicable jurisdictional law, both sets of records must be provided when patient records are requested.

Before trial and in the absence of a subpoena, the psychiatrist should never produce medical records without the signed, dated authorization of the patient, the patient's guardian, or the executor or administrator of the patient's estate.[5] The patient's signature on the authorization should be compared with the patient's signature in the psychiatric record. If the executor or administrator signs the authorization, the psychiatrist should insist on being supplied the court order appointing the representative of the estate.

The patient's record should never be altered to put the psychiatrist in a "better" position in the lawsuit. Aside from the obvious dishonesty of such an approach, the chances of being found out are great. Often there are many sets of the same records, and no plaintiff's lawyer could hope for anything more advantageous than clear proof that a psychiatrist has changed the records. Even in the best of liability cases, from the defendant-psychiatrist's point of view, the alteration of records alone may be enough for a jury to decide against the psychiatrist.

At times, lawyers will not advise the psychiatrist that they are investigating a malpractice claim but will merely request records. Certainly every request for records should not send a psychiatrist scurrying to the phone to call the malpractice carrier. But, it's better to be on the safe side. If a psychiatrist believes that a patient may sue and receives a seemingly innocuous request for records, turning to a lawyer, whether the physician's personal lawyer or the insurance company's attorney, is a good idea.

Once the psychiatrist is aware that a lawyer is considering bringing a lawsuit, the *only* people with whom the physician should discuss the patient's care are the insurance company's representative and the personal lawyer. The psychiatrist should *not* talk to the potential plaintiff, his or her lawyer or family, or a private investigator. The psychiatrist should also not talk to other patients, other defendants, and their lawyers, friends, and family. An innocent discussion before the suit is filed may be a breach of confidentiality and could result in scathing testimony during the trial.

Responding to the Summons and Complaint

After the patient's lawyer has completed the evaluation and determined that a lawsuit will be brought, suit papers are filed with the appropriate court. Jurisdictions differ as to whether a complaint—the long form that gives notice of the reasons for suit or gives detailed facts—or summons—the short-form notification of a lawsuit—or both need to be served on the defendant. The service may be made, according to the court's rules, by a sheriff, by any adult person, or by certified mail. Many times the summons and/or complaint will be the first notice a psychiatrist has that a lawsuit is pending. The initial suit papers should never be ignored. Most states and the Federal system require the defendant to answer the complaint or summons within a short time, usually 20–30 days, after it is served. Holding on to the summons and complaint or ignoring it may result in an adverse judgment being entered and in the insurance company's refusal of coverage for any losses that arise due to the suit.

Note the date and time the summons or complaint was served, by whom it was served, in what manner (by mail or by person) it was delivered, who received the process, and where it was served. All that information may be important if the manner in which the process was served is contested. Cases can be dismissed for improper service.

Soon after the psychiatrist reports the receipt of the summons or complaint and forwards the complaint to the insurance company, a lawyer will be hired by the insurance company to represent the psychiatrist, who is now officially a defendant in a lawsuit. The lawyer will interview the psychiatrist concerning the facts of the case so that a response to the complaint can be filed.

Establishing Rapport and Cooperating With Your Lawyer

The psychiatrist must accept from the outset that the lawyer will be in charge of the lawsuit, "running the show" in the legal arena. Therefore, the psychiatrist must cooperate fully with the lawyer.

The first requirement is unfailing honesty between the psychiatrist and the lawyer representing him or her, even if the defendant-physician perceives his or her rendition of the facts makes the case less favorable than it would be under a different factual scenario. A lawyer's work can be effective only when he or she knows what really happened.

All information and records requested by the lawyer should be provided expeditiously. The advantage of keeping complete records will be evident when years of treatment need to be reconstructed. All questions the lawyer asks should be answered quickly and candidly.

Whenever the psychiatrist has a question about the lawsuit or any papers received in connection with the case, those inquiries should be directed to the lawyer. It is better to have the lawyer's input than to do or say something to endanger the outcome of the case. A lawyer would be far happier to answer a volley of questions than to be surprised by the actions of a client who made an independent decision.

The psychiatrist should establish a good rapport with the lawyer from the outset, although it may not be easy. In most cases, the insurance company hires the lawyer, not the psychiatrist. Still, rapport is crucial. Human nature dictates that a lawyer who likes and respects a particular client will work harder and respond more quickly than for a client toward whom the attorney feels more ambivalent. If the psychiatrist encounters problems in his or her relationship with the lawyer, those problems should be confronted gently and directly. Lawyers are notorious for failing to return phone calls but would probably alter their behavior if directly confronted about this failing. If the lawyer continues to be elusive after a frank discussion, try again. Sometimes a client can get needed information by consulting a paralegal or a young associate. If the psychiatrist's senior lawyer is elusive, establishing contact with a younger, less harried attorney or paralegal may help.

If the psychiatrist has attempted on many occasions to establish rapport but has failed, other strategies may be necessary. One strategy may be to advise the lawyer that if problems are not solved, the matter will be discussed with his or her superiors. Such an approach may ensure that the psychiatrist's needs are met, but it could anger the attorney and backfire. Establishing rapport with the next lawyer assigned to his or her case may be difficult.

Another approach is to hire a personal attorney who is knowledgeable in malpractice to monitor the case and intercede with the insurance company's lawyer. Lawyers often tend to be more responsive to other lawyers than to their own clients. In addition, the psychiatrist's personal lawyer will speak the same language as the lawyer hired by the insurance company and will know the correct questions to ask when information is not readily volunteered. Although hiring a personal lawyer to oversee the litigation may anger the insurance company's lawyer, engaging a personal lawyer may also make the carrier's lawyer more responsive.

On rare occasions, the lawyer and the firm that the insurance company hires seem not to be on the psychiatrist's side, appear to be pushing a rapid settlement, or seem incompetent. If the psychiatrist's personal lawyer also reaches any of those conclusions, the psychiatrist should first ask the insurance company for new counsel. Failing that, permission to hire his or her own attorney to handle the litigation should be requested. If the insurance company gives permission for substitution of a personal attorney for the one hired by the carrier, the psychiatrist can expect to pay substantial amounts to the personal lawyer for defense of the claim. Should the psychiatrist's malpractice insurance be inadequate to cover the possible judgment in the case, or should the insurance company disclaim coverage, the physician should certainly hire independent counsel.

Participating in the Discovery Process

The portion of the lawsuit that follows complaint and answer, usually called the pleading stage, is discovery. Each party to the lawsuit can ask questions of the others in written or oral form to get necessary information for trial. The written questions are interrogatories. The oral questions are posed at depositions. Each side can also make requests for production of documents, such as medical records and hospital protocols. The defendant may be asked by his or her lawyer to prepare first-draft answers to interrogatories and to gather documents in response to requests for production. The psychiatrist should be scrupulous in assembling all of the requested documents and in providing honest answers to the questions asked. Because of various technical objections that can be made to those inquiries, the psychiatrist's lawyer may or may not answer the interrogatories or requests for production exactly as the physician has. The doctor will be given an opportunity to review the answers to interrogatories before they are filed or sent to the plaintiff's attorney. The psychiatrist may receive subpoenas for records or other information in connection with the lawsuit. If a subpoena is received, the lawyer should be advised and consulted about how to handle it.

The defendant's deposition may be taken early in the litigation, sometimes even before written interrogatories are propounded. The deposition of a defendant-psychiatrist is a crucial aspect of the litigation. The purpose of the plaintiff in taking the defendant's deposition is both to get information about the case and to assess the psychiatrist's demeanor. The physician's deposition may be used at trial as both substantive evidence and to contradict the doctor's direct testimony. At deposition, the psychiatrist's testimony is frozen for later, more crucial use. The psychiatrist should not be lulled by the apparent informality of the deposition process, which takes place in the presence of just a few people sitting around a table with a stenographer.

In the usual procedure, the psychiatrist's lawyer prepares his or her client for the deposition. Some firms now use videotapes to teach some of the following aspects of depositions and deposition testimony. When the defendant's deposition is taken, lawyers, the defendant-witness, and a stenographer are present. At the deposition, which is usually held in a lawyer's office, the dress and demeanor are extremely important. Conservatively dressed, the defendant should be candid and assured—not hostile, tentative, or pretentious. The psychiatrist-defendant should seem compassionate, not cold. When testifying, three rules in particular are important. One, tell the truth; two, answer only the questions that are asked; and three, if you don't know or don't remember the answers to any questions, say so. An excellent way to prepare a witness for a deposition is to conduct a mock examination; the defense lawyer questions in the way that he or she assumes the plaintiff's lawyer will ask.

The psychiatrist-defendant should insist on being fully and adequately prepared for his or her deposition. Often lawyers assume that physicians are acquainted with the deposition process. The psychiatrist who is new to litigation procedures must be sure the lawyer is aware of that fact. If the lawyer prepares the physician quickly and casually for the deposition, the psychiatrist must insist on more rigorous preparation. Many cases are won or lost at the defendant's deposition. At the end of the preparation session, the psychiatrist should ask to read, correct, and sign the transcript after the deposition is taken.

Many defendants are amazed at the breadth and depth of questions asked at depositions. Federal discovery rules, which govern the scope of discovery generally in federal cases, allow broad latitude and require only that questions be reasonably calculated to lead to information that may be admissible at trial.[6]

To Settle or Not to Settle

At some point during discovery, after discovery, before trial, during trial, or even after trial, the psychiatrist's lawyer may broach the possibility of settling the lawsuit by paying monetary damages to the plaintiff. Settlement ends the case, so most malpractice insurance policies require the approval of the physician before a case can be settled. The psychiatrist's lawyer should explain the advantages and disadvantages—economic, social, and psychological—of settling and proceeding to trial before asking the doctor to decide on settlement. The psychiatrist should then make a decision based on those options. If the defense lawyer does not fully discuss the pro's and con's of settlement, the psychiatrist should insist on such a counseling session. The psychiatrist should find out how the settlement will affect future malpractice insurance premiums, his or her standing in the psychiatric community, and finances. If the psychiatrist has already retained a personal attorney, that attorney should also be consulted about settlement. If the psychiatrist has questions about the advice to settle proposed by the insurance company's attorney, he or she should consider, perhaps for the first time, consulting a personal lawyer.

Proceeding to Trial

A trial is a very emotionally charged experience for all the participants, particularly for the defendants. Very often, criminal trials are confused with civil trials. The defendant in a civil malpractice trial cannot be found guilty—only negligent. The only punishment is financial, and only rarely will the damages come out of the defendant's own pocket. The trial is nonetheless a public airing of a charge of professional negligence, and such charges, even if unfounded, can be very embarrassing.

Ordinarily, malpractice cases are tried before a judge and jury. The jury, composed of lay people, determines the facts and the credibility of witnesses and applies the law given by the judge to the facts. In some Federal lawsuits and in those where neither side requests a jury trial, the case will be tried before a judge who performs the functions of both judge and jury. The first step in a jury trial is the selection of the jurors. The physician should be at jury selection to help decide who is an appropriate juror for the case and to begin an early relationship with the jury. After the jury is selected, the attorneys for plaintiff and defendant give their opening statements to the jury. The opening statements are outlines of the evidence to be presented during the trial. The plaintiff presents its witnesses, who are then cross-examined by the defense; the defense then presents its witnesses, who are cross-examined by the plaintiff. Finally, the lawyers present closing arguments, during which they persuasively present their versions of the case to the jury. The judge instructs the jury on the law of the jurisdiction in his charge, and then the jury deliberates and renders its verdict.

The rules for the psychiatrist-defendant testifying at trial are the same as those at deposition. Dress must be conservative. The doctor must be honest and straightforward, never arrogant or angry, and appear compassionate. The psychiatrist should use plain English so that the judge and jury can identify with and understand the defendant. The psychiatrist should use few words of art. Attendance at each court session is not mandatory; however a jury will probably be more kindly disposed toward a doctor who is so concerned about the case that he or she is there every day than to the psychiatrist who attends court only sporadically.

Appeal

If the verdict is in favor of the plaintiff, the psychiatrist will be required to decide whether to appeal. The lawyer should fully counsel the doctor on the merits of appeal. The psychiatrist should insist on such counseling if it is not forthcoming from the attorney. If the doctor decides not to appeal, the judgment must be paid and the case must be left behind emotionally. The psychiatrist should learn from the experience—either from the error that was made or from the trial of enduring the legal process.

Countersuit

Depending upon the jurisdiction in which the psychiatrist practices, a defendant who wins the case may have the option of bringing a countersuit against the plaintiff.[7] The countersuit will allege that the plaintiff and/or the plaintiff's lawyer had no reasonable basis for bringing the lawsuit and will ask for damages for the cost of defense and for the emotional distress occasioned by the prosecution of the case. Countersuits are rare, possibly because the last thing a defendant wants is to begin another protracted legal matter.

Summary

Being aware of how to protect one's assets from the threat of a malpractice judgment is necessary for every psychiatrist. Knowledge of the stages of a malpractice lawsuit and how to respond at each stage is also crucial. The psychiatrist who is knowledgeable about the legal process and wise about how and when to consult legal counsel will be in an excellent position to present an effective defense to a malpractice claim.

References

1. *Model Rules of Professional Conduct,* American Bar Association, Rule 3.1.
2. 42 *Pennsylvania Consolidated Statutes* §8351 *et seq.*
3. *Federal Rules of Civil Procedure,* Rule 11.
4. *Model Rules of Professional Conduct,* American Bar Association, Rule 4.2.
5. *Guidelines on Confidentiality,* American Psychiatric Association, "Release of Record to a Third Party," p. 9.
6. *Federal Rules of Civil Procedure,* Rule 26(b)(1).
7. 42 *Pennsylvania Consolidated Statutes* §8351 *et seq.*

7

Personal Consequences for the Psychiatrist Being Sued for Malpractice

JARRETT W. RICHARDSON, M.D.

Editor's Note

There should be ways in which patients who have not been properly treated by doctors and other health professionals and have suffered damages as a result should have access to compensation. But there are serious questions as to whether the present system to attend to such grievances is really appropriate, especially when one considers that the accused physician, whether he is subsequently found to have been at fault or not, often suffers great emotional anguish in the process. His family does, too.

In this lesson the author highlights the emotional, physical, social, and professional effects of living through malpractice suits on physicians in general and psychiatrists in particular. The experience is a combination of acute and chronic post-traumatic disorder syndrome. Some of the strategies which have helped survivors of other arduous stresses also work for beleaguered psychiatrists: group support systems, resilient personality and family attributes, and, when necessary, psychiatric care.

Introduction

In the title of her somewhat autobiographical book, *Defendant—A Psychiatrist on Trial for Medical Malpractice,* Sara C. Charles quickly focuses on one of the central personal issues for all physicians who are involved in malpractice litigation and most particularly the psychiatrist: the identity as "the defendant." It is imposed by external forces and a process initiated by either a patient to whom the psychiatrist has been personally committed in a doctor-patient relationship or by a grieved family member whose hostility and desire for retribution is often driven by guilt. As a result, the core sense of identity of the psychiatrist is changed forever. Perhaps typical of psychiatrists involved in this process, Charles offers very little direct revelation of her own thoughts and feelings in recalling her own experience as a defendant. Many aspects of a psychiatrist's response to such a circumstance are revealed indirectly in the attempted objectivity shown by presenting the case transcript and more directly by observations made by her co-author and husband, Eugene Kennedy, such as ". . . What hung in the balance I painfully realized was Sara's whole sense of herself as a physician, her identification with the profession at which she works so conscientiously . . . found negligent she would never be the same again—and maybe we wouldn't either—for charges of professional malpractice aimed finally at the soul and spirit." In a more general way, Charles's production of this book and continued professional interest in the area of malpractice (to the point at which she has published more information in this area than any other single individual) symbolize the deep and lasting personal effect of this experience.[1]

As I have reviewed the literature and walked with colleagues through the experience of medical malpractice litigation, the fact that this is a life-changing experience has been confirmed. This section will focus on the reality of the current malpractice litigation environment, summarize what has come to be known as malpractice stress syndrome, describe what is known about the natural history for individuals and families involved in the process, present theoretical models that are proposed to help understand the process, and summarize the counsel that is available to those who are victims of this process.

Malpractice Stress Syndrome

Briefly summarized, the malpractice stress syndrome is as follows:

1. "Almost in every case [the accused doctor] shows signs of emotional disequilibrium, depression, frustration, irritability, sleep difficulties, appetite disturbance, and headache."[2]
2. "15% to 18% of patients report either new or exacerbated cases of duodenal ulcer, hypertension, coronary heart disease, and colitis."[2]
3. "Symptoms recur in periodic cycles for periods of four or even five years."[2]

This oversimplified description summarizes anecdotal and large group surveys of information from physicians who have been involved in medical malpractice litigation. In a growing literature largely produced by Charles and her colleagues, the personal impact of malpractice litigation is being thoroughly documented. Although no studies are specific to psychiatry as a specialty, most of what is described about physicians in general would logically apply to the reactions of psychiatrists.

Anecdotal Literature

Individual and anecdotal reports emphasize that the experience of being sued is one of the worst experiences of a lifetime,[3] is experienced as a "death in the family,"[4] and contain descriptions commonly heard from those who have been victimized, such as "Physician felt he was being jerked around by the plaintiff's attorney, malicious, inconsiderate behavior."[5] Emotions such as shame, rage, and a sense of being assaulted, devastated, and overwhelmed occur frequently in personal descriptions. A common experience is the loss of trust in "the system"—a disruption of the general sense and expectation that if you do your best, things will be okay. Resentfulness, bitterness, humiliation, and frustration build during the time of preparation for and the experience of a malpractice trial, and even the most self-assured clinician becomes doubtful and develops an ambivalence that undermines the basic sense of security important for active clinical practice.

The degree to which an individual physician's personal identity is co-existent with his or her professional identity is brought into focus during that time: the accusation of negligence is experienced as an accusation of being bad, not just professionally but personally. Most defendants are alarmed at the degree to which they develop intense hostility and resentment. They describe the trauma of involvement in medical malpractice litigation as a time of a desperate sense of loss of control and intense soul-searching about whether or not to continue trying to sustain an identity as a physician. Of the many factors that contribute to the type and degree of emotional reaction, one of the most important is the conflict between the physician's expectation of a doctor-patient relationship based on trust and emotional support, and the reality of his or her being the target of attack by the legal system and being accused as "the vendor of a defective product."[6] Although lawyers consider the process to be just business, physicians usually experience it as a personal assault.

The extreme of the individual and anecdotal responses includes suicide.[4] The experience of a sensitive physician who feels trapped in a situation that is personally degrading can quickly lead to a malignant and eventually fatal circumstance, particularly in those who develop feelings of powerlessness and hopelessness, a progressive sense of unworthiness, and a sense of being overwhelmed.[7] The physician's general personality characteristics—sensitive; empathetic; compulsive; having an exaggerated sense of responsibility; desiring to be omnipotent, needed, loved, and admired; and maintaining a self-expectation to make no mistakes and live up to society's expectation of perfection—render him or her particularly vulnerable to devastation by malpractice litigation.[8]

The physician's initial response to receiving a summons alleging negligence is disbelief and shock.[7] Since the suit often represents feelings of broken trust, betrayal, hurt, and misunderstanding, a significant disruption of emotional equilibrium occurs and is accompanied by feelings of anger and rage.[7] As will be described subsequently, a significant percentage of physicians who are sued experience clinically significant symptomatology prior to and during the malpractice trial; however, perhaps the most destructive part of the process is the change in the way in which physicians relate to their patients and the practice of medicine. The loss of satisfaction in work, the increase in defensive medical practice, and the realization that every patient (even those for whom particular time and effort are spent) is a potential plaintiff leads to a significant loss in the unique intimacy and healing power of the doctor-patient relationship for all future patients. For the psychiatrist, whose practice is almost entirely based on the development of a trusting and intimate relationship with the patient and whose clinical practice is dependent on self-awareness and a high degree of confidence in one's own ability to elicit, understand, process, integrate, formulate, and interpret information that is not easily quantifiable or reproducible with numbers or photographs, the experience of being a defendant is a devastating personal and professional loss.

Effect on Spouse and Family

The physician's spouse and family are also significantly affected. In addition to experiencing some degree of helplessness as the physician is subjected to the process of malpractice litigation, the spouse and family may be subjected to public embarrassment and humiliation. Even if the verdict is in favor of the defendant, ". . . the years of worrying and waiting and being angry and scared are over, but there was no sense of triumph, just the wastefulness, degradation, and sheer senselessness of the whole procedure."[9] "Our home life was like a dream during this time. We were obsessed with the trial and could think of little else. We weren't with the children much during those days. When we were the preoccupation with the trial made family matters seem far away. Sleep came only in bits and pieces and naturally added to our exhaustion from the experience."[9] Because the physician frequently has difficulty with openness and vulnerability at home, the spouse often feels placed in the position of having to stand at a distance and watch. Comments frequently heard from spouses include: "Our lives would never be the same;" "Our lives were on hold for the time being;" "It was a bittersweet ending for there really were no winners. The hurt and feelings of futility are still there;" "We continue to live life on the edge since my husband is so much more anxious and careful."[10] "It was as if everyone internalized the lawsuit, as if we were all being sued."[5] The physician's withdrawal from family and colleagues, a sense of isolation induced by the need "not to talk with anyone about the case," and progressively diminished self-esteem and increased self-doubt often lead the spouse to describe the malpractice litigation process as a "terrible and brutalizing ordeal especially if it goes to trial because of the public nature of the trial, the attempts to discredit the physician (spouse) and the open attack in public on the professional and personal integrity of the loved one. The physician's spouse frequently feels a sense of rejection, notices regression on the part of the physician, and experiences uncertainty and shame in public resulting in their own social withdrawal within the community."[8]

Survey Literature

The first large survey to be published on the effects of a malpractice suit upon physicians was based on interviews of all Connecticut physicians who had been sued for malpractice between July 1, 1947, and September 30, 1959.[11] According to the authors who conducted the interview, those physicians who had been sued were indistinguishable from their colleagues in terms of appearance, age, mannerisms, diplomas, and other aspects which might characterize physicians sued for malpractice. "They do not constitute the lower crust of physicians but appear to be almost uniformly spread across the physician spectrum with a concentration at the upper level if anywhere. Many of the most distinguished and honored physicians of great competence were included in this group. A large number of the physicians sued were chiefs of services or even chiefs of staff in some of the best hospitals in Connecticut."[11] The aspects of the process of a malpractice suit discussed by Wyckoff included the impact on the physician of first learning about the lawsuit, the impact of the extent of publicity, the impact of the process on the physician's practice and doctor-patient relationships, and subjective effects. Of the 58 doctors interviewed, 40 felt the malpractice suit against them had no significant effect upon their pleasure and satisfaction in practice, 12 reported a slight adverse effect to their pleasure in medical practice, and 4 reported a moderate adverse effect. One physician reported the effects were so severe that he would no longer accept serious cases or make a night call.

The authors continue: 'While some conscientious exceptions to the rule were found a fair general statement of the observations in this study is that anxiety and subjective symptoms vary in direct proportion to the threat the doctor perceived to himself. Publicity increased both the anxiety and the threat by placing his status before his patients on the entire populace for them to pass judgment on him. His fear of publicity is in part justified because of the reporter's temptation to write the sensational, the frequently inaccurate and misleading articles printed, together with the inability of the general public to understand the medical facts basic to a fair decision." Wyckoff concluded that, objectively, the effects of a malpractice suit upon a physician appear to be much less than generally believed.

It would appear the greatest damages to the doctor who is sued for malpractice were subjective in origin. The author states, ". . . It is sincerely hoped that this study . . . will provide a reliable standard of what the doctor can expect from a malpractice suit and indicates to the medical profession as a whole, that a view of the malpractice suit has been taken which is too pessimistic. It is my hope that this study will reduce the ethereal to the concrete which can be realistically, honestly, and confidently appraised and mastered."[11]

More than 20 years passed before another large survey of physicians was published. In their survey work with physicians who have been sued for malpractice, Charles and colleagues found a 500% increase in the frequency of malpractice suits against physicians in northern Illinois between 1977 and 1983, and only 4% of sued physicians say that they had no physical or emotional reaction to being sued.[12-14]

In the first of three studies,[12] approximately 40% of physicians acknowledge symptoms suggestive of major depressive disorder that lasted longer than two weeks. These individuals had dysphoric mood and at least four additional symptoms included in a DSM-III diagnostic criteria for major affective disorder. Twenty percent acknowledged a syndrome which included pervasive anger accompanied by at least four of eight symptoms, including change in mood and attention, frustration, irritability, insomnia, fatigue, gastrointestinal symptoms, or headache. Eight percent noted onset of physical illness; three experienced myocardial infarction during the time of litigation. Seven percent experienced an exacerbation of a previously diagnosed medical condition such as angina, duodenal ulcer, spastic colon, or hypertension. Between 2 and 10% of physicians acknowledged misuse of alcohol and somewhat less than 1%, misuse of drugs. Suicidal ideation during the process of litigation occurred in 2–7% of the physicians surveyed.[14]

In the second survey that Charles and colleagues conducted, 4.5% (401) of the 8900-member Chicago Medical Society were psychiatrists. Of the survey respondents, 6.1% (21) were psychiatrists, and

2.6% (5) of respondents who had been sued were psychiatrists, indicating that 23.8% of the psychiatrists who responded to the survey had been sued.[13] No specific information is available about the symptomatic response of the psychiatrists as differentiated from the physician group as a whole. Perhaps one of the most telling comments from Charles's conclusions was that only 1.6% of the sued physicians had received adverse trial verdicts, suggesting that a significant degree of morbidity suffered by physicians involved in malpractice litigation is based on very minimal justification with regard to favorable financial outcome for the plaintiff patient.

The Process of Medical Malpractice

The medical malpractice litigation process strikingly molds the thinking of the defendants involved. The defendant's clinical openmindedness often becomes a victim of the need to demonstrate certainty in the courtroom; openness to seeking the truth evolves to a position in which vindication is most important. An initial sense of a desire to not have the process interfere with life often evolves to a circumstance in which the physician seriously questions his or her continuation of the practice of medicine. Dramatic changes occur in the feeling and thinking of physicians between the time they enter the adversarial-legal culture and the time they are finally brainwashed and ready for a courtroom battle. The cross-cultural move from the familiar territory of scientific inquiry in an empathetic doctor-patient relationship to the foreign territory of courtroom combat bring about extremely stressful adaptations from which most defendants never completely recover. Instead of the open, reflective, and cooperative mentality that characterizes clinical medicine, the rules become those of certainty, closure, and competition. The world view of the physician is shifted by the experience, and re-entry from the artificial courtroom culture to the real world of clinical practice usually leaves the defendant much more guarded, vigilant, and insecure. For those who are able to include their spouses in this cross-cultural experience by having them involved in the preparatory sessions and courtroom, re-entry to the "real world" is more tolerable, since there are certain aspects of the experience that are extremely difficult to explain to someone who has not "been there." For instance, most defendants are later alarmed at the degree to which they allowed themselves to be drawn into the legal mentality and find themselves resenting the embarrassment and insecurity that resulted from their capitulation to that alien influence. If the spouse has experienced this with the defendant, both have a better chance of survival—as does the relationship. The legal actors may achieve a sense of closure to the process and then move on to other business after what seems to them to have been "just another good day's work." On the other hand, physicians are unable to walk away so simply: having experienced assault, abuse, injury, and manipulation, most will never be the same again.

Because physicians are a strange blend of idealism and pragmatism and are committed to what is considered a high purpose—the discovery and use of scientific information and the application of that knowledge and technical skill toward the care of the patient—they are truly unprepared for the courtroom culture. When the needs of individuals or patients compete with the needs of society or even the physician's own needs, doctors have traditionally championed the patient's cause. They are committed to "facing the facts" about health, disease, dying, and human imperfection and then trying to provide the best solution possible for the patient. Physicians generally expect others to profess these same beliefs and are shaken to the core if they don't, particularly if there is no external standard or if the only court of appeal for these conflicting values is the legal system. Physicians are used to combating death and suffering but are not trained to do battle with people who appeal to different goals, such as "the bottom line," or "the greatest good for the greatest number," or "entitlement to a good outcome." The spouses of physicians are likewise subject to extreme self-sacrifice and commitment in support of the values and careers of medicine, and their destiny is very tightly bound to the physicians'. A doctor becomes the object of betrayal by a patient for whom he or she has sacrificed time and energy and often personal needs.

Spouses and families are also betrayed and experience their own dismay and anger. If they are included in the suffering, an alliance can be formed that strengthens and heals. If, as is common, the physician suffers alone, the attack divides and destroys even the most intimate of relationships. Unfortunately, the unique intimacy and healing power of the doctor-patient relationship is severely undermined for all future patients after former patients become plaintiffs and use the painful language of negligence to place the physician on the defensive. For the physician and his or her family and patients, it is the legal adversarial process of the malpractice trial that actually becomes the enemy. The process also divides the profession, pitting physician against physician not only with combative expert testimony on the witness stand but also within the medical literature.[15] The distress also extends to relationships with paramedical staff members who are closely involved with the physician in day-to-day practice.[16]

Theoretical Models for Intervention

One specific theoretical model that has been proposed presents an analogy between the physician's reaction to a malpractice suit and the stages of grief described by Elizabeth Kübler-Ross.[17] Thinking about the evolution of response to a malpractice suit, through the stages of denial, anger, bargaining, depression, and acceptance, cannot only provide a framework for understanding what is happening but also help individualize the implementation of appropriate intervention by the physician or others who are concerned. Janssen proposes the four psychological factors in his formulation of this process: self-analysis and soul-searching; regression and withdrawal; isolation and despair; and resolution and rebounding (regaining objectivity).[8]

Charles suggests several separate aspects to intervention. First is sharing the experience, particularly with the spouse. A second is involvement in peer support, as is often available through a medical society or its auxiliary. Third is understanding and optimizing usually effective coping strategies such as denial, reaction formation, suppression, rationalization, and sublimation, as well as resumption of recreational activities and other forms of relaxation. The fourth is active involvement in one's defense by mastering all medical aspects of the incident in question, demanding that legal counsel communicate regularly, and working actively with counsel in the preparation of the case.

For the 15% who develop or exacerbate physical disorders, active medical intervention is indicated; for those whose psychological symptomatology does not respond to the above strategy, psychiatric consultation is appropriate.[14] Perhaps the most valuable of all suggestions for handling malpractice stress is involvement in one of the many support groups being specifically developed for physicians involved in medical malpractice.[18,19] Specific assistance and advice about how to give a deposition or prepare for trial is available not only from individual attorneys but in the medical literature as well.[20,21] Preparation for this whole process actually may need to begin in residency, since for the foreseeable future all practicing physicians will be vulnerable to this potentially devastating occurrence.[22]

A specific psychological assessment tool has been developed to help assess the degree of psychological vulnerability an individual may have to excessive fear of litigation.[23] Scales such as that litigaphobia scale have well become valuable in prospectively identifying and providing support to the most vulnerable practitioner. For the psychiatrist, it may well be that the best preparation in dealing with the personal impact of malpractice litigation would begin with reading Charles's account and actively discussing with psychiatric colleagues the book and the issues and feelings it generates.[1] That process of cognitive assessment, the experience of commonality, the identification of emotional conflict, and working through specific and individual vulnerabilities are what is recommended to patients dealing with issues of assault, victimization, and helplessness similar to what physicians are likely to experience if forced into the identity of "the defendant."

References

1. Charles SC, Kennedy E. *Defendant—A Psychiatrist on Trial for Medical Malpractice*. New York: The Free Press; 1985.
2. What happens to you when you're sued? *J Med Assoc Ga*. 1986; 75:629.
3. Tillman RA. You and malpractice stress: II. One physician's story. *J Med Assoc Ga*. 1986;75:659.
4. Fokes EC. You and malpractice stress: V. A death in the family. *J Med Assoc Ga*. 1987; 76:115–116.
5. Ross SM. Eight who survived. *Va Med*. 1987; 114:218–221.
6. Covi L: Physicians' emotional reactions to being sued. *Md Med J*. 1987; 36(6):478.
7. Charles SC. Malpractice suits: Their effect on doctors, patients, and families. *J Med Assoc Ga*. 1987; 76:171–172.
8. Janssen E. Presentation at the American Medical Association Auxiliary 1987–88 Leadership Confluence—"Family Stress During Malpractice Litigation."
9. Montgomery M. You and malpractice stress: III. Two spouses' views. *J Med Assoc Ga*. 1986; 75:723–724.
10. Unpublished comments by Janet R. Ebersold, R.N.

11. Wyckoff RL. The effects of a malpractice suit upon physicians in Connecticut. *JAMA*. 1961; 176(13):1096–1101.

12. Charles SC, Wilbert JR, Kennedy EC: Physicians' self-reports of reactions to malpractice litigation. *Am J Psychiatry. 1984;* 141(4):563–565.

13. Charles SC, Wilbert JR, Franke KJ. Sued and nonsued physicians' self-reported reactions to malpractice litigation. *Am J Psychiatry*. 1985; 142(4):437–440.

14. Charles SC. Malpractice litigation and its impact on physicians. *Curr Psychiatric Ther*. 1986; 23:173–180.

15. Sandmire HF. Malpractice—the syndrome of the 80s [letter]. *Obstet Gynecol*. 1989; 73(1):145–146.

16. Blum R. You and malpractice stress: IV. The office staff's perspective. *J Med Assoc Ga*. 1987; 76:61–62.

17. Lavery JP. The physician's reaction to a malpractice suit. *Obstet Gynecol*. 1988; 71(1):138–141.

18. Reineck MC. Handling malpractice stress: Suggestions for physicians and their families. *Instr Course Lect*. 1988; 37:285–287.

19. Charles SC. Physician support group formed. *IMJ*. 1985; 167(6):454–455.

20. Quinn NK. How to give a deposition. *Orthop Rev*. 1986; 15(7):479–481.

21. Stone ML. How to prepare for a trial: Medical viewpoint. *Clin Obstet Gynecol*. 1988; 31(1):184–189.

22. Bredfeldt RC, Ripani A, Cuddeback GL. Emotional response to malpractice suits: Should residents be prepared? *Fam Med*. 1987; 19(6):465–467.

23. Breslin FA, Taylor KR, Brodsky SL. Development of a litigaphobia scale: Measurement of excessive fear of litigation. *Psychol Rep*. 1986; 58(2):547–550.

8

Recent Developments in Clinical Psychiatry and the Law

ROBERT L. SADOFF, M.D.

Editor's Note

With the growth of managed care, psychiatrists must give serious thought to their legal vulnerabilities. For example, under the administrative mandate of a managed care company, if a psychiatrist reluctantly discharges a patient who is not safe to discharge, the psychiatrist is nevertheless vulnerable to any subsequent malpractice charges. Therefore, the psychiatrist should stay true to his or her own clinical judgment.

The author of this lesson suggests that a psychiatrist who absolutely believes a patient to be dangerous to self or others and who cannot procure more time for hospitalization should demand to speak to the medical director of the managed care company; being a physician as well, the director also can be held liable and, hence, may be more understanding of and sensitive to the clinical issues involved. Breaching of confidentiality is never justified to maintain economic or fiscal support of a patient's treatment. However, it must be breached in the event of a threat on the life of a third party or when there is a serious

CME questions for this chapter begin on page 353.

threat of suicide. Two other areas of legal vulnerability addressed in this lesson include boundary crossings and the recollection of repressed memories of childhood sexual abuse.

Introduction

Litigation has spawned an increased regulation of psychiatric practice, resulting in profound changes of which psychiatrists must be astutely aware to practice confidently and safely. As patients have gained a greater degree of autonomy in the therapeutic relationship, they have developed specific rights that psychiatrists have had to learn—especially psychiatrists who previously had assumed a paternalistic role in treating their patients. Beginning with cases involving the right to treatment and cases declaring a right to refuse treatment under certain conditions, psychiatrists have had to modify their practices to remain consistent with changes in the law. Issues of confidentiality, informed consent, and privacy of medical records also have modified psychiatric practice.

Perhaps one of the most important changes in psychiatric practice involves the clinician's ability to predict "dangerousness" (i.e., the degree to which a particular patient is deemed dangerous to self or others). For a patient to be committed involuntarily for psychiatric treatment, psychiatrists in all states must abide by involuntary commitment regulations that impose a standard of "clear and present danger" because of mental illness. Psychiatrists must be aware of potential danger to third parties because the *Tarasoff* decisions of the mid-1970s imposed on clinicians a "duty to protect" identifiable third parties when a specific threat has been made by a patient.[1] Unfortunately, some jurisdictions have held psychiatrists liable for the damage to third parties even when there was no specific threat or identifiable third party.[2] In a recent case, the United States Supreme Court[3] declared that psychiatrists are able to predict the dangerousness of a psychiatric patient even when they have never examined that patient.

Believing that psychiatrists can accurately predict dangerousness has led to a number of malpractice suits when patients have been discharged from hospitals and then killed themselves or harmed third parties. Such cases share the rationale that because the psychiatrist either knew or should have known the patient was "dangerous," the psychiatrist should not have discharged the patient. Furthermore, psychiatrists who treat patients in an outpatient setting may be held liable for the violent or self-destructive behavior of their patients.

With the advent of managed care regulating the practice of psychiatry in many areas, questions have arisen about psychiatrists' authority, as opposed to their liability, regarding their patients. What are psychiatrists to do when they are told by nonphysicians of a managed care company that they must discharge their patients? If all appeals have failed, what should psychiatrists do when they are mandated to release a dangerous patient? Who, then, is liable if such a patient were to commit an act of violence or to engage in self-destructive behavior after a premature discharge from the hospital? Who really has the authority in such cases?

Issues of confidentiality also arise when third parties regulate psychiatric care. Should confidentiality be modified or breached because third-party payers demand information that therapists believe is not germane to administrative decisions often made by third-party payers?

Another significant issue in contemporary malpractice cases involves psychiatrists who cross boundaries with their patients, boundaries including not only sexual behavior but also dual relationships between patients and psychiatrists. What are other boundaries, and when exactly is each crossed?

Arguably the most notable new issue in forensic psychiatry is the controversial concept of "repressed memories" or "false memory syndrome." What risks do repressed memory patients pose for the treating psychiatrist? How can psychiatrists protect themselves from liability in the event that their patients begin to remember early childhood sexual abuse by a parent or both parents?

Managed Care

As the economics and financing of psychiatric treatment continues to evolve, the practice of psychiatry undoubtedly will continue to be changed by policies of managed care companies. Some therapists view this development as a positive measure that will adequately pay for the increasing costs of medical and psychiatric treatment; others are concerned about the regulation of psychiatric practice by nonphysician administrators who set limits on psychiatric treatment, especially with regard to time in the hospital and use of various treatment modalities.

Who really makes the final decision about psychiatric hospitalization: the therapist or the administrator?

Consider a hypothetical case of a patient with paranoid schizophrenia who has a history of violent behavior and of medication noncompliance. The patient is hospitalized; it typically takes 2–3 weeks to stabilize the patient on his medication. The managed care company tells the therapist that she has 5 days to stabilize the patient, but the psychiatrist knows the patient cannot be stabilized that quickly. After 4 days, the psychiatrist requests an extension of another week; the managed care company allows 3 more days. The extensions continue for a total of 10 days until a final mandate is given that the patient must be discharged from the hospital or the company will not pay for further hospital stay.

If the therapist discharges the patient under the administrative mandate and the patient kills himself or injures a third party as a result of his mental illness, the psychiatrist faces liability in malpractice charges for prematurely releasing the "dangerous" patient. In some cases, psychiatrists who acted in accordance with regulatory guidelines have attempted to bring in the third-party payer or managed care company as a codefendant. Thus far, all courts have held psychiatrists liable for discharge decisions and have exonerated the managed care company. The courts have stated that the managed care company attempted to limit the cost of care by telling the psychiatrist that the company would not pay for a longer stay in the hospital but did not make the clinical decision to discharge. Legal precedence forewarns psychiatrists to take clinical responsibility and assume liability for the decisions they make in releasing or discharging patients irrespective of the cost-containment measures of managed care firms. In response to psychiatrists' complaint that their hands are tied and they have no alternative but to discharge, the courts have stated that psychiatrists can make a decision to keep the patient in the hospital even if the policy of a managed care company recommends otherwise; because human life is more important than money, financial issues can be litigated or argued subsequently. Therefore, the courts believe that the psychiatrist has the final say in holding a patient in the hospital if, in the psychiatrist's clinical judgment, the patient continues to be potentially self-destructive or violent.

If the psychiatrist absolutely believes that, once released, the patient will be harmed or others will be harmed and if the psychiatrist can get no extension for hospitalization of the patient, the psychiatrist should demand to speak to the medical director of the managed care company. There is always a medically responsible person (a physician) within such health care companies that can be approached as a clinician as well as an administrator. If the medical director of the managed care company reviews the clinical situation and decides that the patient must be discharged, then logic would dictate that the responsibility and liability would ultimately rest with the medical director, who would be making not only a financial, economic, and administrative decision, but also a clinical decision because of his or her physician's training.

It is likely that the medical director of a managed care company would agree with the therapist and recommend that an extension of time be granted. This situation has never been tested and may not be considered legally valid. However, such a scenario might help the practicing psychiatrist who is faced with the dilemma of treating a "dangerous" patient in a hospital after a managed care company has discontinued all extensions.

Confidentiality Within Managed Care:

As with all third-party payers, managed care companies also require certain information about the patient to make administrative and economic decisions regarding his or her treatment. Longstanding regulations in the insurance industry have maintained the confidentiality of medical records. However, some managed care companies routinely request information that goes beyond the scope of these accepted regulations.

Breaching confidentiality is never justified to maintain economic or fiscal support of a patient's treatment. The patient has a right to maintain confidentiality of information that need not be divulged because a managed care company has requested it. The psychiatrist should use sound clinical judgment in deciding what information is appropriate and what information should be withheld. It is definitely not unreasonable to expect managed care companies to adhere to industry standards regarding confidentiality.

If withholding information leads to a discontinuation of payment by the managed care company, the psychiatrist can appeal to the medical director of the company for a clinical decision. Should that fail, the psychiatrist still has access to the agencies within his or her state that regulate the insurance industry.

Confidentiality

In other areas of practice, the confidentiality of the patient's treatment and the privacy of his or her records is paramount. However, confidentiality does not entail absolute secrecy. As in the *Tarasoff* case, confidentiality must be breached in the event of a threat on the life of a third party. The patient's right to confidentiality also is breached when he or she threatens to kill him- herself. Thus, breach of confidentiality per se is not unethical. Petrila and Sadoff[3] have expanded the concept of confidentiality to include information that can be shared with caretakers (i.e., family members to whom the hospitalized psychiatric patient will be returned).

With the development of the National Alliance for the Mentally Ill, family members have assumed a much greater role in the treatment of psychiatric patients. When a patient returns home, caretakers need specific information to maintain the quality of care. The psychiatrist should discuss with family members the importance of any medication the patient is taking, including its side effects and ways to ensure maximum medication compliance. In the event the patient becomes noncompliant with the medication regimen, the psychiatrist also should describe for family members the symptoms of deterioration associated with the patient's mental illness. By sharing such information with family members, psychiatrists share some of the liability. For example, a patient is discharged from the hospital, goes home, does not take his or her medication, shows signs of deterioration that the family notices but does not report to the follow-up (i.e., outpatient) therapist, and becomes violent or self-destructive. The psychiatrist, having shared the necessary information and documented it properly, may not be liable for any violent behavior that might occur during the next 2 or 3 months. By not sharing the information, the psychiatrist insulates the patient's family members from their responsibility because they cannot be expected to have professional knowledge.

Boundary Violations

A number of recent malpractice cases have concerned the dual relationship between a psychiatrist and his or her patient that is sometimes referred to as boundary crossing, or mishandling, of the transference within the therapeutic process. Boundary crossing does not always refer to sexual behavior between a therapist and his or her patient. Of course, this type of behavior is prohibited by all professional organizations. The American Psychiatric Association recently prohibited sexual contact even with former patientsl. Some authorities have argued that this prohibition is excessive and should be limited to 2 years after the termination of treatment. However, a more reasonable approach would forbid a psychiatrist from becoming sexually involved with a former patient if such involvement might harm the former patient. Time limits appear to be irrelevant in this regard.

A boundary violation may involve touching, sharing information, inappropriately socializing with patients, or entering into business or financial relationships with patients. Although these and other dual relationships are prohibited by ethical standards, some therapists believe that such a broad ban borders on puritanical policy. For instance, in some small communities, it can be difficult for physicians not to be social friends of patients. In general, however, socializing with patients is deemed imprudent because of the intimacy of treatment and the information that is shared during the course of psychiatric treatment. Perhaps the major risk in such dual relationships is a potential breach of confidentiality that may negatively affect the patient.

Studies have shown that the patient most often harmed by boundary crossing is one who suffers from borderline personality disorder.[5] Patients with borderline personality disorder typically tend to test boundaries that other types of patients typically respect. Statistics prove that most of the false accusations against psychiatrists come from patients with borderline personality disorder, and, without corroborating evidence, it is difficult either to prove or disprove such inappropriate behavior.[5]

To avoid the risk of malpractice accusations, psychiatrists should maintain therapeutic boundaries, especially with patients with borderline personality disorder, and refuse to humor the patient in a seemingly innocuous test. Although it may be tempting for a psychiatrist, who usually listens to the plight of others, to share some of his or her own experiences or personal difficulties with an interested patient, the temptation should be avoided. Patients may use this personal information as "proof" in court that there existed extratherapeutic experiences that are prohibited in the practice of psychiatry.

Repressed Memories

One of the most controversial issues in contemporary psychiatry involves the emergence of repressed memories of patients during the course of therapy. These memories usually focus on early childhood sexual abuse by family members. The patient allegedly has no memory of any such experience before entering therapy; however, during the course of therapy, the patient begins to remember them, either through dreams or often through subtle or overt encouragement by the therapist.

The patient, usually a young woman, typically presents with symptoms of an eating disorder or of a sexual disorder. The therapist states that many of his or her previous patients with these symptoms had experienced early childhood sexual abuse. The therapist encourages the patient to try to remember if she was ever abused as a child. Initially, the patient fails to recall such abuse, but the therapist's continued encouragement may lead to a wish to please the therapist by relating either dreams or memories of such experiences that, in reality, may never have occurred.

Without corroborating evidence, which often is missing, the courts will not support such memories as facts. The therapist may wish to believe that these experiences occurred because they would fit the diagnostic formulation and psychodynamics often consistent with such symptoms. However, the memories may not be based on "fact," which is different from perceived "truth." Nevertheless, during the course of treating the patient, the therapist should deal with the memories as though they are true and help the patient manage the effects of such memories. Believing the patient may be part of the therapy and helpful to the patient.

Encouraging the patient to take the memories out of the realm of the consultation room and into the environment of the courtroom may prove disastrous. Cases have shown that "true" memories that are "false" (i.e., not based on objective fact) may harm the persons who are accused of such behavior. They also may harm the therapist, who may be sued by the accused and sometimes by the patient when he or she realizes that the memories are not real but were "iatrogenically induced" during the course of therapy.

There are numerous published cases of women who accused their fathers of sexually abusing them as children and later recanted their accusations because they came to realize that these memories were fabrications as a result of therapy. Thus, therapists must be very cautious about the nature of such memories before accepting them as veritable.

Guidelines are available to help therapists determine whether repressed memories are likely to be "false." In a comprehensive article on the subject of repressed memories, Wakefield and Underwager[6] noted: "When there is no corroborating evidence, and the alleged behaviors are highly improbable, it is unlikely that the abuse actually happened." Generally, they stated that the only likelihood that the allegations are correct or real is when supporting evidence is found.

Therapists should not encourage or suggest various alternatives when such memories arise. For example, they should not recommend group attendance with verified incest survivors because such information tends to be "contagious." Also, the memory should not be encouraged by use of hypnosis or relaxation techniques. The therapist should observe the memory's genesis, consider its content and its probability or improbability, and try to seek confirmation of the memory.

The psychiatrist should treat the entire clinical presentation and look for other reasons that might explain the presence of such symptoms. The risk of bringing a repressed memory case to court is exemplified by the Ramona case,[7] which resulted in the father successfully suing the therapist for stimulating memories of alleged sexual abuse in his daughter, which led to damage to the father when his daughter sued him.

The American Psychiatric Association issued a statement[8] regarding repressed memories: "Psychiatrists should refrain from making public statements about the veracity or other features of individual reports of sexual abuse, and psychiatrists should vigilantly assess the impact of their conduct on the boundaries of the doctor–patient relationship."

The American Medical Association (AMA) stated:

The AMA recognizes that few cases in which adults make accusations of childhood sexual abuse based on recovered memories can be proved or disproved, and it is not known how to distinguish true memories from imagined events in these cases. The AMA encourages physicians to address the therapeutic needs of patients who report memories of childhood sexual abuse and that these needs exist quite apart from the truth or falsity of any claims. The AMA also considers recovered memories of childhood sexual abuse to be of uncertain authenticity which should be subject to external verification.[7]

Conclusions

Recent developments in forensic psychiatry have indeed affected the practice of psychiatry. These changes have occurred primarily in the areas of managed care, confidentiality, boundary violations, and repressed memories. Other issues, such as emergency psychiatry, involuntary commitment of the mentally ill, and inappropriate use of psychotropic medications, also may provide risks for the practicing psychiatrist. It is especially reasonable to expect increased litigation in the realm of psychopharmacology, as new medications continue to proliferate and the use of combination drug therapy (usually involving an off-label indication) enjoys even more widespread practice.

With regard to emergency psychiatry or involuntary commitment, cases still in litigation have charged psychiatrists with involuntarily committing patients who do not have a mental illness but who may be dangerous to society. It is important for practicing psychiatrists to remember that the concept of dangerousness is fraught with risk for the psychiatrist. If the patient is deemed dangerous, that danger should be related to a mental illness and not merely to intoxication, anger, or jealousy. The latter cases may be more appropriately managed by law-enforcement officials than by psychiatrists.

Courts require therapists to act in a reasonable manner consistent with the guidelines, ethics, and standards of the mental health profession. The basic tenet of "first, do no harm" is an important consideration in reducing the risk of malpractice for psychiatrists. Because of the rapid changes in the mental health profession, psychiatrists must keep up with the literature, not only in psychiatry but also in the regulatory cases that affect the practice of psychiatry.

References:

1. Tarasoff v. Regents of University of California, 33 Cal App 3d 275, 108 Cal Rptr 878 (1973), rev'd, 13 Cal 3d 177, 529 P 2d 553, 118 Cal Rptr 129 (1974), modified, 17 Cal 3d 425, 551 P 2d 334, 131 Cal Rptr 14 (1976).
2. Schuster v. Altenberg, 144 Wis 2d 233, 424 NW 2d 159 (1988).
3. Barefoot v. Estelle, 463 US 880 (1983).
4. Petrila J, Sadoff R. Confidentiality and the family as caregiver. *Hosp Community Psychiatry.* 1992;43:136–139.
5. Simon RI. Sexual exploitation of patients: how it begins before it happens. *Psychiatr Ann.* 1989;19:104–112.
6. Wakefield H, Underwager R. Recovered memories of alleged sexual abuse: lawsuits vs. parents. *Behav Sci Law.* 1992;10:483–507.
7. Recent developments in health law: false memory syndrome and sexual abuse cases. *Am J Law Med.* 1994; 22:287.
8. American Psychiatric Association. *Psychiatric Times.* February 1994:26.

PART II

Specific Psychiatric Liabilities

9

Malpractice Liability Prevention in Hospital Psychiatry

JAMES E. ROSENBERG, M.D.

Editor's Note

Common malpractice claims relevant to hospital psychiatry include improper diagnosis, improper use of medication and other somatic therapies, patient self-injury or suicide, harm by patients to third parties, improper supervision of other hospital staff, and abandonment. In this lesson, the author discusses the issues surrounding involuntary civil commitment, which, in all states, requires the presence of a mental illness, and patient refusal to enter the hospital when he or she poses a significant risk of harm to self or others because of mental illness. Such refusal also can stem from the patient's inability to recognize the need for hospitalization.

Once the patient has been hospitalized, the psychiatrist must carry out a sufficient, though not all-inclusive assessment, which includes, among other things, identifying and attempting to obtain essential outside sources of information and formulating an adequate disposition or treatment plan. Keep in mind that psychiatrists can be held liable for negligent acts committed by other members of the treatment team under their

CME questions for this chapter begin on page 354.

supervision; thus, they should read all notes placed in the chart by such staff. Reasonable efforts must be made to obtain past records, and a release of information must be signed by the patient to obtain these records.

Physical disorders must be appropriately diagnosed and treated. The risk of self-harm and harm to others must be carefully assessed and managed. Issues of confidentiality, informed consent, the maintenance of accurate and sufficient progress notes, and conditions for discharge must be carefully considered.

Introduction

Compared with clinics, private offices, and other settings, hospitals pose unique medicolegal benefits and hazards for treating psychiatrists. The advantages include a greater degree of control, closer monitoring, and the availability of a wider array of services and databases. However, inpatient psychiatry is fraught with potential malpractice liabilities. By definition, hospitalized patients are sicker and more difficult to manage than are outpatients. Ward psychiatrists are held to a higher standard for the protection and improvement of their charges. Third-party payers, hospital utilization reviewers, and courts monitoring the care of involuntarily committed patients regularly pressure psychiatrists to discharge patients who may still constitute a substantial risk of assault or suicide.

The goals of this lesson are twofold. First, it will attempt to identify common areas of potential malpractice liability in hospital psychiatry. Second, the lesson will provide practical, clinically oriented guidelines designed to minimize these risks. The focus will be on the evaluation and treatment of patients admitted to acute psychiatric wards, not medical-surgical wards, chronic long-term care facilities, or other qualitatively different inpatient situations.

Scope of Malpractice Liability

The core issue in psychiatric malpractice, as in other areas of medical malpractice, is whether the evaluation or treatment provided by the psychiatrist was negligent (i.e., whether it fell below the standard of care). This standard is defined as what a psychiatrist, acting in his or her professional capacity, would reasonably and diligently do in similar circumstances.[1]

Common malpractice claims relevant to hospital psychiatry include improper diagnosis, improper use of medication and other somatic therapies, patient self-injury or suicide, harm by patients to third parties, improper supervision of other hospital staff, and abandonment.[2] These potential problem areas will be addressed in the course of considering the three basic, overlapping elements of inpatient psychiatric care: evaluation, treatment, and patient discharge. Emphasis will be placed on the adequacy of the care rendered during each phase and the appropriateness of the documentation that flows from that care.

Inpatient Evaluation

In this era of cost-containment, less expensive alternatives to psychiatric hospitalization are pursued whenever feasible. Third-party payers reserve authorization for patients for whom less intensive therapies have failed, patients who are unable to meet their basic necessities of life, or patients who pose a significant threat to themselves or others. Financial pressures and the high levels of patient acuity demand that the initial evaluation process unfold with utmost efficiency so definitive treatment may begin. Evaluation begins at admission with the decision of whether to hospitalize a patient, and, if so, whether involuntary civil commitment is required.

Involuntary Civil Commitment:

Although the initial commitment criteria and process vary considerably from state to state, psychiatrists and other selected professionals are empowered by statute to hold mentally ill persons for brief periods for further evaluation. If a psychiatrist proceeds with further holds, the commitment criteria and legal safeguards become more stringent.

Admitting psychiatrists must understand the involuntary commitment criteria for their state and must use these criteria to establish the basis on which a person should be held. In all states, the threshold criterion is the presence of a mental illness. The definition of mental illness is defined by statute or case law and may exclude, for example, acute substance intoxication or personality disorders. A requirement of involuntary commitment may be that a patient refuses hospitalization or lacks the capacity to recognize the need for it.

The next step involves establishing that a patient poses a significant risk of harm to self or others because of mental illness. The danger may arise from an act that a patient does not recognize as potentially harmful (e.g., a manic patient who drives recklessly at high speeds). Some states include grave disability or the patient's lack of ability to meet his or her own basic day-to-day needs as an alternative criterion. Several jurisdictions require admitting psychiatrists to determine that hospitalization would constitute the "least restrictive alternative" compatible with community or patient safety.[3]

Two types of patients who require acute hospital care should be admitted on involuntary holds: patients who refuse voluntary hospitalization and patients who lack the capacity to give informed consent for voluntary hospitalization. In the latter situation, patients who lack such capacity must be admitted on a hold, regardless of their consent to hospitalization, to set legal due process in motion and to protect their civil rights.[4]

The assessment of capacity is task specific. Thus, a patient may be psychotic, demented, or retarded and still retain the capacity to give informed consent to voluntary hospitalization. In general, the capacity to consent to admission to a psychiatric facility includes four elements[5]: (1) awareness or insight into the mental illness, (2) factual understanding of the nature and consequences of hospitalization, (3) the ability to use these facts rationally in arriving at a decision whether to accept or refuse admission, and (4) the ability to adhere to a choice. Patients who waver between accepting or refusing admission should be strongly considered for involuntary commitment. Otherwise, psychiatrists may risk liability for a patient who requires inpatient care, momentarily assents, and is placed in an unrestricted setting only to elope or demand discharge shortly thereafter.

Psychiatrists should understand the process by which a third party can authorize the hospitalization of a patient in their jurisdictions. If guardianship papers are presented as third-party authorization, admitting psychiatrists should confirm that these papers have not expired and that they include admitting powers. If the validity of the papers is in question, or they are not currently available, the safest course of action is to admit the patient on an involuntary hold until proof of guardianship is established.

Furthermore, psychiatrists should be aware that, in addition to traditional malpractice claims based upon negligence, they may be sued for false imprisonment and other intentional wrongs. Coverage for intentional torts is not included in many medical malpractice plans.

Admission Criteria:

If psychiatrists perform a reasonable, diligent assessment of the need for admission and commit a patient in good faith, the risk of subsequent liability is low. The assessment needs to be sufficient, not all-inclusive. Five steps are included: (1) identifying and attempting to obtain essential outside sources of information, (2) eliciting an adequate history from the patient, (3) performing an adequate mental status examination, (4) considering (if relevant) the possible organic causes or concomitant physical disorders, and (5) formulating an adequate disposition or treatment plan. Potential outside sources of information include the patient's medical chart; family, friends, or co-workers; or an outpatient therapist. Psychiatrists potentially incur liability for releasing a patient from the emergency department solely on the basis of the person's history when a glance at a discharge summary or conversation with a family member would have raised substantial safety concerns. If a patient refuses to give consent to a psychiatrist to speak with a relevant third party or to obtain an important record, the threshold for involuntary commitment should be reduced accordingly.

New-Patient Intake Evaluations and Reports:

Negligent evaluation of a patient during the intake process on a ward can produce an array of potential medicolegal traps. These pitfalls include most of the major areas of liability previously addressed: choice of medication and other somatic therapies, assessment of self-injury risk, assessment of risk of danger to others, and diagnosis of underlying or concomitant physical disorders. In addition, misdiagnosis and its consequences may lead to premature termination of authorization for continued hospitalization by third-party payers.

Ward psychiatrists can protect themselves during the intake process through a three-step process. The first two steps assure that the standard of care is met. The third step involves the proper documentation of the first two steps. First, psychiatrists must make a reasonable and diligent effort to collect sufficient information about a patient. Second, psychiatrists must be appropriately trained, up-to-date, and careful in using this information to arrive at a reasonable preliminary assessment from which further evaluation and treatment can flow. Third, psychiatrists must adequately chart the data collected, efforts to collect other relevant information that remains pending, and the reasoning process by which the conclusions have been reached.

Psychiatrists all too frequently write at length about what was learned during the interview and then jot down a few brief lines about the preliminary assessment and plan, as if they were exhausted by the data section of their reports. Documentation of the reasoning process (i.e., weighing of positive and negative factors), of the evaluation process, and of treatment plans is absolutely essential to sound malpractice liability prevention. Psychiatrists are not liable for errors or misfortunes that befall a patient, provided it is clear that steps one and two were followed. Courts look for reasonableness and diligence, not perfection.[5]

Preparing a Sound Intake Report
Gathering Information from Comprehensive Sources:

The art of medicine demands that psychiatrists have latitude, within reason, to pick and choose among acceptable alternatives in providing patient care. Thus, courts should not show a preference for a particular approach, but rather measure the standard of care against what a reasonable and diligent psychiatrist from the same school of thought would do in similar circumstances.[6]

The suggested format for a psychiatric intake report elaborated herein can be rearranged and expanded as the practitioner sees fit. However, the elements described are essential to sound malpractice liability prevention and should be included in every intake report. They reflect both the needs of a patient in crisis, in an era when anything less is relegated to outpatient status, and the primary areas in which malpractice claims are filed. Although psychiatrists may have a special interest (e.g., in family issues) and may paint this section of the report with broad strokes, they must save enough time and energy to address all the essentials in the history and explicate adequately the reasoning of the assessment and plan sections of the report.

A sound intake report must reflect that psychiatrists have taken into account relevant sources of information in addition to their own interview of a patient. These sources should include reports of other members of the treatment team; chart materials generated up to the time of the intake; conversations with third parties (e.g., a parent or spouse); available outside records (e.g., discharge summaries); and vital signs, laboratory test results, and other "hard" medical data. Otherwise, if clinicians make a decision that runs contrary to what most psychiatrists would do given the same data, and if an untoward event occurs, they may be portrayed by opposing counsel in court as having acted recklessly by ignoring other relevant information.

The Treatment Team

Although advantageous in several ways, the team or multidisciplinary model of patient care causes a bidirectional increase in liability for ward psychiatrists. On the one hand, the doctrines of vicarious liability, such as *respondeat superior* ("let the master answer"), impose potential liability upon psychiatrists for negligent acts committed by other members of the treatment team who are under their supervision or control.[2]

On the other hand, observations or opinions charted by other members of the treatment team automatically become the burden of psychiatrists either to accept or reject. Psychiatrists may accept such writings by ignoring them, referring to them in their own notes, or initialing or cosigning them. Psychiatrists may reject them by mentioning the specific entries and explaining why these entries are incorrect. Psychiatrists cannot afford to let pass unread notes that are deleterious to their own assessment or plan. The classic example is the clinician who discharges a patient as "much improved," unaware that the nurse on the night shift wrote that the patient's suicidal ideas had resurfaced (e.g., after an upsetting phone call).

Information recorded by other members of the treatment team is a subset of the next, more general issue: reviewing the materials generated in the chart prior to psychiatrists' intake evaluation. These documents may include emergency department records, involuntary commitment forms, pharmacy computer printouts of medications, photocopies of records from the transferring hospital or admitting clinic, and other vital and not-so-vital paperwork. Crucial documents should probably be initialed and dated by psychiatrists or listed in their intake report (e.g., under the "Sources of Information" section).

Generally, clinicians can register sufficiently in their report that the existing chart, including notes of other treatment team members, has been incorporated into the present evaluation by including a phrase such as, "Patient interviewed and discussed with treatment team. Chart reviewed." Again, critical items can be mentioned specifically (e.g, "Chart reviewed, including letter dated 1/1/97 from outpatient therapist, Dr. Smith").

Third Parties

Psychiatrists are obliged to make a reasonable attempt to contact third parties who might be expected to be of potential relevance to their evaluation of a patient. Examples include a patient's outpatient therapist, roommate, significant other, parent, board-and-care operator, conservator, or another person who presumably has special knowledge of the patient's prior psychiatric history or who has spent considerable time with the patient during the days prior to hospital admission. When not contacted, third parties may serve in court as witnesses for the plaintiff, stating, "I would have told Dr. Johnson that the last seven times my son was admitted with those feelings he tried to kill himself, but Dr. Johnson never called, and I didn't know how to reach him."

As a rule of thumb, at least one key third party should be contacted, either to obtain additional information or to corroborate a patient's story. Start by contacting the third party who brought the patient to the hospital or therapist's office. Psychiatrists should document in the intake report that they requested a patient's consent to contact an identified third party for specific reasons. If a third party knows the patient professionally, a release-of-information form signed by the patient will have to be sent by fax or other expeditious means as well. If a patient initially refuses to give consent, and the third-party information is crucial, psychiatrists are likewise obliged to document further attempts during the hospitalization to obtain consent. A patient later may yield such objections, as the patient-psychiatrist relationship builds or as he or she responds to treatment and becomes less guarded.

Past Records

Analogous to a psychiatrist's duty to seek essential third parties, clinicians are obliged to make a reasonable effort to obtain outside records that would likely be relevant to their current evaluation and plan. The yardstick remains the same: what would a prudent psychiatrist reasonably think and do in similar circumstances? The records of past psychiatric hospitalizations and outpatient treatments are obvious candidates. Again, psychiatrists must document their attempts to obtain a patient's consent for release of information as well as their attempts to obtain that information. If initial attempts are thwarted, additional attempts must be recorded.

In the case of Bell v. New York City Health and Hospital Corp, the psychiatrist in charge was held liable for a patient's attempted suicide 1 week after hospital discharge. The psychiatrist made no attempt to obtain past records. Prior records from a Veterans Administration hospital documented three suicide attempts that would have been relevant to the decision to release the patient from the current hospitalization.[7]

Psychiatrists must choose a method of acquiring information that matches the circumstances. A request by phone and then by follow-up fax is one useful approach. It does not make sense to send a letter by mail to a large county hospital that one hopes will be answered in 8 weeks when a patient is currently in crisis. When reasonable attempts have been made but to no avail, psychiatrists have nevertheless met their obligation and can proceed with a clear conscience.

Psychiatrists who find daunting a stack of records of past psychiatric hospitalizations should find solace in the standard of care: unless there are special circumstances, current treating psychiatrists are required only to read prior hospital discharge summaries, not other details of the record (P.J. Resnick, personal communication, July 1995). It is the responsibility of the discharging psychiatrist from the prior hospitalization to include all relevant information that a future treating psychiatrist would need in preparing the discharge summary.

Physical Disorders

Physical disorders are relevant at hospital admission (and follow-up) in at least three ways. First, the physical disorder may explain the psychiatric symptoms. Second, the physical disorder may be unrelated but potentially serious if not detected. Third, the psychiatric treatment contemplated may need to be modified to avoid exacerbating complications related to the disorder.

The following guidelines should be followed to avoid liability because of negligent misdiagnosis or lack of diagnosis of physical conditions:

1. Acquire an up-to-date, fundamental knowledge of the signs of organicity in psychiatric disorders. This knowledge includes understanding the patterns and ages of onset of the functional disorders

and recognizing atypical symptoms, such as olfactory or gustatory hallucinations.

2. Elicit an adequate history of major medical conditions, including head injuries and infection with HIV. Use pertinent negatives or something akin to "no major medical in detail" to indicate that the various major categories were actually addressed with a patient.

3. Obtain adequate general medical and neurologic histories and physical examinations as part of the intake process. This can be accomplished through an internist or other consultant.

4. Use basic laboratory tests, electrocardiography, and other studies in a manner appropriate to the patient.

5. Obtain specialized studies, such as head imaging or electroencephalography, when indicated.

6. Seek consultation from other specialists as needed.

Once psychiatrists are aware that laboratory tests or other studies are pending, the burden is upon them to verify the results and act upon them within a reasonable period. In an acute hospital setting, "reasonable period" may mean the first working day the results are available. Available test results left unchecked invite disaster. Clinicians also should document repeated attempts to obtain tests or specialized evaluations from uncooperative patients and the fact that their patients understood the risks implied by their refusals.

Psychiatrists should be able to screen every new patient for delirium and, in turn, embark upon an emergency evaluation for the underlying physical condition that caused it, whether personally or through consultation. Psychiatrists may choose to use the standard Mini-Mental State Examination[8] or at least should address attention span, concentration, and other cardinal features of delirium as part of every intake mental status examination.[9]

Other Information

Several other items are essential to every intake interview. Sufficient questions should be asked regarding the time course, severity, and multitude of psychiatric symptoms to allow for a reasonable differential diagnosis according to DSM-IV diagnostic classifications.[9] A history of substance abuse is relevant not only as a separate problem to be addressed but also because of its etiologic significance for mood, psychotic, and other symptoms as well as the withdrawal risks engendered by abstinence in the hospital. Other core questions should focus on current medications, medication compliance, drug and food allergies, and a history suggestive of mania.

Expanding the assessment portion of the intake report beyond the diagnosis to issues such as danger to self and others as a matter of policy serves two valuable functions: it demonstrates that clinicians have given the matter special attention and focuses the attention of psychiatrists on the issue, forcing them to evaluate these high-liability areas every time.

Assessing Risk:
Patient Self-Harm

In a study of more than 2,000 closed malpractice claims, suicide constituted an impressive 10% of the cases.[10] Psychiatrists are not expected to predict suicide; they are required to make a reasonable and diligent assessment of the risk of suicide.[11] Akin to an appendectomy for acute appendicitis, the assessment should err in good faith on the side of safety, incorporating a significant class of false-positive persons who ultimately do not make an attempt.

Malpractice claims involving suicides by psychiatric inpatients fall into three general classes: failure to diagnose that a patient was a significant suicide risk, failure to act appropriately once a patient's suicide risk was appreciated, and negligent release of a suicidal patient. The legal test has two arms: Was the patient's risk of suicide recognized or should it have been recognized (i.e., was it foreseeable)? Were proper steps taken to reduce that risk through observation and treatment? Inpatient psychiatrists are held to a higher standard than clinicians in other settings. When admitted to a hospital, a patient has largely relinquished responsibility for his or her safety to the special environment and expertise offered by the hospital and its staff.[1]

Proper diagnosis (i.e., risk assessment) of suicidality involves using the principles elaborated previously. Psychiatrists must uncover and incorporate into their assessment significant information obtained from other treatment team members, outside records, and third parties. Contrary observations by other staff members in the chart must be addressed.

The intake interview of a patient must be comprehensive to address major suicide risk factors relevant to the situation. In addition to formulating the most likely diagnosis, psychiatrists must focus in detail on anxiety, mood, and psychotic symptoms that individually confer a high suicide risk on a patient. For example, if a patient has command auditory hallucinations to kill him- or herself, follow-up questions should include if he or she has an associated delusion that the hallucinations are true, how he or she responded to similar hallucinations in the past, whether the voices are appealing or repulsive, and other relevant issues. The portion of the interview that addresses the past psychiatric history should incorporate the number of past suicide attempts, methods used, dates, if the circumstances were similar to a patient's current situation, and if he or she had ever made a suicide attempt in the hospital.

Thus, the risk assessment section of every psychiatric intake report should address separately the risk of suicide. Clinicians should indicate that the assessment is based on an overall evaluation of relevant factors rather than on opinion derived simply from a subset of available data. The manner in which the suicide risk assessment is written also should be taken into account; the use of terms such as "high" or "moderate" percentage risks only invites retribution by the plaintiff's attorney at trial. Appropriate phraseology that conveys information while affording the author maximal liability protection follows: "On the basis of my overall evaluation, the patient's risk of danger to self is low," ". . . is not sufficiently increased to warrant 1:1 observation," or ". . . is sufficiently increased to warrant 1:1 observation at the present time." The phrase "no risk" is never appropriate.

Psychiatrists should provide two different risk assessments: one applies to a patient's present condition in the hospital setting and the other involves a patient's risk of suicide following hospital discharge. The latter considers additional factors such as lack of a social support network, history of medication noncompliance, or likelihood of a return to substance abuse.

Danger to Third Parties

The assessment of a patient's risk of danger to others similarly deserves separate recognition in that section of the intake report. Clinicians can rely upon the same basic principles of sound care and malpractice liability prevention that were employed in assessing the risk of danger to self:

1. Formulate an assessment of risk of danger to others, not a prediction.[12] Err on the side of safety.

2. Perform a sufficiently comprehensive interview to ascertain symptoms, past history of violence, and other factors relevant to a reasonable and diligent evaluation.
3. Pay sufficient attention to third parties, outside records, and the observations and conclusions of other team members.
4. Focus on particularly relevant symptoms and the value of past behavior in determining the risk of future behavior.
5. Demonstrate that the assignment of risk flowed from a careful, overall weighing of factors.
6. Avoid specifying the degree of risk in poorly defined terms, such as "moderate" or "high," or in unrealistically precise terms, such as percentages. Favor instead statements such as "unacceptably increased risk" or "significantly increased risk" of danger to others.

As with an assessment of suicide, the risk assessment of violence toward others should distinguish between current in-hospital risk and factors that will alter risk after discharge. In addition to a clinical assessment of dangerousness, psychiatrists must be able to apply the legal test in their jurisdiction for what constitutes a violent patient to proceed with involuntary commitment, reporting duties, and other actions.[13] It is essential to maintain a current, basic understanding of risk assessment for potentially violent patients.[14]

In summary, the assessment section should cover separately the five axes of DSM-IV diagnoses, risk assessment of danger to self and others, substance-withdrawal risk, delirium, and unstable or acute physical disorders. The assessments of these particular areas may be as brief as pertinent negatives but should always be noted.

Confidentiality and the Duty to Protect Others
Background:

Patient confidentiality in the context of inpatient psychiatry refers to the right of a patient to expect that information disclosed during the course of the patient-psychiatrist (or, more generally, patient-therapist) relationship will not be divulged without his or her consent. A variety of civil remedies are available to a patient whose confidentiality has been breached. Confidentiality differs from privilege; privilege constitutes a specific legal construct that limits testimony in court about information that was acquired in confidences of certain fiduciary relationships.[2]

Psychiatrists should be aware of the specific exceptions to confidentiality in the patient-therapist relationship in their state. Exceptions may include, for example, emergencies, involuntary commitment proceedings, danger to third parties, reporting requirements, and discussions with fellow caregivers or clinical supervisors.[2] Government agencies may require that clinicians report child abuse, elder abuse, gunshot wounds, certain categories of unsafe drivers, inappropriate conduct by physicians and other professionals, and specific infectious diseases. Mandatory reporting laws provide immunity for appropriate, good-faith reporting as well as substantial penalties for failures to report.

Protecting Third Parties:

The statutory and case law that governs *Tarasoff*-type exceptions to patient confidentiality because of foreseeable danger to third parties varies widely across states. The landmark *Tarasoff* case in California has been widely misunderstood as expressing a duty to warn. In its 1976 *Tarasoff* decision, the California Supreme Court expanded the duty to warn to a duty to protect.[15] Hence, a variety of options are available to clinicians in fulfilling the duty to protect, including involuntary commitment, increase in medication, removal of potential weapons, and the like.

Psychiatrists should choose the means of protecting a third party that least intrudes upon a patient's confidentiality.[11] For example, most patients would consider a brief period of involuntary hospitalization to be less intrusive than notifying their employers of threats against them. If a patient threatens to harm a third party while involuntarily committed to a psychiatric facility, it would not be appropriate, in most cases, to issue a warning at that point. A patient is no longer a threat while under civil commitment in a locked hospital unit. There is time to observe whether the threat resolves prior to hospital discharge with proper medication and other interventions. If so, a warning is no longer necessary, and a patient has been saved that intrusion into his or her confidentiality. The identified victim also has been spared needless emotional anguish.

Most jurisdictions have restricted the duty to protect and warn to identifiable third parties. Some courts have expanded the doctrine to include the general public or another broad class of potential victims. Psychiatrists have been held liable in a limited number of cases for motor-vehicle accidents caused by patients whom they discharged. Thus, the duty to protect and warn has been expanded to include unintentional injuries to third parties.[1] Only a handful of states have authorized breaches of confidentiality because of the risk of patient suicide or destruction of property.

An emerging area of controversy in *Tarasoff*-type duties is the unsafe practices of HIV-seropositive patients. The American Psychiatric Association (APA) has issued a position statement regarding this dilemma.[16] The APA Commission on AIDS states that, in limited circumstances where all less-intrusive means have failed, it is permissible ethically for a psychiatrist to notify at-risk third parties or a public health agency. Because legal requirements vary from state to state, it is advisable to obtain legal advice and to consider resolving a patient's release through an involuntary commitment hearing for danger to others.

Treatment Issues

Malpractice liability may arise in a multitude of ways at the initiation of treatment. The most crucial element is the procurement of inadequate informed consent from patients. Other potential pitfalls include the correct treatment of the wrong diagnosis, the wrong treatment of the correct diagnosis, and insufficient medical clearance prior to initiating therapy.

Informed consent:

Informed consent arises from the triad of information, voluntariness, and capacity (avoiding the legal term competence).[17] Appropriate information includes the nature of the mental illness; risks and benefits of the proposed treatment; risks and benefits of alternative treatments; and risks and benefits of no treatment, which includes a prognosis. The legal yardstick here is what a reasonable person in a patient's situation would want to know in making an informed decision about the proposed treatment.[18]

Voluntariness refers to a patient being free to make a choice without coercion. A patient also must have the capacity to understand the factual information presented, to use it rationally in arriving at a decision, and to reach a conclusion and be able to express it. Although preprinted consent forms are helpful in reducing liability, the optimal combination is an adequate discussion of the treatment issues with a patient followed by a progress note to that effect in the chart.[17] It is prudent to describe the general discussion that occurred, the questions answered, and the risks of greatest concern to liability prevention that were addressed (e.g., the risks of tardive dyskinesia in cases where neuroleptics were prescribed).

Exceptions

There are four exceptions to informed consent: (1) lack of a capacity to consent, (2) emergencies, (3) therapeutic privilege, and (4) a waiver.[19] If a patient lacks the capacity to give consent (e.g., because of delirium or dementia), then a substitute decisionmaker must be sought, in accordance with requirements of that jurisdiction. The decision-maker may be the court, a guardian, or another third party. The legal system views the purpose of involuntary commitment as protection, not treatment.[20] A patient preserves his or her right to refuse treatment unless decided otherwise in a manner that varies from state to state. Clinicians should request approval from the court and hospital ethics committee before administering medication via hiding it in food, forcibly using a nasogastric tube, and other less conventional means.

Courts will generally allow ward staff to medicate or restrain a patient against his or her will in an emergency situation (i.e., if he or she poses an immediate threat of injury to self or others). Psychiatrists should document the circumstances that arise, clarifying that no less intrusive method of controlling the patient is feasible, which may be especially important if the patient suffers any adverse outcome from the imposed treatment. In addition to a malpractice claim, the unnecessary imposition of seclusion and restraint or a somatic therapy invites suits alleging assault and battery, civil rights violations, and other intentional torts that may not be covered by the malpractice insurance carrier.[11]

In the case of therapeutic privilege, psychiatrists can temporarily withhold parts of the discussion about diagnosis and treatment if a fuller disclosure would be deleterious to a patient's well-being. As a patient improves, additional information must be "titrated" to suit the clinical situation. Obviously, clinicians must document in detail the reasoning behind withholding information essential to the informed-consent process.

Patients also can waive their rights to being informed or participating in the consent process if it would be too upsetting for them and if they would prefer to leave themselves in a psychiatrist's hands. Again, as treatment proceeds and a patient becomes more autonomous, clinicians should document additional attempts to provide sufficient information for bona fide informed consent. The consent process is dynamic and continues to unfold until patient discharge.

Additional Considerations

More intrusive or atypical treatment regimens require more extensive justification and documentation of the informed consent process. At one end of the spectrum, the risk of a successful civil suit for negligent psychotherapy is remote because of the wide variation in acceptable methods of psychotherapy and the lack of demonstrable physical injury.[21] Exceptions include sexual indiscretions or deprivation of necessary somatic therapy because of an overreliance on psychotherapy alone.

At the other end of the spectrum, liability considerations become substantial with electroconvulsive therapy and less conventional pharmacotherapy. Examples of the latter include starting medications without baseline medical clearance, employing higher-than–usual blood levels or dosages, continuing medication despite significant side effects, prescribing psychotropic medication inappropriately during pregnancy, using benzodiazepines chronically, employing unapproved uses or routes of administration of a medication, and unnecessary polypharmacy.

Psychiatrists must take great care to explicate the reasoning process (i.e., the weighing of positive and negative factors) leading to their decision. Furthermore, it should be documented that the dilemma was shared with the patient, who agreed to proceed. Liability concerns should not trump patient-care needs but, rather, alert psychiatrists to the importance of tightening their consent and documentation practices.

One element of this documentation process is to explain why a particular case warrants deviation from hospital policy, published treatment guidelines, or other standards. Each "authority" constitutes a suggested standard of care that should be considered in the overall risk-benefit analysis. The final clinical decision flows from the weighing of multiple factors.[11]

A major area of malpractice liability in psychopharmacology involves tardive dyskinesia that results from neuroleptic medication. The legal system focuses on the risks of such medication, whereas clinicians perceive mainly the benefits.[22] This disparity emphasizes the need for careful and appropriate justification, use, and documentation. The APA has published guidelines regarding the prevention and management of tardive dyskinesia when prescribing neuroleptic drugs.[23] The justification for neuroleptic use and the informed-consent process should be viewed as responsibilities that continue throughout hospitalization.[24]

In difficult cases, an important resource is the formal consultation by a colleague or a hospital medical director, which should be documented in the patient's chart. It would be more difficult for plaintiff's counsel to claim that the standard of care was breached when two psychiatrists agreed upon the same care.

Inpatient Follow-Up Care:

Once the initial assessment has been completed and treatment is under way, psychiatrists must employ similar liability prevention strategies in their follow-up evaluations. Progress notes should contain the following elements:

- Attention to vital signs, diabetic blood glucose monitoring, new laboratory results, and other parameters of physical functioning
- Review of the case with the treatment team as well as awareness of the observations and conclusions of other team members as recorded on the chart
- Follow-up of outside information from requested records and third parties
- Monitoring of progress through consistent attention to specific target symptoms
- Monitoring of adverse reactions to hospitalization and treatment
- Ongoing risk assessment for danger to self and others
- Need for continued involuntary commitment and use of the inpatient setting

In other words, every progress note should address physical well-being, medication side effects, cognitive functioning, and suicidality.

These recommendations are not meant to imply that clinicians should write excessively long notes three times a week under the specter of malpractice liability risk. One useful strategy is to write a detailed progress note each Monday, with brief follow-up notes on the following days. A note might read: "Vital signs stable, afebrile. Patient seen in detail and discussed with treatment team. Chart reviewed. No med side effects in detail. Otherwise no major change. Continue present plan."

Discharge Issues

In discharging patients or transferring them to less restrictive settings, courts recognize the value of maximizing independent functioning in exchange for accepting a certain level of risk to a patient and the community. When a patient is granted a pass, grounds privileges, or transfer to an open unit, the transferring psychiatrist should be as comfortable with the patient's risk of suicide or violence as if the patient were being discharged outright. A substantial percentage of inpatient suicides occur during a pass or following an elopement.

Transferring clinicians have three essential duties: to ascertain that a patient is appropriate for transfer, to ensure safe transfer of a patient, and to ensure that the receiving psychiatrist is made aware of all essential information regarding a patient's current state and of any warning signs of decompensation.

Malpractice claims involving negligent release from the hospital center around suicide potential, violence potential, and unintentional harms possibly perpetrated by a patient. One rule of sound liability prevention is to avoid last-minute surprises. The patient's chart should reflect that he or she was interviewed on the day of hospital discharge and that the discharge plans remain appropriate. Notes by other team members should be checked with extra care. The discharging psychiatrist should avoid the classic nightmare: everyone but the clinician was aware that in the past 24 hours, the patient received a tragic phone call, made a threat, or refused medications, etc.

Comprehensive risk assessments of danger to self and others should be restated near the time of patient discharge, accounting for the commonsense factors that will potentially increase risk after discharge: return to substance abuse, medication noncompliance, psychosocial stressors, and other factors specific to a patient. With a less cooperative patient, the psychiatrists should document that key interventions to reduce risk were offered and refused and that the patient was aware of the risks of refusal. These interventions might have included decanoate neuroleptic medication, an outpatient follow-up appointment, or referral to an alcohol-drug treatment program. Whenever possible, clinicians should formally enlist a responsible third party to supervise a discharged patient, monitor medications, and ensure that he or she attends the first follow-up appointment.

Although the legal system should not be exploited indiscriminately, the involuntary-commitment hearing process serves a valuable function in reducing a psychiatrist's personal liability upon patient discharge. In rare cases of equivocal or unpredictable risk of harm, it may be advisable to hold a patient in the hospital until the court orders his or her release. In such situations, it is imperative for psychiatrists to document that they have presented an adequately detailed description of factors that increase and decrease a patient's risk. Otherwise, if psychiatrists and the court rely on two different bodies of information to determine patient release, no reduction in liability will result. In contrast, clinicians will be held liable for prematurely discharging a patient because of denial of coverage by a third-party payer or because of other financial pressure.[25]

Unintentional harm by a discharged patient toward self or others can be mitigated, in part, by appropriate discharge instructions. Although patients should be provided with a written copy to take with them, clinicians also should document the discussion in the progress notes. After patient discharge, the instructions will serve as both guidelines for patients and a quick reference for outpatient psychiatrists. Patients should sign that they have read the discharge instructions, understand them, and agree to abide by them. The following six elements should be covered:

1. Final diagnoses of mental and physical disorders.
2. Follow-up plans, including the date, time, and location of an appointment, and parameters under which the patient should return to the emergency room.
3. Medications and brief lay descriptions of their purposes (e.g., "Haldol, 5 mg three times per day, for voices, paranoia").
4. Caveats, where appropriate, regarding restrictions on driving or operating dangerous devices.

5. Prohibitions regarding weapons and substance use.
6. Other caveats, such as those regarding specific medications.

As mentioned previously, psychiatrists may be liable for injuries caused by their discharged patients while operating motor vehicles. In some cases, it is appropriate to notify the state department of motor vehicles regarding a dangerous patient. However, this will confer no short-term protection. If the risk of dangerous driving is substantial, valuable interventions include enlisting a third party in hiding a patient's keys (or car) or making this risk the basis of further involuntary commitment.

Caveats for specific medications alert patients to the risks of stopping the medications on their own or other behaviors that may place them at risk. Examples include warning patients that abruptly stopping an anticonvulsant prescribed as a mood stabilizer could lead to withdrawal seizures, emphasizing the dangers of mixing alcohol and benzodiazepines, and stressing that discontinuing haloperidol (Haldol) and benztropine mesylate (Cogentin) can cause dystonia because of the persisting binding effects of haloperidol.

Summary

Clinicians are obliged to exercise reasonable and diligent care in their evaluation, treatment, and release of hospitalized patients. Inpatient psychiatrists can enjoy a marked reduction in malpractice liability risks by following the author's useful principles regarding evaluation, treatment, and accompanying documentation. In short, obtain sufficient information and use it in an explicit reasoning process to guide patient care.

References

1. Macbeth JE, Wheeler AM, Sither JW, Onek JN. *Legal and Risk Management Issues* in the Practice of Psychiatry. Washington, DC: Psychiatrists' Purchasing Group; 1994.
2. Appelbaum PS, Gutheil TG. *Clinical Handbook of Psychiatry and the Law.* Baltimore: Williams & Wilkins; 1991.
3. Melton GB, Petrila J, Poythress NG, Slobogin C. *Psychological Evaluations for the Courts: A Handbook for Mental Health Professsionals and Lawyers.* New York: The Guilford Press; 1987.
4. Zinermon v Burch, 110 S Ct 975 (1990).
5. Gutheil TG. Legal issues in psychiatry. In: Kaplan HI, Sadock BJ, eds. *Comprehensive Textbook of Psychiatry.* Baltimore: Williams & Wilkins; 1995;2;2748.
6. Roberts v Tardiff, 417 A2d 444 (Me 1980).

7. 456 NYS 2d 787 (App Div 1982).

8. Folstein MF, Folstein SE, McHugh PR. Mini-mental state: a practical method for grading the cognitive state of patients for the clinician. *J Psychiatr Res.* 1975;12:189–198.

9. American Psychiatric Association. *Diagnostic and Statistical Manual of Mental Disorders.* 4th ed. Washington, DC: American Psychiatric Association; 1994.

10. Slawson P. Psychiatric malpractice: the low frequency risks. *Med Law.* 1993;12:673–680.

11. Simon RI, Sadoff RL. *Psychiatric Malpractice: Cases and Comments for Clinicians.* Washington, DC: American Psychiatric Press; 1992.

12. Litwack TR, Kirschner SM, Wack RC. The assessment of dangerousness and predictions of violence: recent research and future prospects. *Psychiatr Q.* 1993;64:245–273.

13. Leong GB, Silva JA, Weinstock R. Dangerousness. In: Rosner R, ed. *Principles and Practice of Forensic Psychiatry.* New York: Chapman & Hall; 1994:432–437.

14. Simon RI. *Concise Guide to Psychiatry and Law for Clinicians.* Washington, DC: American Psychiatric Press; 1992.

15. Tarasoff v Regents of the University of California, 17 Cal 3d 425, 551 P2d 334, 131 Cal Rptr 14 (1976).

16. American Psychiatric Association Commission on AIDS. AIDS policy: position statement on confidentiality, disclosure, and protection of others. *Am J Psychiatry.* 1993;150:852.

17. Gutheil TG. Medicolegal psychopharmacology. In: Gelenberg AJ, Bassuk EL, Schoonover SC, eds. *The Practitioner's Guide to Psychoactive Drugs.* New York: Plenum Press; 1991:473–486.

18. Canterbury v Spence, 150 US App DC 263, 464 F2d 772 (1972).

19. Rozovsky FA. Consent to Treatment: A Practical Guide. Boston: Little, Brown & Co; 1984:87–125.

20. Appelbaum PS. The right to refuse treatment with antipsychotic medications: retrospect and prospect. *Am J Psychiatry.* 1988;145:413–419.

21. Klein JI, Glover SI. Psychiatric malpractice. *Int J Law Psychiatry.* 1983; 6:131–157.

22. Bursztajn H, Chanowitz B, Kaplan E, Gutheil TG, Hamm RM, Alexander V. Medical and judicial perceptions of the risks associated with use of antipsychotic medication. *Bull Am Acad Psychiatry Law.* 1991;19:271–275.

23. Kane JM, Jeste DV, Barnes TRE, et al. *Tardive Dyskinesia: A Task Force Report of the American Psychiatric Association.* Washington, DC: American Psy-chiatric Association; 1992.

24. Beck JC. Determining competency to assent to neuroleptic drug treatment. *Hosp Community Psychiatry.* 1988;39:1106–1108.

25. Wickline v State of California, 192 Cal App 3d 1630; 239 Cal Rptr 810 (1986).

1 0

The Risk of Misdiagnosing Physical Illness as Depression

MARK S. GOLD, MD, FCP, FAPA

Editor's Note

Key Points

- *Many clients have a remarkably low response to the initial treatment of mental disorders. One of the major reasons for this is that they are misdiagnosed; they are actually suffering from a physical illness or from drug or alcohol abuse.*
- *Some common reasons that mental health professionals mistake physical illnesses for mental disorders are: their inability to deal with physical illness, lack of knowledge and continuing professional education, educational lag in training programs, and resistance to new information. Many disorders are on the borderline between mental health/illness and internal medicine and neurology.*
- *Various physical illnesses and nutritional deficiencies that frequently appear to be mental disorders are reviewed.*
- *No matter how closely the first presentation of a mentally disabled client may conform to classic DSM-IV descriptive criteria, one cannot assume that the client is suffering from a psychiatric disorder.*
- *To reduce misdiagnosis and mistreatment of depression and other*

CME questions for this chapter begin on page 356.

mental disorders, a complete physical, neurological, and endocrino-logical examination should be performed by a physician who is fluent in both psychiatry and internal medicine.

Introduction

One of the more recent discoveries of modern mental health care is that the majority of mental disorders show a remarkably low response to initial treatment (Shapiro & Keller, 1981). The rates of relapse of clients who are systematically followed for a period of a year or more is disconcerting (Hamilton, 1982; Shapiro & Keller, 1981). Such relapses are troublesome for both the client, who must ask for further treatment or switch therapists, and the professional, who must encounter a less cooperative client while trying to determine why the initial treatment failed. One of the major reasons for treatment failures is that many clients are being treated for mental disorders when, in fact, they are suffering from physical illness, drug or alcohol abuse (Hall et al., 1978; Herridge, 1960; Koranyi, 1979), or dependence (Gold, 1992a, 1994; Gold; Gold & Gleaton, 1994; Gold & Miller, 1994; Miller & Gold, 1992). Psychiatric symptomatology can be, and frequently is, the first manifestation of a reversible physical illness.

Contrary to the beliefs of most medical professionals, clients whose mental symptoms mask physical illness are not rare. Although many psychotherapists contend that they have never seen cases of this sort, it has, in fact, been repeatedly documented by many different authors that pysical illness needs to be vigorously excluded before a diagnosis of a mental illness can be made.

The Diagnostic and Statistical Manual of Mental Disorders (DSM-IV) (American Psychiatric Association, 1994) committee assumes that physical illnesses must be ruled out before proceeding through the decision tree (this is clear from looking at the DSM-IV differential diagnosis trees). If a physical illness is found, the diagnosis must then move into the section on organic mental disorders. Unfortunately, the most common misdiagnoses and the state-of-the-art workup for each are never addressed.

Misdiagnosis: Is It Really a Problem?

Hall and associates (1978) studied 658 consecutive psychiatric outpatients; they found that 9.1% had medical disorders that produced mental, emotional, and behavioral symptoms. In an additional group of patients, medical disorders were mostly or partially causative. Forty-six percent of these patients could have been identified by their initial treating physicians, but they were not. In another study of outpatients, Koranyi (1979) excluded all patients who were immediately hospitalized as well as patients who failed to complete a comprehensive assessment. He started with an initial sample of 2670 patients; a final sample of 2090 patients who had been completely evaluated was examined. Forty-three percent of these patients were suffering from one or several major physical illnesses, 46% of which were undiagnosed at the time of referral; 7.74% of the total population had a physical illness that directly caused their psychiatric symptoms. Herridge (1960) studied 209 consecutive admissions to an inpatient unit and found that at least 5% had major physical illnesses that were causative of and presented as a psychiatric disorder. Hall and associates (1978) studied 658 consecutive psychiatric outpatients; they found that 9.1% had medical disorders that produced mental, emotional, and behavioral symptoms. In an additional group of patients, medical disorders were mostly or partially causative. Forty-six percent of these patients could have been identified by their initial treating physicians, but they were not. In another study of outpatients, Koranyi (1979) excluded all patients who were immediately hospitalized as well as patients who failed to complete a comprehensive assessment. He started with an initial sample of 2670 patients; a final sample of 2090 patients who had been completely evaluated was examined. Forty-three percent of these patients were suffering from one or several major physical illnesses, 46% of which were undiagnosed at the time of referral; 7.74% of the total population had a physical illness that directly caused their psychiatric symptoms. Herridge (1960) studied 209 consecutive admissions to an inpatient unit and found that at least 5% had major physical illnesses that were causative of and presented as a psychiatric disorder."

Hall and colleagues (1981) conducted a prospective study of 100 admitted state hospital patients. Patients with known physical disorders along with sociopathic personality disorders and patients with significant histories of alcohol or drug abuse were omitted. An intensive search for causative physical illness revealed that 46% of the patients had a previously unrecognized and undiagnosed physical illness that was specifically related to their psychopathological symptoms and either caused these symptoms or substantially exacerbated them. Hall noted, ". . . 28 of 46 patients evidenced dramatic and rapid clearing of their mental/emotional symptoms when medical treatment for the underlying physical disorder was instituted. Eighteen patients were substantially improved immediately following appropriate medical treatments." The study of Hoffman (1982) yielded similar results: of 215 patients referred to a specialized medical psychiatric inpatient unit for further evaluation, the referring diagnosis was inaccurate in 41% of the cases, and 24% of the cases were changed from physical to psychiatric or from psychiatric to physical illness.

Both medical and mental health professionals fail to diagnose physical illness. Koranyi (1979) reported that of all the sources referring clients to his outpatient clinic, medical personnel failed to find 32% of physical illness in referred clients, whereas psychiatrists missed 48% of physical illness in referred patients. Most striking was that 83% of all clients referred by social agencies or who were self-referred had undetected physical illness at the time they were seen in the outpatient department. Physicians are better than the patients themselves and other mental health workers in diagnosing physical illness, but their overall performance is poor by any standards (Dackis & Gold, 1984, 1986a; Extein & Gold, 1986; Gold, 1992b, 1993; Gross, Extein, & Gold, 1986; Miller, Mahler, & Gold, 1991).

These studies clearly show that physical illness is either a precipitant or associated condition that needs to be considered in any diagnostic formulation. More sophisticated and provocative testing techniques have been used successfully to help diagnose thyroid disease (Gold & Pearsall, 1983b) and identify low-dose drug and alcohol abuse among mental health clientele (Estroff & Gold, 1986b; Gold, 1989a, 1989b; Miller & Gold, 1991; Verebey, Gold, & Mule, 1986). These new tests will increase the percentage of detected medical illnesses (Extein & Gold, 1986; Gross, Extein, & Gold, 1986; Verebey, Martin, & Gold, 1987).

Why Misdiagnosis Exists

The factors leading to diagnostic errors are important and need to be scrutinized in detail. Many mental health professionals are unequipped to deal with physical illness in their clients. Klein and associates (1980) believed that errors in diagnosis "cannot be attributed to random sloppiness, bad faith, or lack of desire to help a patient to the utmost." They proposed a variety of reasons for why misdiagnosis occurs, including simple lack of knowledge, educational lag in training programs, lack of continuing professional education, and resistance to new information. This can lead to a selective rejection of certain facts of the case so that the client will more easily fit into the caregiver's specialty or orientation, which often results in a distortion and misperception of the client and his or her sometimes obvious physical illness. McIntyre and Romano (1977) found that less than 35% of practicing psychiatrists give their patients a physical examination. Thirty-two percent of psychiatrists admitted that they did not feel competent to perform even a rudimentary physical examination. However, these numbers may be much greater. Mental health professionals tend to consult either the client's family doctor, internist, pediatrician, or gynecologist for a medical clearance to rule out physical disorders.

The previously cited studies refer only to physical illnesses that presented as mental disorders and were, in whole or in part, causative of the mental symptoms. Physical illness can cause or worsen the symptoms of mental illness to a variable extent. Some disorders that present exclusively with symptoms of a mental disorder are wholly causative of the psychopathologic symptomatology. These disorders, if they are treated properly and have not progressed to an irreversible stage, should result in a total clearing (a cure) of all such symptomatology without institution of nonphysical treatment. Other disorders exacerbate or, in part, cause the observed mental symptomatology, and, when treated, result in a significant but only partial clearing of the psychiatric symptoms. Still other illnesses are concomitant with and unrelated to the mental disorders, and, when treated, produce no effect on the mental symptoms. The group of psychopathologic symptoms that develop in reaction to previously existing illness will be considered only in passing. Finally, some mental illnesses are often treated incorrectly as medical disorders by nonpsychiatric practitioners.

Many disorders are truly on the borderline between mental health/illness and internal medicine and neurology. Most of these disorders are not detectable by physical examination or by "routine" laboratory screening alone. The correct diagnosis may not be made until the consulting physician is aware of the existence of these diseases and actively pursues the diagnosis through aggressive specialized testing.

As many as 50 or 100 patients with apparently similar symptomatology may have to be tested to find 1 patient with a physical disorder. This search is always worthwhile.

Misdiagnosis exists in the Prozac era because depression has been destigmatized and illicit drug addictions and alcoholism are seen as "abuses" and grounds for termination. Also, pharmacologic treatment advances have been rapid in affective, panic, obsessive compulsive disorder (OCD), and other psychiatric disorders, yet the current treatment of choice for alcoholics is evaluation, detoxification, Alcoholics Anonymous (AA), and abstinence. Many alcoholics and drug abusers are treated for "depression" with antidepressants or other agents out of treatment bias.

Specificity of Presenting Psychopathologic Symptoms

From the previously cited studies, and many others, it becomes clear that no matter how closely the first presentation of a mentally disabled client may conform to classic DSM-IV descriptive criteria, one cannot assume that the client is suffering from a psychiatric disorder.

This nonspecificity of medical disease causing specific syndromes is particularly true for depressive disorders. The differential diagnosis of depression is long and involved. Giannini, Black, and Goettsche (1978) listed 91 possible disorders that can present as depression. Hall (1980) listed 24 medical illnesses that frequently induce depression and 77 medical conditions that can present as depression.

To summarize thus far, many clients who present with mental/emotional symptomatology actually have medical illnesses. The psychiatric symptoms are merely the first and most obvious manifestation of the physical illness. No psychopathologic sign or symptom is pathognomonic of a mental disorder to the extent that it cannot be caused by a physical disorder. Many nonpsychiatric physicians and mental health professionals, including psychiatrists, are either unaware of these facts or choose to ignore them. A diagnosis of a mental disorder is only made by exhaustive evaluation. Simply meeting descriptive criteria does not confirm such a diagnosis at any time. Most clients who present with mental/emotional symptoms are not given a thorough physical examination and medical workup to detect possible medical causes of the psychiatric symptoms, which would then be reversed by treating the primary disease.

Medical Illnesses that May Present as Mental Disorders

The following section will review various medical disorders that can present psychopathologically and mimic any depressive illness.

The Carcinoid Syndrome:

Carcinoid tumor may be confused with major depression, hypomania, major depression with psychosis, or anxiety. It may not always be accompanied by spontaneous flushing of the upper body precipitated by consuming certain foods or alcohol, epinephrine administration, excitement, or exertion. An attack may be accompanied by abdominal pain and diarrhea. The syndrome accompanies a variety of tumors that can occur in the gastrointestinal tract and lungs and that secrete various biologically active substances, including dopamine, histamine, corticotropin (ACTH), and serotonin. Serotonin-secreting tumors are most common.

If this disorder is included in the differential diagnosis, the diagnosis may be confirmed by an increased urinary excretion of 5-hydroxyindoleacetic acid (5-HIAA), which normally does not exceed 9 mg daily.

Cancer:

Many patients with malignant tumors may present to the mental health professional with depressive symptomatology, often meeting DSM-IV criteria months or even years earlier than physical symptoms or signs. Of all the malignant tumors that present psychopathologically, pancreatic carcinoma is the most notorious (Jefferson & Marshall, 1981). The first signs of the tumor are often severe depression with crying spells, insomnia unresponsive to sleeping medication, and anxiety associated with the fear that the patient has a very serious illness.

Central nervous system (CNS) tumors present with mental/emotional symptomatology, especially if they occur in the temporal and frontal regions. The most common symptom is a change in personality. Left-sided tumors present more frequently as irritability or depression, whereas tumors of the parietal and occipital lobes tend to be relatively silent. Limbic system tumors can present as depression, delusions, assaultive behavior, and confusional states. Human immunodeficiency virus (HIV) infection in the central nervous system and right-sided cerebrovascular accidents (CVAs) can mimic depression, anxiety, and panic attacks. A high index of suspicion is indicated when the client presents in an atypical fashion with a personality change, depression with a weight loss greater than 20 pounds, or is unresponsive to a first trial of standard mental health care.

Diabetes Mellitus:

In a study by Hall and colleagues (1981), certain clients with diabetes mellitus presented psychiatrically and met the diagnostic criteria for major depression, and for other disorders as well. Diabetes may present as depression, sexual dysfunction, and/or marital problems (Gold, 1995). The diagnosis is made by demonstrating an elevated fasting blood sugar or an abnormal response to a glucose load at 1 and 2 hours.

Illicit Drugs:

Drug (Gold, 1995) and alcohol abuse (Dackis and Gold, 1986b) and withdrawal may imitate depressive illnesses. Furthermore, hospitalized psychiatric patients sometimes abuse drugs in the hospital, resulting in confusing changes in function and severe exacerbations of their illnesses (Miller, Hoffman, & Gold, 1994). The only way to make the drug abuse diagnosis is to be constantly aware of the frequency of drug and alcohol problems. Simply questioning the client without formal testing is both naïve and dangerous. Drug intoxication, drug withdrawal, and the sequelae of drug abuse should be actively eliminated from consideration (Gold, Pottash, & Extein, 1982). Such clients commonly present with symptoms of depression, and they may meet the DSM-IV criteria for major depression. Drug abuse can, however, resemble any known condition from psychosis to mild anxiety states and must be considered in all psychiatric disorders no matter how classic the presentation. Asking the client about the existence and extent of drug use is essential; however, anecdote should never be confused with fact. Drug use, drug intoxication, and drug withdrawal diagnosis should be confirmed whenever possible by blood or urine testing.

Nicotine and alcohol abuse, dependence, and involvement are also common causes of misdiagnosis and failure to respond to treatment. Nicotine dependence is decreasing in response to widespread public education and the availability of successful smoking cessation programs. This decrease has been most pronounced among the most well-educated citizens in the United States. When a cigarette-smoking nurse, therapist, or physician is identified and detoxified (or fail in detoxification), underlying depression may be found to be the cause. Patients with depression who smoke cigarettes may be found to be nonresponders because their nicotine dependence has not been treated. Cigarette smoking can interfere not only with medication response by altering the metabolism of the antidepressant; it can make treatment difficult in many cases.

Alcoholic patients generally meet DSM-IV criteria for major depressive disorder. If a person does not know that he or she is an alcoholic, treatment will fail. Alcoholics often have depressed moods and disturbed sleep and appetite symptoms commonly associated with naturally occurring depression.

Many frequent users of marijuana experience anxiety and complain of memory loss and affective changes. This is becoming more true as the THC (tetrahydrocannabinol) level has increased in the typical marijuana cigarette. MDMA, or ectasy, the use of which is widespread at "raves," or all-night dance parties packed with participants fueled by various hallucinogenic drugs (Gold, in press), is associated with panic and anxiety which can persist long after MDMA use is discontinued. Similarly, the resurgence in LSD (lysergic acid) use has made the diagnosis of psychosis all the more difficult (Gold, in press).

Prescription Drugs:

Psychopathological symptoms occur in at least 2.7% of patients taking prescription medication on a regular basis, according to the Boston Collaborative Drug Surveillance Study of 9000 patients (Extein & Gold, 1986).

Hyperadrenalism (Cushing's Syndrome) and Hypoadrenalism (Addison's Disease):

Cushing's syndrome may present as an affective illness with or without psychosis, euphoria, or anxiety. In one study using structured interviews and RDC criteria, depression was present in 83% of patients with endogenous Cushing's syndrome who met RDC criteria for either mania or hypomania prior to the depression (Gold, 1995).

Hypoadrenalism commonly presents as depression or organic brain syndrome. The diagnosis is usually made on the basis of low diurnal serum cortisol and low 24-hour urine cortisol excretion. Hypoadrenalism is easily treated with steroid replacement therapy.

Hypoglycemia:

Many people diagnose themselves as hypoglycemic in order to explain their depressive symptomatology. There is little proof that all such clients have symptomatic hypoglycemia. However, there are several conditions that can cause symptomatic hypoglycemia. The most prominent are insulinoma and the exogenous administration of insulin. Insulinoma is probably the most frequent cause of symptomatic hypoglycemia and may produce bizarre behavior that can be indistinguishable from schizophrenia, depression, dementia, or anxiety attacks.

Hyperparathyroidism and Hypoparathyroidism:

The mental/emotional disturbances seen in hyperparathyroidism are directly related to serum calcium levels. Serum calcium levels of 12 to 16 mg/100 mL are associated with psychopathological changes (Extein & Gold, 1986; Gross, Estein, & Gold, 1986). Hypoparathyroidism with resultant low serum calcium levels most commonly presents as an organic brain syndrome, but it may appear to be delirium tremens or depression with psychosis. Diagnosis of both hyperparathyroidism and hypoparathyroidism is first suspected upon seeing an abnormal serum calcium level on routine blood screening or from a history of thyroid or parathyroid disorders in the family and/or previous thyroid or parathyroid surgery.

Hyperthyroidism and Hypothyroidism:

Hyperthyroidism may resemble panic disorder, anxiety, neurosis, or mania. People fail to realize that hyperthyroidism frequently presents as depression. The diagnosis of hyper-thyroidism is made by the classical symptoms of hyper-thyroidism, along with elevated T3 and T4, a depressed level of thyroid-stimulating hormone (TSH), and a low TSH response to thytroprin-releasing hormone (TRH) administration.

Hypothyroidism has been classically associated with psychosis in the form of "myxedema madness." It is also associated with depression and organic brain syndromes. Gold and Pearsall (1983b) demonstrated that there is a subtle form of hypothyroidism, "subclinical hypothyroidism," in which all the thyroid function tests, including T3, T4, and T3 uptake, and TSH are normal in the presence of exaggerated TSH response to the administration of intravenous TRH. Patients with an augmented TSH and titers of thyroid autoantibodies have successfully been treated with thyroid hormone alone. Furthermore, symptomless autoimmune thyroiditis (SAT), a discrete syndrome, exists in 7%-15% of inpatients and outpatients who meet DSM-IV criteria for major depression (Gold, 1995). Thyroid abnormalities and subclinical hypothyroidism have been identified as a cause of rapid cycling in bipolar disease (Extein & Gold, 1988; Goodnick, Estein, & Gold, 1988; Gross, Extein, & Gold, 1986; Gold, 1994; Miller & Gold, 1994).

Metal Poisonings:

Heavy metal poisoning can occur with environmental exposure to or ingestion of a wide variety of metals, including magnesium, copper, zinc, manganese, lead, mercury, thallium, bismuth, aluminum, arsenic, and bromides. Most consistently, these metals produce an organic brain syndrome but can also mimic major depression.

Unless they are actively looked for with heavy metal screens by atomic absorption or plasma emission spectroscopy of urine and blood, these metals will not be found and properly treated. If such conditions are detected and treated early enough, the mental and emotional symptoms are, for the most part, reversible.

Huntington's Disease:

A high incidence of symptoms resembling both mania and depression is common in patients with Huntington's disease. This was noted even in Huntington's original article of 1872: "The tendency to insanity and sometimes that form of insanity which leads to suicide is marked." Like other diseases from hypothyroidism to folate or B12 deficiency, psychiatric manifestations of this disease can occur well before any of the choreiform movements or any of the signs of dementia.

Infectious Mononucleosis:

Infectious mononucleosis may be followed by a syndrome that is identical to a major depressive episode. The diagnosis of infectious mononucleosis is made by a positive heterophile or mono spot test. A single negative test never excludes the diagnosis.

Infectious Hepatitis:

Mental and emotional symptoms before, during, or after infectious hepatitis of any type, A, B, or non-A non-B, can range from mild lethargy to major depression. There are even some reports of suicide and acute delusional mania following hepatitis.

Multiple Sclerosis:

Multiple sclerosis (MS) is a demyelinating neurologic disease characterized by lesions that are separated in space and time within the central nervous system. MS has been associated with a wide variety of psychopathological symptomatology, including mania and depression.

Panhypopituitarism:

Psychiatric presentations are common in pituitary failure and usually present with depression and/or lack of libido.

Postconcussion Syndrome:

The postconcussion syndrome occurs as the aftereffects of brain damage from severe head injury. It may present as anxiety, depression, excess anger, loss of emotional control, mood swings from euphoria to depression, and social disinhibition. Lesions of the left hemisphere, especially the left temporal lobe, tend to produce more intellectual deficits, whereas affective and behavioral symptoms are more frequently observed in right-hemisphere damage.

Syphilis (General Paresis):

At one time, syphilis accounted for 10%ñ20% of all admissions to state hospitals for the insane. This makes penicillin one of the most important psychiatric treatments of all time (Estroff & Gold, 1986a; Extein & Gold, 1987). "At one time, syphilis accounted for 10%ñ20% of all admissions to state hospitals for the insane. This makes penicillin one of the most important psychiatric treatments of all time (Estroff & Gold, 1986a; Extein & Gold, 1987)."

Systemic Lupus Erythematosus:

Systemic lupus erythematosus is a relatively uncommon disease that occurs in 2ñ3 per 100,000 population, with a 9:1 ratio favoring females (Gross, Extein, & Gold, 1986). It can present any time between ages 10 and 70 and may be accompanied by a wide variety of psychiatric symptoms, including mania, depression, schizophreniform or schizophrenic psychosis, and organic brain syndrome; it may even be labelled as a conversion disorder (Gross, Extein, & Gold, 1986). Systemic lupus erythematosus is too often overlooked in young women presenting with emotional symptoms and complaining of arthralgias, despite the fact that arthralgias are the most common first presentation of this disorder. "Systemic lupus erythematosus is a relatively uncommon disease that occurs in 2ñ3 per 100,000 population, with a 9\:1 ratio favoring females (Gross, Extein, & Gold, 1986). It can present any time between ages 10 and 70 and may be accompanied by a wide variety of psychiatric symptoms, including mania, depression, schizophreniform or schizophrenic psychosis, and organic brain syndrome; it may even be labelled as a conversion disorder (Gross, Extein, & Gold, 1986). Systemic lupus erythematosus is too often overlooked in young women presenting with emotional symptoms and complaining of arthralgias, despite the fact that arthralgias are the most common first presentation of this disorder."

Vitamin Deficiencies:

Among the better known vitamin deficiencies associated with mental and emotional symptoms are folate (Hall et al., 1981; Jefferson & Marshall, 1981), vitamin B_{12} deficiency (Jefferson & Marshall, 1981), and niacin (nicotine acid). Folic-acid deficiency presents with depression, fatigue, and lassitude. Marked deficiency can present with burning feet, restless leg syndrome, and/or a depression that is unresponsive to antidepressant therapy. Coppen and Abou-Saleh (1982) found a higher rate of affective morbidity in patients with low folate levels than patients with normal folate levels in patients treated in a lithium clinic. Hall and colleagues (1981), in a prospective study of hospitalized state psychiatric patients, found three cases of folate deficiency, two of which presented as RDC schizophrenia and one as RDC schizoaffective disorder. Normal CBC (complete blood cell count) folate deficiency occurs frequently and is often misdiagnosed and mistreated.

A deficiency of vitamin B12 may also present psychopathologically in the absence of any signs of anemia or bone marrow changes. It may present neurologically as a peripheral neuropathy or myelopathy (subacute combined degeneration). It has been known to present with a wide spectrum of mental and emotional disorders, including apathy, irritability, depression, dementia, confusional states, paranoid states, and schizophreniform psychosis (Jefferson & Marshall, 1981).

Patients who develop a zinc deficiency may become depressed, complain of lost interest in food, and show weight loss.

The Relative Frequency of Occurrence of NonPsychiatric Illness Presenting as Psychopathological Symptoms

Symptoms of depression caused by the use of drugs, alcohol, and other substances appear to be the most common cause of psychiatric misdiagnosis and mistreatment. As a general category, endocrine disorders present most frequently in association with depressive symptoms. Provocative testing will make that point even more evident in the future. The second most commonly involved organ system is the central nervous system. Toxic and withdrawal disorders were found third most commonly. Nutritional disorders and infectious diseases are the fourth most common. Cancer and metabolic disorders, such as Wilson's disease, acute intermittent porphyria, G6 PDase deficiency, and polycystic ovaries, exist but are rare unless the client has an unusual presentation, recent treatment failure, atypical features, or 20 pounds or more weight loss.

Summary

To reduce misdiagnosis and mistreatment of depression and other mental disorders, a complete physical, neurological, and endocrinological examination should be performed by a physician who is fluent in both psychiatry and internal medicine. This examination should be directed toward finding possible addictive, physical, or other illnesses that might cause or exacerbate mental and emotional symptoms (Gold, 1992a, 1994; Gold & Gleaton, 1994; Gold & Miller, 1994; Miller & Gold, 1992).

The laboratory is becoming an important component of any evaluation (Gold, 1995), but it does not replace the physician. Lab tests are ordered to correspond to and confirm the major issues in the differential diagnosis, and they may reveal unsuspected diagnostic clues.

A common model of care is to establish a clinical diagnosis and then treat the patient. For example, patients who meet DSM-IV criteria for major depressive episode may be treated with the selective serotonin reuptake inhibitors (SSRIs) by primary care and other physicians. Failure to respond to the appropriate psychopharmacological treatment of the diagnosis, therefore, is a very important indicator; it suggests that the diagnosis is incorrect and that the patient is in a high-risk group for underlying and undiagnosed exacerbating or precipitated illness.

The mental health practice is likely to change radically in the future. We hope that the information contained in this chapter and reported elsewhere in greater detail (Gold, Lydiard, & Carman, 1984) will help present and future mental health professionals make this change to more easily.

References

1. American Psychiatric Association. (1994). Diagnostic and statistical manual of mental disorders (4th ed.). Washington, DC: Author. "American Psychiatric Association. (1994). Diagnostic and statistical manual of mental disorders (4th ed.). Washington, DC: Author."

2. Coppen, A., & Abou-Saleh, M. T. (1982). Plasma folate and affective morbidity during long-term lithium therapy. British Journal of Psychiatry, 141, 87–89.

3. Dackis, C. A., & Gold, M. S. (1984). Depression in opiate addicts. In S. M. Mirin (Ed.), Substance abuse and psychopathology (pp. 20–39). Washington: American Psychiatric Press, Inc.

4. Dackis, C. A., & Gold, M. S. (1986a). The self-medication hypothesis of addictive disorders: Focus on heroin and cocaine dependence. [Letters to the editor.] American Journal of Psychiatry, 143(10), 1309.

5. Dackis, C. A., & Gold, M. S. (1986b). Evaluating depression in alcoholics. Psychiatry Research, 17, 105–109.

6. Estroff, T. W., & Gold, M. S. (1986a). Medication-induced and toxin-induced psychiatric disorder. In I. Extein & M. S. Gold (Eds.), Medical mimics of psychiatric disorders (chap. 7, pp. 163–198). Washington, DC: American Psychiatric Press.

7. Estroff, T. W., & Gold, M. S. (1986b). Psychiatric presentations of marijuana abuse. Psychiatric Annals, 16(4), 221–224.

8. Extein, I., & Gold. M. S. (Eds.) (1986). Medical mimics of psychiatric disorders. Washington, DC: APA Press.

9. Extein, I., & Gold. M. S. (1987, April). Endocrinological diseases mimicking affective disorders. Paper presented at the International Conference on New Directions in Affective Disorders, Jerusalem, Israel.

10. Extein, I., & Gold. M. S. (1988). Thyroid hormone potentiation of tricyclics. Psychosomatics, 29(2), 167–174.

11. Giannini, A. J., Black H. R., & Goettsche, R. L. (1978). Psychiatric, psychogenic, and somatopsychic disorders handbook. New York: Medical Examination Publishing Co.

12. Gold, M. S. (1989a). Drugs of abuse: A comprehensive series for clinicians. Vol. I. Marijuana. New York & London: Plenum.

13. Gold, M. S. (1989b). The good news about panic, anxiety, and phobias. New York: Villard & Bantam Books.

14. Gold, M. S. (1992a). Seeking drugs/alcohol and avoiding withdrawal: The neuroanatomy of drive states and withdrawal. Psychiatric Annals, 22, 430–435.

15. Gold, M. S. (1992b). Cocaine (and crack). In J. Lowinson, P. Ruiz, & R. Millman (Eds.), Clinical aspects in substance abuse: A comprehensive textbook. (2nd ed., pp. 205–221). Baltimore: Williams & Wilkins.

16. Gold, M. S. (1993). Distinguishing psychiatric syndromes in alcoholism. In M. Aronson, Alcoholism: Recognition of the disease and considerations for patient care (pp. 24–27). Rancho Mirage, CA: Betty Ford Center.

17. Gold, M. S. (1994). The epidemiology, attitudes, and pharmacology of LSD use in the 1990s. Psyciatric Annals, 24(3), 124–126.

18.. Gold, M. S. (1995). The good news about depression. New York: Bantam Books.

19. Gold, M. S. (in press). Trends in hallucinogenic drug use: LSD, Ecstasy, and the rave phenomenon. In The Hatherleigh Guide to Substance Abuse I. New York: Hatherleigh Press.

20. Gold, M. S., & Gleaton, T. J. (1994). Marked increases in USA marijuana and LSD: Results of an annual junior and senior high school survey. Biological Psychiatry, 35(9), 694.

21. Gold, M. S., & Herridge, P. (1988). The risk of misdiagnosing physical illness as depression. In F. Flach (Ed.), Affective disorders (chap. 7, pp. 64–76). New York: W. W. Norton & Co.

22. Gold, M. S., Lydiard, R. B., & Carman, J. S. (Eds.). (1984). Advances in psychopharmacology: Predicting and improving treatment response. Boca Raton, FL: CRC Press.

23. Gold, M. S., & Miller, N. S. (1994). The biology of addictive and psychiatric disorders. In N. S. Miller (Ed.), Treating coexisting psychiatric and addictive disorders (pp. 35–52). Center City, MN: Hazelden.

24. Gold, M. S. & Pearsall, H. R. (1983a). Depression and hypothyroidism. JAMA, 250(18), 2470–2471.

25. Gold, M. S., & Pearsall, H. R. (1983b). HypothyroidismóOr is it depression? Psychosomatics, 24, 646–654.

26. Gold, M. S., Pottash, A. C., & Extein, I. (1982). The psychiatric laboratory. In J. G. Bernstein (Ed.), Clinical psychopharmacology (pp. 29-58). Boston: John Wright PSG.

27. Goodnick, P. J., Extein, I., & Gold, M. S. (1988, March). Subclinical moods in substance abuse. American Psychopathological Association poster session. New York: American Psychopathological Association.

28. Gross, D. A., Extein, I., & Gold, M. S. (1986). The psychiatrist as physician. In I. Extein & M. S. Gold (Eds.), Medical mimics of psychiatric disorders (pp. 1–12). Washington, DC: American Psychiatric Association.

29. Hall, R. C. W., et al. (1978). Physical illness presenting as psychiatric disease. Archives of General Psychiatry, 35, 1315–1320.

30. Hall, R. C. W. (1980). Psychiatric presentations of medical illness. New York: Spectrum.

31. Hall, R. C. W., et al. (1981). Unrecognized physical illness prompting psychiatric admission: A prospective study. American Journal of Psychiatry, 138, 629–635.

32. Hamilton, M. (1982). The effect of treatment on the melancholias (depressions). British Journal of Psychiatry, 140, 223–230.

33. Herridge, C. F. (1960). Physical disorders in psychiatric illness: A study of 209 consecutive admissions. Lancet, 2, 949–951.

34. Hoffman, R. S. (1982). Diagnostic errors in the evaluation of behavioral disorders. Journal of the American Medical Association, 248, 964–967.

35. Jefferson, J. W., & Marshall, J. R. (1981). Neuropsychiatric features of medical disorders. New York: Plenum.

36. Koranyi, E. K. (1979). Morbidity and rate of undiagnosed physical illness in a psychiatric clinic population. Archives of General Psychiatry, 36, 414–449.

37. Klein, D. F., Gittelman, R., Quitkin, F., & Rifkin, A. (1980). Diagnosis and drug treatment of psychiatric disorders: Adults and children. Baltimore: Williams & Wilkins.

38. McIntyre, J. W., & Romano, J. (1977). Is there a stethoscope in the house (and is it used)? Archives of General Psychiatry, 34, 1147–1151.

39. Miller, N. S., & Gold, M. S. (1991). Drugs of abuse: A comprehensive series for clinicians. Vol. II. Alcohol. New York & London: Plenum.

40. Miller, N. S., & Gold, M. S. (1992). The psychiatrist's role in integrating pharmacological and nonpharmacological treatments for addictive disorders. Psychiatric Annals, 22(8), 436–440.

41. Miller, N. S., & Gold, M. S. (1994). LSD and ecstacy: Pharmacology, phenomenology, and treatment. Psychiatric Annals, 24(3), 131–133.

42. Miller, N. S., Hoffmann, N. G., & Gold, M. S. (1994). Comorbid depression, drug dependence, and alcoholism. Society for Neuroscience Abstract, 20, 1609.

43. Miller, N. S., Mahler, J. C., & Gold, M. S. (1991). Suicide risk associated with drug and alcohol dependence. Journal of Addictive Diseases, 10(3), 49–61.

44. Shapiro, R. W., & Keller, M. B. (1981). Initial 6-month follow-up of patients with major depressive disorder. Journal of Affective Disorders, 3, 205–220.

45. Verebey, K., Gold, M. S., & Mule, S. J. (1986). Laboratory testing in the diagnosis of marijuana intoxication and withdrawal. Psychiatric Annals, 16(4), 235–241.

46. Verebey, K., Martin, D., & Gold, M. S. (1987). Interpretation of drug abuse testing: Strengths and limitations of current methodology. Psychiatric Medicine, 3(3), 287–297.

11

The Suicidal Patient

MICHAEL L. PERLIN, ESQ.

Editor's Note

Suicide is a major source of all tort litigation against mental health professionals. The standard against which the courts will assess culpability is whether a psychiatrist who exercised reasonable care would have predicted the risk of suicide and taken steps to prevent it. Legitimate concern over whether a patient represents a risk is compounded by the fear of liability, giving rise to situations in which the treating psychiatrist may be torn between playing it safe and taking intelligent chances to facilitate a patient's recovery.

Certainly it is clear that patients who present any degree of suicide risk should be as carefully monitored as possible. Periodic assessments and assessments at times when undue stress arises should be carried out and carefully documented. One should also note what measures one has taken to reduce the risk and protect the patient, including, in severe instances, involuntary hospitalization.

Still, every clinician is only too familiar with the dilemma presented by the suicidal patient who will not comply with treatment recommendations. Even as patients have a right to treatment, so, too, do they enjoy the right to refuse treatment. Thus, more than ever, we must know what we can and cannot do under such trying conditions.

Suicide: A Major Source of Tort Litigation

Suicide, a major cause of death,[1] is also a major source of all tort litigation against mental health professionals.[2] Given the fact that suicide

CME questions for this chapter begin on page 357.

predictions are particularly "fraught with uncertainty,"[3] that the treatment of suicidal patients involves the balancing of "several indeterminate variables,"[4] and that, especially in the setting of a large, public institution, the "logistics of preventing [a] suicide may be formidable,"[5] courts have traditionally been reluctant to impose civil liability for such an act.[6] However, more recently liability has been found in a variety of fact situations.[7] In this type of case, perhaps even more than in other psychiatric tort areas, courts will scrutinize carefully and rigorously "the facts and circumstances of the particular case" to determine whether there has been a breach of duty toward a plaintiff.[8]

Hospitalized Suicidal Patients[9]

In cases where hospital doctors have failed to foresee that an institutionalized patient was likely to harm himself, courts will ask whether a psychiatrist who exercised reasonable care would have predicted the risk of harm.[10] Since this is an extremely difficult prediction to make accurately,[11] courts will generally find liability only where the doctor's treatment decision was not a reasonable one (as opposed to where it is an *inaccurate* one).[12] According to Klein and Glover, "Psychiatrists are not insurers of their patients' well-being, and should not be held liable for a mere error in judgment."[13]

Another paradox makes decision-making in this area even more difficult. While such prophylactic measures as increasing frequency of observation, use of seclusion, and use of restraints might appear to reduce the risk of suicide, such measures "may also disturb the patient, cause anxiety, and aggravate feelings of worthlessness."[14] Again, as Klein and Glover have noted:

> Indeed, although such precautions may reduce the short-term risk of suicide, they may prolong the patient's illness, delay his release from the hospital, and increase the likelihood that he will harm himself at some point in the future.[15]

Thus, in *Topel v. Long Island Medical Center,*[16] the New York Court of Appeals rejected the argument made on behalf of the deceased patient that it was negligent for defendants not to have placed the patient under continuous observation in light of his previous suicide attempts, explaining:

[The patient's] reaction to constant surveillance, the possibility that his heart condition would be aggravated by continuing such surveillance, the gesture-like nature of his prior suicidal indications, the rehabilitative aspects of open ward treatment and the enhanced probability of obtaining [the patient's] consent to electroshock therapy in the more relaxed open ward atmosphere were all factors which defendant doctor could properly consider in reaching the judgment whether, on balance, the prescribed program was worth the risk involved.[17]

In short, "there is a limit to the degree of care required of a hospital in protecting a patient against him or herself."[18]

In other representative cases, no liability was found (1) (in an "open door" case involving a "walk away" patient who committed suicide by throwing himself in front of a passing truck) where there was evidence that the patient would not have been found even if "[appropriate] search procedures" had been followed by the hospital,[19] (2) where the hospital staff *had* provided protective measures in an attempt to thwart suicide,[20] (3) where the patient had not previously exhibited such "unusual behavior" as to give reason to the hospital staff to depart from the orders given by the treating psychiatrist as to degree of supervision required,[21] and (4) where the psychiatrist had never been told about a specific delusion of the patient's (that he could breathe under water) which caused his death.[22]

On the other hand, a number of courts have either reversed dismissals or grants of summary judgment or have found liability in similar cases where the defendant either underestimated the seriousness of the suicide risk,[23] failed to take appropriate precautions,[24] failed to obtain the patient's relevant prior records,[25] or was unable to satisfactorily explain why he deviated from his normal practice in an individual case.[26]

Formerly-Hospitalized Suicidal Patients

Although the questions faced here are conceptually similar to those regarding institutionalized individuals, resolution is even more difficult. This is especially true in cases where the defendant has agreed to release the patient following a determination that prolonged hospitalization—and the iatrogenic illness that sometimes accompanies it—may reduce the likelihood that the patient will be able to resume a normal life outside of the institution.[27] The therapist's decision in such a case will thus depend on the assessment of several factors, including "the individual patient's dangerousness, the patient's ability to care for himself or receive assistance from others, the extent to which his illness is in remission, and the extent to which it can be controlled by medication and/or outpatient treatment."[28]

Generally, in such cases, courts are relatively deferent to the psychiatrist's judgment, noting the difficulties in predicting dangerous behavior,[29] the lapse in time between treatment and suicide,[30] the implicit possibility of some added peril as an outcome of the adoption of an "open door" policy,[31] and the potentially negative social results of the imposition of liability in such situations (e.g., long-term institutionalization of a greater number of patients, and fewer rehabilitation opportunities for patients in the community).[32] On the other hand, at least one reported case has affirmed a trial court verdict finding negligence where a patient was prematurely released because the examining physician failed to conduct a proper medical examination in failing to investigate the nature of the patient's delusions.[33] The court noted pointedly:

> A decision that is without proper medical foundation, that is, one which is not the product of a careful examination, is not to be legally insulated as a professional medical judgment . . . Stated otherwise, "[p]hysicians are not liable for mistakes in professional judgment, provided that they do what they think best *after careful examination*. . . . However, liability can ensue if their judgment *is not based on intelligence* and thus there is a failure to exercise any professional judgment."[34]

Conclusion

Psychiatrists and their lawyers have expressed considerable concern over the imputation of liability in suicide cases. Thus, Rachlin has suggested that strict standards can "thwart treatment and lower the quality of care by forcing the adoption of antitherapeutic restrictions" and lead to "obsessive overconcern [by therapists and administrators] about legal minutiae to the detriment of the clinical perspective."[35]

Klein and Glover add that a liability rule "may well affect psychiatric behavior in perverse ways":

> To avoid liability, psychiatrists are likely to become extremely cautious. They will increase their supervision of inpatients, and rely more extensively on chemical and physical restraints. They may also seek to delay the release of inpatients and hospitalize outpatients. Yet, for many of these patients, the risk of suicide may actually be quite low, and the therapeutic benefits of increased freedom substantial. These individuals, and society as a whole, will suffer as a result of the increased caution. Indeed, the liability rule could conceivably encourage psychiatric conduct that leads to more suicide. Cautious psychiatrists may decide not to provide any treatment at all to potentially suicidal patients.[36]

Although this concern is understandable, it appears to paint too pessimistic a picture, given the reality of cases already litigated and decided on appeal. Almost all of those few cases in which liability was found and upheld reveal scenarios of obvious negligence and clear errors in treatment and supervision.

While Klein and Glover express fear that juries will not be able to distinguish between suicides in cases of high-risk and low-risk patients,[37] it would seem that some of the combinations of social and clinical factors militating against the finding of psychiatric malpractice—e.g., difficulties of proof as to causation and standard of care, stigma[38]—generally are exacerbated in suicide cases where predictivity is so much more difficult, and the standard of care thus an "easier" one to meet.

References

1. See Perr, "Liability of the Hospital and Psychiatrist for Suicide," 122 *Am. J. Psych.* 631 (1965). Subsequently, "the suicide rate has not declined and suicide remains a leading health problem." Drukteinis, "Psychiatric Perspectives on Civil Liability for Suicide," 13 *Bull. Am. Acad. Psych. & L.* 71, 80 (1985).
2. As of 1977, cases involving patients who committed suicide or attempted to do so accounted for 15% of all reported psychiatric malpractice decisions. See 3 Hogan, *The Regulation of Psychotherapists* 406 (1979).
3. Dr. Karl Menninger, *e.g.,* has concluded that assigning a cause or multiple causes to the ultimate act of suicide is "grossly misleading." Menninger, "Fore-

ward," in Schneidman & Faberow, eds., *Clues to Suicide* vii (1957); see also, *e.g.*, Capstick, "The Methods of Suicide," 29 *Medico-Legal J.* 33, 35 (1961). But see, Lesse, "Editorial Comment," 19 *Am. J. Psychother.* 105 (1965) (therapist is "inescapably responsible for all his severely ill patients").

4. Klein & Glover, "Psychiatric Malpractice," 6 *Int'l J. L. & Psych,* 131, 141 (1983).

5. Beresford. "Professional Liability of Psychiatrists," 21 *Defense L.J. 157* (1972).

6. See Note. "The Liability of Psychiatrists for Malpractice," 36 *U. Pitt. L. Rev.* 108, 110 (1974); Schwartz, "Civil Liability for Causing Suicide: A Synthesis of Law and Psychiatry," 24 *Vand. L. Rev.* 217 (1971). Professor Schwartz distinguishes carefully between the historical development of cases involving conduct designed to cause severe emotional distress, *id.* at 222–226, and negligently-inflicted harm, *id.* at 226–232.

7. See, *e.g., Cohen v. New York,* 51 App. Div. 2d 494, 382 N.Y.S. 2d 128 (App. Div. 1976).

8. *Ray v. Ameri-Care Hospital,* 400 So. 2d 1127, 1138 (La. Ct. App. 1981).

9. While this article will focus solely on the legal issues which apply to the suicides of *hospitalized* and *formerly hospitalized* patients, it should be emphasized that there may be differing duties on therapists in cases involving outpatients. Such issues are beyond the scope of this article. See generally, Chapter 12 of Perlin, *Mental Disability Law: Civil and Criminal* (©Kluwer Law Books 1988).

10. Klein & Glover, *supra* note 4, at 141.

11. See *id.* n.36 (citing sources).

12. See *Katz v. New York,* 46 Misc. 2d 61, 258 N.Y.S. 2d 912, 914 (Ct. Cl. 1965) (failure to predict an "honest error of professional judgment").

13. Klein & Glover. *supra* note 4, at 142.

14. *Id.* at 143.

15. *Id.* See also. Slawson, Flinn & Schwartz, "Legal Responsibility for Suicide," 48 *Psych. Q.* 63 (1974) ("in the matter of suicide, stricter liability for clinical management may thwart treatment by compelling a conservative posture which subordinates innovative treatment to safe custody").

16. 55 N.Y. 2d 682. 446 N.Y.S. 2d 932, 431 N.E. 2d 293 (Ct. App. 1981) .

17. *Id.,* 446 N.Y.S. 2d at 934.

18. McCafferty & Meyer, *Medical Malpractice: Bases of Liability* (1981), §10.20, at 263. See, *e.g., Hirsh v. State,* 8 N.Y. 2d 125, 202 N.Y.S. 2d 296, 298, 168 N.E. 2d 372 (Ct. App. 1960): "An ingenious patient harboring a steady purpose to take his own life cannot always be thwarted."

19. *Saporta v. State,* 220 Neb. 142, 368 N.W. 2d 783, 787 (Sup. Ct. 1985).

20. *Johnson v. Grant Hospital,* 32 Ohio St. 2d 169, 291 N.E. 2d 440, 446 (Sup. Ct. 1972).

21. *Payne v. Milwaukee Sanitarium Foundation,* 81 Wis. 2d 264, 260 N.W. 2d 386, 391 (Sup. Ct. 1977).

22. *Ray v. Ameri-Care Hosp.,* 400 So. 2d 1127, 1132 (La. Ct. App. 1981).

23. See, *e.g., Breese v. Indiana,* 449 N.E. 2d 1098 (Ind. Ct. App. 1983); *Stallman v. Robinson,* 364 Mo. 275, 260 S.W. 2d 743 (Sup. Ct. 1953).

24. *Meier v. Ross General Hospital,* 69 Cal. 2d 420, 71 Cal. Rptr. 903. 445 P. 2d 519 (Sup. Ct. 1968); *Brown v. State,* 84 App. Div. 2d 644 444 N.Y.S. 2d 304 (App. Div. 1981) (placing patient in room with openable window despite former suicide attempts); *DeMontiney v. Desert Manor Convalescent Ctr.,* 144 Ariz. 6, 695 P. 2d 255, 259 (Sup. Ct. 1985) (placing patient in room with bed linens and exposed pipe); *Dow v. State,* 183 Misc. 674, 50 N.Y.S. 2d 342 343 (Ct. C 1. 1944) (failure to visit restrained patient for 3 hours where hospital had "ample warning" of patient's suicidal tendencies and where its policies mandated a two-hour limit on unattended use of restraints).

25. *Psychiatric Institute of Washington v. Allen,* 509 A. 2d 619, 623 (D.C. Ct. App. 1986) (records would have revealed that teenage patient had been previously hospitalized for "escalating firesetting [which was] potentially life-threatening").

26. *Weatherly v. United States,* 109 Misc. 2d 1024, 441 N.Y.S. 2d 319 (Ct. Cl. 1981) (psychiatrist could not explain why she failed to return patient to "suicide precaution status"). See also, *Abille v. United States,* 482 F. Supp. 703 (N.D. Cal. 1980) (stressing doctor's failure to make notes so as to justify transferring patient from suicide-precaution ward to one appropriate for less dangerous purposes). Dr. Rachlin points out that the importance of written documentation supporting the decision to grant a potentially-suicidal patient less restrictive conditions of hospitalization "cannot be overemphasized." Rachlin, "Double Jeopardy: Suicide and Malpractice," 6 *Gen'l Hosp. Psych.* 302, 306 (1984), citing Halleck, "Malpractice in Psychiatry," in Halleck, ed., *New Directions for Mental Health Services: Coping with the Legal Onslaught* (1979); Waltzer, "'Malpractice Liability in a Patient's Suicide," 34 *Am. J. Psychother.* 89 (1980).

27. See Klein & Glover, *supra* note 4, at 145.

28. *Id.* On the other hand, some patients become *more* violent (either to themselves or others) after receiving psychotropic medication. See, *e.g.,* Perlin, *supra* note 9, at §5.11, note 199.

29. See, *e.g., Johnson v. United States,* 409 F. Supp. 1283, 1293 (M.D. Fla. 1981).

30. *Maier v. Roosevelt Hospital,*—Misc. 2d—,—N.Y.S. 2d—(Sup. Ct. 1986), reported in *N.Y.L.J.* (July 8, 1986).

31. *Johnson,* 409 F. Supp. at 1293.

32. *Fiederlein v. City of New York Health & Hospitals Corp.,* 80 App. Div. 2d 821, 437 N.Y.S. 2d 321 (App. Div. 1981); see also, *Centeno v. City of New York,* 48 App. Div. 2d 812, 369 N.Y.S. 2d 710 (App. Div. 1976), aff'd 40 N.Y. 2d 932, 389 N.Y.S. 2d 837, 358 N.E. 2d 527 (Ct. App. 1976).

33. *Bell v. New York City Health & Hosp. Corp.,* 90 App. Div. 2d 270, 456 N.Y.S. 2d 787, 795 (App. Div. 1982).

34. *Id.* at 794 (citations omitted; emphasis supplied in cited case).

35. Rachlin, *supra* note 26, at 305.

36. Klein & Glover, *supra* note 4, at 149 (emphasis in original).

37. *Id.*

38. See generally, Chapter 1, *supra* (this volume).

COMMENTARY

The Suicidal Patient

ROBERT L. SADOFF, M.D.

Editor's Note

As Dr. Sadoff points out, clinicians are obliged to carefully and systematically assess the level of suicidal risk in all patients, although primarily among those such as depressed patients where such a risk is common. The risk can mount from (1) simple ideas of killing oneself to (2) consideration of a particular way to do so to (3) possession of the means to do so to (4) practicing the method to commit suicide.

Other information is also pertinent. Has the patient made prior attempts? Demographics enter the picture: Is the patient in a particularly vulnerable age or population group? For example, men experiencing divorce seem especially suicide-prone.

Then, too, what acceptable measures can be taken to prevent suicide? The fact that a patient may wish for and even has a right to the least restrictive environment for treatment should not stand in the way of the treating physician insisting as strongly as he can for a protective environment when he believes such is indicated. He should not hesitate to involve family members if the seriousness of the risk warrants.

Historically, the psychiatrist has been charged with the responsibility of caring for severely depressed patients who are prone to suicide. Psychiatrists have the responsibility, when alerted to the potential for suicide, to protect the patient from self-destructive behavior. A patient may have little or no control over his behavior and require assistance from the professional to keep from acting on urges related to his illness that can be reversed with time and treatment. The psychiatrist is not always able to keep the patient from committing suicide, but the law requires that he act in a reasonable manner to prevent suicide whenever possible. That is what is meant by the standard of care practiced by the average psychiatrist in that community. One cannot guarantee a person will not kill himself, even under reasonable medical treatment conditions, but every effort must be made to protect the patient, whenever possible, from his own self-destructive behavior.

Translating those concepts into specifics, the psychiatrist must question the patient about suicidal ideation, previous suicide attempts, specific means by which the patient proposes to kill himself, and whether the patient has the means by which to destroy himself. The psychiatrist must also ask the patient if he has practiced the method he has chosen to kill himself. Those questions may reflect the various levels of suicidal potential for the patient.

Level One is the thought of suicide by the patient. Many people think about killing themselves or feel they and others would be better off if they were dead. An individual with a Level One potential is at low risk for committing suicide.

Level Two adds the dimension of focus. The patient has thought of a particular method of killing himself. For example, the patient may have said he is going to shoot himself. At this level, the risk of suicide is greater than at Level One.

Level Three involves a still higher risk of suicide. The patient states that he has the means by which to carry out the specific method in which he intends to kill himself. For example, he states he has a gun at home, with bullets, and intends to use it to kill himself. Guns are very common instruments of suicide. Psychiatrists should make every effort to inquire about the accessibility of guns to depressed and/or suicidal patients. Once they have ascertained that guns are available, they should make every effort to have the guns removed from the reach or availability of the suicidal patient.

Finally, Level Four involves the attempt by the patient to "practice" what he intends to do. For example, a patient indicates that he has put the unloaded gun to his head and pulled the trigger, or a patient who intends to cut his throat practices by cutting his wrist to see how it feels. That patient is at a very high-risk level for suicide and should be hospitalized.

Those levels are not intended to suggest that all patients go from Level One to Level Four until they kill themselves—many do not. Some begin at Level Three.

The other major criterion for determining suicidal potential is a history of one or more suicide attempts. Lawyers tend to use previous suicide attempts, no matter how far back in history, to indicate that the patient is suicidal because he or she has tried to kill himself before. Lawyers are not clinicians. They are advocates for their position. Therefore, if a patient has a history of prior suicide attempts but is not currently actively suicidal, that patient must be regarded as a higher risk than a patient who has not attempted suicide before.

Demographic data are also important in assessing risk of suicide. Statistics have shown that various age groups of men or women, at various stages of their lives, involved in particular occupations, and experiencing specific life situations or crises may be more prone to suicide. All those factors must be taken into consideration by the practicing psychiatrist in assessing suicidal potential or risk.

Even though the patient has a right to the least restrictive environment for treatment, the added clause, which is often omitted, states that the least restrictive environment for treatment be "consistent with the needs of the patient at that time." Therefore, the means by which treatment is afforded and the place in which it is given is a medical or psychiatric decision, not the patient's decision. Potentially suicidal patients should not be treated as outpatients if the psychiatrist feels that hospitalization is required. Patients and their lawyers may argue against hospitalization, but neither will be present to support the psychiatrist in the event the patient kills himself and has to justify the less-restrictive alternative of treatment at the time of death. The psychiatrist then stands alone to defend his decision to treat that person as an outpatient when more restriction was obviously required. Thus, the psychiatrist is in a position to make a medical decision about the place of treatment for the patient. With that decision, the psychiatrist must weigh the risks of suicide or violence against the potential gain for the patient by reducing the restrictions placed on him.

Sometimes one cannot tell prospectively that a patient is going to commit suicide because he has none of the criteria generally used to denote suicidal risk. His suicide may be a complete surprise to everyone, with no signals before his death. If the psychiatrist used clinical judgment in assessing the suicidal risk of his patient and made medical decisions consistent with that assessment, no malpractice case would be successful because no negligence or deviation from the standard of care could be proved. An error in clinical judgment without negligence does not lead to successful malpractice suits. Only retrospectively do we find that something went wrong. A death or suicide does not always indicate negligence or malpractice. Sometimes there is a bad result to good clinical practice.

12

Management of Suicidal Patients

JEROME A. MOTTO, M.D.

Editor's Note

The practicing psychiatrist is repeatedly confronted with patients representing various degrees of suicide risk. A review of the principles involved in determining the nature and degree of such risk is valuable. The physician's own intuitive judgment is commonly an important element in this evaluation. The steps that he can take in the management of suicidal patients, whether as inpatients or outpatients, can be identified, as well as the special problems he or she faces in dealing with families of potentially suicidal patients and patients who are not cooperative with the physician's recommendations.

Introduction

Social and legal as well as therapeutic implications of self-destructive behavior imbue the suicidal patient with a special position in clinical practice. As the most visible source of mortality from psychiatric disorders, and frequently a matter of intense concern to family members, the high-risk suicidal patient often brings a sense of increased urgency to many questions involved in clinical areas. Developing a sound approach to these questions will not always preclude a suicidal death, but

CME questions for this chapter begin on page 358.

it will help to minimize those unnecessary and preventable suicides that constitute a tragic human loss and can be so traumatic to vulnerable survivors, especially children.

Treatment plans are carried out within the context of management decisions. The importance of management, which should provide optimal conditions for effective treatment, is exaggerated in the case of a suicidal patient because all other efforts are contingent on the patient's survival. Thus, management decisions have a certain priority in the treatment plan because they are geared to assure survival, sometimes at the expense of optimal treatment. Though a sharp distinction is implied here between management and treatment, it should be understood that, in practice, all interactions with patients have treatment implications, and in some situations management decisions can have greater therapeutic impact than formal treatment measures. Some aspects of this matter have been discussed elsewhere.[1-5]

The present discussion focuses on how a therapist can best handle the problem of suicide. Many opportunities for intervention with patients in suicidal states occur in the clinical work of persons whose experience with this problem is relatively limited. This chapter is intended as a pragmatic answer to the question, What should I do when faced with the need to make critical decisions and why?

Recognition and Assessment of Suicidal States

The presence of high suicide risk often makes itself unmistakably known, but the exceptions are so numerous that there is no substitute for a direct, matter-of-fact inquiry in every patient. This applies to medical-surgical as well as to primarily psychiatric problems. When any degree of positive response is elicited, the presence and intensity of self-destructive ideas require careful assessment and subsequent reassessment as the clinical picture dictates.[4-8]

The tendency to identify depressive states with suicide has led to underemphasis of nondepressive conditions that are conducive to suicide. Personality disorders and schizophrenic, paranoid, manic, and organic states are most pertinent here, though no diagnostic category is free of risk. Observations of suicidal persons who have gone on to complete the act indicate that age (over 45), race (white), sex (male), a history of prior suicide attempt, chronicity of self-destructive behavior, progressively severe health problems, loss of previously stabilizing resources (e.g., spouse, job, home), presence of a detailed suicide plan, and termination behavior (making out a will, etc.) carry special weight.[4-7] In depressed patients there is evidence that the intensity of feelings of hopelessness is more closely related to suicidal intent than is the intensity of depression.[9]

In any given patient, however, the numerous predictive variables correlated with subsequent suicide give us only limited assistance. The common denominator of all the factors conducive to suicide is psychic pain, and since every person experiences a given situation in a unique way it is necessary first to determine the level of pain created by the patient's situation and second to ascertain how close that level is to the person's limit of tolerance. Those with a low threshold may thus be highly suicidal with only moderate stress, while others are not at high risk in spite of severe stress. This largely accounts for the absence of any generally accepted "predictive scale," psychological test, or other measuring device for the assessment of suicide risk.

Empathic and intuitive judgments, based on an understanding of the patient's unique pathology and strengths, provide the most dependable criteria of risk and deserve priority when traditional risk factors are inconsistent with those judgments.

Management Decisions

The first management decision concerns treatment setting. Characteristics of both the patient and therapist must be taken into account; a careful evaluation, including a clear definition of the risks and the rationale for the decision made, is essential.

The clearest indication for hospitalization is the judgment that the patient is not likely to survive as an outpatient. The option of a day-care hospital exists, although in the author's experience this setting has an unsatisfactory record with patients at high risk for suicide. The judgment regarding chances of survival is largely intuitive, even when aided by specific criteria.[1] Emotional pressures can be intensified in both the work and home settings, culminating in frantic efforts at relief. These efforts may be in the form of increasing alcohol intake during the day and taking large amounts of sleeping medication at night, accompanied by suicidal preoccupation. At times, high-risk persons with near-psychotic levels of disorganization have been treated as outpatients because in work situations they seemed able to use their defenses—especially obsessive patterns—effectively; suicidal impulses were diminished remarkably as long as they were at work. Others can manage at home when home is experienced as a protective environment. When no readily available setting affords relief, a hospital becomes the preferred setting.

A well-established relationship with the patient increases the treatment options. With such a relationship, additional data may be available to bolster the therapist's confidence in his intuition, and the quality of outside support (e.g., friends or family) is usually made clearer. Most importantly, a solid therapeutic relationship can provide the sustaining force that helps the patient get through a painful period when no other sources of emotional support are evident.

The use of contracts is pertinent to this issue. To the extent that a relationship of mutual trust and respect is formed, a patient's agreement to continue in treatment, arrive at appointments, or not kill himself or herself can be negotiated. Many therapists who do not identify their work with behavioral modification techniques often make an implicit contract with the patient through an inquiry such as, Can I count on seeing you next week? or, Can you make it until Thursday? Such agreements require an established relationship to warrant much reliance. It has been advised that with adolescents, it is not reasonable to depend on such implicit contracts even when a good relationship exists.[10] Other special considerations to take into account when dealing with adolescents and children are discussed elsewhere.[11-13]

A power struggle with suicidal patients must be avoided if at all possible. A nonpsychiatric inpatient setting can be a means of buying time to set up a stronger support system. If the patient refuses any form of inpatient care, the examiner must be prepared to accept the risk of outpatient treatment rather than force the issue by initiating a procedure the patient would not agree to.

A serious suicide attempt is generally a clear indication for inpatient care regardless of other factors in the situation. The support system must be solidified before resuming the higher risk of outpatient treatment. Sometimes, the examining psychiatrist, if he has established a good relationship with the patient, may insist on psychiatric hospitalization even if it means relinquishing his potential therapeutic role because of the patient's resentment. This is an example of management taking precedence over treatment—of a potentially antitherapeutic step being deliberately taken in order to ensure survival.

A special obstacle is introduced when the patient is a professional person. It is important to resist the impulse to rationalize higher risks away because of the patient's professional role or position in the community. If forced into compromising optimal management, the decision should be clearly documented; for example, it should be noted that hospitalization is indicated, recommended, and refused, and that the requirements for involuntary measures are not present.

Alternatives to hospitalization are clearly indicated when (1) both the patient and family are firmly opposed to hospital care; (2) the risk is not considered high, and responsible caring persons are available; (3) a firm relationship has been established with the patient, and assurances can be accepted on the basis of trust; (4) the patient is primarily seeking a place to be cared for, and the suicidal behavior is consciously or unconsciously serving to request such a place; or (5) use of a psychiatric hospital would impose an insurmountable psychological burden by virtue of the social-cultural setting in which the patient lives. At times the hospital must be used simply because no alternatives are available or the patient refuses to accept those that are. In such a case, it is essential that the therapist and hospital staff be free of handicapping defensiveness about "manipulative behavior" or "playing into the patient's dependency needs."

When the patient refuses indicated hospitalization and involuntary measures are not appropriate, it may be best for the therapist to settle for less than the ideal, inform the person of his serious concern, offer what help the person will accept, assure him of the therapist's availability and desire to be of continued assistance, and ask that if he changes his mind about hospitalization to let the therapist know.[4] Intensified, even daily, outpatient contact with the patient and family can be an effective alternative.

Finally, if nothing but unresolved doubts are generated by available information, the most conservative available alternative is indicated, along with as much equanimity as can be mustered. It is important to avoid a power struggle with the patient, since the patient ultimately has all the power. Whatever potential there is for therapeutic work can be sacrificed by such struggles. In rare instances one may be forced to take this course, nonetheless, and trust that the pieces can be put back together later.

Decisions Regarding Treatment

Decisions concerning treatment are largely determined by the philosophy and personality of the therapist. Attitudes about death, concerns about therapeutic competence, fear of vulnerability to legal action, and anxiety about criticism by family members, colleagues, or community may determine treatment planning even more than strictly clinical matters.

A realistic approach to treating high-risk patients requires that the therapist be emotionally and professionally prepared to lose the patient to suicide. This implies an acceptance of his own limitations as well as a certain fortitude without which a psychotherapeutic effort is seriously handicapped. If the therapist is intimidated by the threat of a suicidal act, he may deny himself the opportunity to obtain the very experience that would reduce that intimidation. Such experience would foster full appreciation that: a very small proportion of suicidal people go on to kill themselves; suicidal persons respond readily and positively to a caring, interested, and concerned therapist; the ambivalence regarding life and death can be influenced by already-learned therapeutic techniques; and, in the exceptional instance when the patient is lost, family members and colleagues can be understanding, supportive, and appreciative of the efforts expended. Further, considerable personal and professional growth is stimulated by working with these patients, who are so often thoughtful and perceptive persons. Their conflicts can profoundly enhance our appreciation of the human condition as well as provide an opportunity for effective therapeutic intervention.

It is important to judge the patient's capacity to collaborate with a given plan, even when he has readily accepted it. Persons who have a compulsive need to be reasonable, rational, grateful, and cooperative may agree to arrangements that they cannot fulfill, precipitating an unbearable crisis. When such needs and the accompanying vulnerability to guilt feelings are recognized by the therapist, the role they play in agreeing to a treatment plan requires careful scrutiny. This scrutiny can blend imperceptibly into the psychotherapeutic process itself.

The Treatment Process

Awareness that all aspects of clinical care have therapeutic implications takes on exaggerated importance in suicidal states. Especially if a suicide attempt has been made, the patient tends to perceive the world as rejecting and contemptuous. The careful exploration of the patient's emotional life during the initial assessment is a crucial first step in generating the all-important sense of relatedness and the feeling of being both understood and accepted that exert an essential stabilizing influence on subsequent therapy.

The optimal therapeutic approach varies so much with different therapists and with different patients that the only clear guideline is that each therapist has the responsibility "to treat his patient as best as he knows how."[14] There is general consensus among specialists in the field, however, that the therapist should maintain an "active relatedness" to the patient as opposed to a more reflective approach; the therapist should be willing to take more initiative with poorly motivated persons than might be appropriate in other situations; the patient-therapist relationship is the primary therapeutic ingredient regardless of technique used; early focus should be on symptom relief and on the underlying state that has given rise to the suicidal impulse; and long-term follow-up is important to optimal care.[5,15]

In pursuing these points, the following have been recognized as pertinent:

(1) The patient's family and other resources (minister, friend, physician, etc.) are potential members of a therapeutic team, each to have a possible role in the treatment plan, which is worked out freely and openly with the patient. Any communication with such resources should be discussed with the patient, and any change in the availability of a team member must be carefully considered. The timing of a therapist's vacation or a spouse's business trip may require special measures to compensate for diminution of support at a critical time.

(2) The importance of clear, supportive communication cannot be overestimated. The telephone can be of great value in touchy situations to maintain almost constant contact with the patient—for example, while awaiting an inpatient bed or when a patient refuses a supportive procedure. In the hospital, communication is more complicated, involving a number of clinical personnel, different shifts, etc.,

and necessitating special attention to clearly written orders and persistent monitoring to assure no communication breakdown.

(3) Vegetative needs, especially sleep, deserve high priority in supporting the person's biological strengths, without which psychological efforts are seriously handicapped.[1,5]

(4) The therapist must have a high tolerance for dependent behavior and be able to maintain an attitude of quiet confidence that the patient's pain will be relieved even though the means of achieving this are not evident. Time alone is the key in some cases, and helping the person to simply endure a crisis period may be lifesaving even though the situation itself appears hopeless. The patient should be cautioned that fluctuations are to be expected, so that resurgence of a painful experience will not be seen as confirmation of hopelessness, precipitating a suicidal act during a period of apparent improvement.

(5) Medications (or procedures such as ECT) that help relieve the underlying pathological process or its symptoms will reduce suicide risk as well. The toxicity of tricyclic antidepressants necessitates caution in outpatients in view of their frequent use for suicide attempts. When they are prescribed, the sedative side effect is often used as a sleeping medication, with the entire daily dose taken at bedtime. Benzodiazepines, trazadone, and fluoxetine appear to have low potential as a means of suicide.

(6) Group therapy is a feasible and potentially invaluable therapeutic adjunct when formed specifically for the treatment of suicidal persons and conducted by therapists with special interest, training, and experience in the problem of suicide.[16]

Treatment Discontinuities

The period of time surrounding the loss or change of a therapist is an especially vulnerable time for suicidal patients and calls for increased support. The impact of the change can be diminished by the absence of prior ongoing treatment or by a new therapist having already established a fairly good rapport with the patient. It bears repetition, however, that any change in the patient's relationship with a therapist, however temporary, may precipitate a crisis. Even in a stabilized situation, a therapist's absence due to illness or vacation can precipitate the interruption of a vital communication process or a resurgence of feelings of abandonment, with accompanying suicidal impulses. Suicide prevention and crisis centers often receive calls from patients in such a situation, and much more persuasive evidence is available from coroners' records. This problem is common to training institutions, since trainees so often move in and out of clinical assignments and frequently move away after completion of their training. A report of four suicides at one such institution reveals that three of them occurred in the context of vacation interruptions.[17]

The patient should be instructed how to reach the therapist at any time, day or night, including weekends and holidays. This includes providing a home telephone number and informing the patient when the therapist would be out of town for a day or more and how to reach him during that time. The term *instructed* is used advisedly. It must be conveyed that the therapist wishes the patient to call if at any time he feels unable to cope. Patients who are oversensitive to appearing dependent or "imposing on the doctor's valuable time" can easily be lost to suicide in an intercurrent crisis. Conveying to such patients that "if they absolutely must call, it will be acceptable to the therapist" is not appropriate because it implies only a willingness to tolerate their needs rather than a desire to respond to them. The ready availability of the therapist is rarely abused; as Mayer points out, the suicidal person's need is not so much to have the therapist immediately available as to know that the therapist's concern extends beyond the ordinary conditions of treatment.[18] The same concept applies to the therapist making special scheduling arrangements. This approach raises questions of a theoretical nature, but it remains a facet of the sound management principle referred to as active relatedness.

Monitoring Suicide Attempts

An important principle of management is that the patient's suicidal impulse should be continuously monitored,[19] but such monitoring cannot be taken for granted as a dependable safeguard. A healthy respect for the patient's need for control requires that no assumptions be made about the adequacy of the information he or she gives. A patient may, for example, resist telling the therapist of resurgent suicidal impulses for fear that it may lead to deterrence. Since the therapist depends, in part, on the patient's ambivalence toward death to obtain information about his self-destructive impulses, information he gives will vary with the degree of conflict he feels.

Pharmacotherapy

The emphasis on adequate sleep may call for the use of flurazepam (Dalmane), 30 to 90 mg, at bedtime. Although there is general agreement that the pathological state underlying the suicidal impulse should be a primary concern of the therapy for suicidal patients, there are divergent views of the definition of that pathological state. It follows that the use of psychotropic drugs with a given suicidal patient can be controversial.

The toxicological properties of tricyclic antidepressants dictate that they be used cautiously in cases of depressed high-risk patients. It is difficult to prescribe a therapeutic dose without providing a potentially lethal supply. Giving frequent small prescriptions is generally preferable to asking a family member to dispense the medication; the latter method expresses clear doubts about the patient's ability to resist suicidal impulses. Even if the therapist does not consider the underlying pathology to be primarily depressive in nature, a trial of antidepressants must be considered because of the current practice and sentiment in the psychiatric community regarding the nature of suicidal states and their relationship to depression. This consideration is more a question of treatment than management. It is common practice to give a therapeutic dose of a tricyclic agent at bedtime to obtain both antidepressant (treatment) and sedative-hypnotic (management) benefits.

Patient Support

The acute, overwhelming suicidal state is a situation requiring massive support for the patient on his or her own terms. Psychological interpretation at such a vulnerable time can generate a feeling of distance that can be lethal. This should not preclude the use of dynamic understanding, but such interpretation should be at a level and in a form that reflects acceptance, caring, and concern rather than intellectual explanation.

The therapist should be in contact with the patient's support system—family, close friends, minister, employer, etc.—and should be available to support and advise them in acute situations. Permission to respond to inquiries made by such friends and relatives or to communicate with them is best obtained from the patient as early in therapy as possible to avoid awkward dilemmas later about confidentiality.

Special Management Problems
Weak or Nonexistent Supports:

When the suicidal patient has a weak or nonexistent support system, the therapist should consider group therapy—especially those groups formed specifically for depressed and suicidal persons—in addition to taking advantage of established mental health resources such as day treatment or residential care programs. For impulsive or labile patients who may not be able to reach the therapist at a given moment but can benefit by having an understanding person to talk with, a suicide prevention and crisis center may be available, providing telephone access to such a person at any hour of the day or night. Some of the trained volunteers in these centers are as skilled in managing suicidal persons—and more experienced—than many professionals. They are trained to support the patient's relationship with a therapist, and they can provide valuable supplemental services. Their effectiveness varies of course, but a trial use of such a facility is warranted in high-risk patients who have no support systems of their own.

In large urban settings there is often a bewildering array of programs to provide help for persons with limited resources. Such programs are usually difficult to keep track of, and their effectiveness is often impossible to assess. An emergency room intake worker or social worker may know about such programs, and suicide prevention centers also should have up-to-date information for therapists about available resources in addition to the counseling help they offer for client callers. When there are no crisis centers or programs available for people in need, a high-risk person may require hospitalization simply because of the lack of resources elsewhere. Despite grumbling from ward staff or utilization-review personnel, there is a sound basis for admission until an alternate resource can be found. Although such a situation does not occur frequently in private practice, it is a common dilemma in public facilities.

Demand for Hospitalization:

Some patients do not seem at high risk for suicide but threaten or imply that suicide will be resorted to "if you don't put me in the hospital," "if the doctor doesn't give me something to get rid of this pain," "if my wife doesn't come back," or "if they reduce my disability payments." Innumerable variants of this situation are known, the common theme being that someone else's specific action, or lack of it, is identified as responsible for the patient's suicidal impulse. Less obvious forms of this situation involve repeated impulsive or unconscious passive-aggressive demands for demonstrations of caring by others in the patient's world.

The first consideration should be a careful assessment of the patient's goals and the reasonableness of his requests. Often the patient wants something that is justifiable, but his request is put in the form of an abrasive, threatening demand. This is experienced by the therapist or by others involved as manipulative, an unreasoning resistance is generated, and the refusal is rationalized as "not playing into the patient's dependent needs." This can easily lead to a power struggle in which the patient has the ultimate power, and a suicidal act may ensue. This power struggle can be critical; often, by the time the patient is seen in a psychiatric setting, the family has exhausted its energies.

If the patient's demands have merit, it should be acknowledged in spite of the irritation created. The treatment plan should include discussion with the patient of how much more readily others would respond to his needs if they were expressed in a different way. Candidates for insight-oriented therapy would have much to work on in this situation, as would patients engaged in cognitive or behavioral approaches.

If the demands do not have merit, the needs that generate them should be identified if possible and an alternative means should be formulated to meet them. For example, a 42-year-old draftsman lost his job, spent his resources on alcohol, and was then evicted from his hotel room. His demand for hospital admission because of his suicidal impulses was seen, after evaluation, as a request for gratification of his legitimate dependent needs. These were identified and validated, and a plan was worked out for providing transportation to a non-hospital setting where he would obtain adequate food, shelter, and medical attention. The patient's uncertainty that his needs would be met were expressed by his asking if the examiner wanted to be responsible for his suicide. The examiner responded that the patient would be the one to decide if he would commit suicide and that the examiner could not prevent that. He did want to help the patient as much as possible, however, and felt that making suitable living arrangements for him would accomplish that. The patient seemed to accept the statement with relief and he left in apparent good spirits.

Lethal Quantities of Medicines:

If the patient has a lethal quantity of medications at home and declines to bring it in or give it to a family member, the significance of the cache should be explored before deciding on any action. At one pole is the control-oriented person, usually with obsessive defenses, for whom access to a way out is a precondition for sustained psychotherapeutic work. In this situation it may be best to support the person's sense of control over his fate and to direct one's efforts toward the sources of psychic pain. In time the cache may lose some of its emotional load and may be relinquished spontaneously. In one instance, a patient needing sleep medication under unusual circumstances offered to borrow some from the cache on the condition that the therapist would later prescribe replacement. This was readily agreed to, and a certain humor was attached to the situation which had a therapeutic value of its own.

At the other pole is the person who is impulsive and unpredictable, for whom ready access to a lethal weapon is not likely to have a stabilizing influence. If the patient is a child or adolescent, or if his situation involves alcoholism, psychotic elements, organic cortical dysfunction, or emotional lability, the therapist should suggest removal of any readily accessible lethal instrument. Each situation deserves evaluation of the issues it presents, with an intuitive judgment as to the ultimate best interests of the patient.

Involuntary Procedures

High-risk patients who refuse professional attention pose questions of social philosophy as well as of psychiatric treatment. The basic question to be resolved is "What limitations should be put on a person's right to kill himself, and is the therapist prepared to both accept and implement those limitations?"

One suggested response to this question[20] is that a person must (1) be able to make a realistic assessment of his life situation, (2) be relatively free of ambivalence, and (3) be of legal age. In clinical terms, if the adult who wishes to kill himself is delirious, psychotic, in a panic, or seeing the world in a grossly distorted way because of an emotional disorder such as depression or schizophrenia, the therapist is acting appropriately if he employs involuntary measures to deter the suicide. Similarly, if the adult comes to the therapist's office, calls on the phone, or writes of his intent, such action can be interpreted, rightly or wrongly, as a request to intervene in the person's ambivalent struggle. There is much room for "what if . . . ?" variations, which can force the therapist into taking a somewhat arbitrary position. However, these criteria have demonstrated their usefulness as general guidelines. Each clinician must eventually find his own best approach, derived from his own experience and temperament. Documented concurrence of family members is, of course, desirable in any involuntary action, even if not a formal requirement. If a patient is held involuntarily, care must be taken to follow the prescribed certification procedure carefully, mindful that failure to do so has been a leading basis for legal action.

If the Patient Commits Suicide

A patient's suicide tends to bring into focus both the realities and fantasies of social and cultural attitudes about death, family reactions to the suicide, professional implications of such an event, and reaction to the personal loss sustained. The painful fantasies—social and professional humiliation, angry relatives, loss of confidence by other patients, lawsuits—are rarely realized. Rather, the world goes on in its inexorable way, and the therapist is left to make what he will of the experience.

Ideally this is the time for careful review, for self-scrutiny, for sharing of questions and doubts, and for sharpening of clinical awareness, skill, and judgment. The next suicidal patient becomes a challenge to pass on the legacy of the one who died, in the form of these enhanced therapeutic resources. In institutional work the process is made easier by the staff-shared setting and an established procedure for discussing clinical matters. In private work it is necessary to rely on colleagues or consultants who, ideally, were also available for discussion of the case before the suicide.[22] Making time for supportive sessions with family members is appropriate in any setting.

Most important is the continued effort to benefit fellow human beings who are in pain and who struggle with feelings of hopelessness and isolation. If our efforts in a given instance are not sufficient, we must accept our limitations and in spite of our dismay take some satisfaction from having done what we were able to do, regardless of whether it met the other's needs.

Sample Case

A 38-year-old male professional spoke of preoccupation with suicide as "the only thing left." He was extremely tense and agitated and he chain-smoked; he showed no psychotic manifestations and no crying or despondency, although he revealed numerous signs and symptoms of extreme anxiety. He was very self-critical, belittling himself for his inability to function effectively, control his feelings, work at his profession, concentrate, or even account for his emotional state. Seeing a therapist was acutely embarrassing for him: it was equated with "wallowing in self-pity." Since the only supportive persons available had exhausted their abilities to cope, the patient was finally persuaded to see the interviewer.

The therapist decided to hospitalize this patient without delay, based on his clinical judgment that the suicide risk was so high that survival outside a protective setting was unlikely. Though the patient had considerable strengths, they were not readily available to him at the time. Some rapport was established, but a firm relationship with the patient could not be accomplished in so short a time. The patient had an adamant resistance to psychiatric hospitalization, so arrangements were made with the patient's internist for admission to the medical ward of a hospital in a nearby city for a thorough physical evaluation. This was an obvious compromise.

While the patient was in the hospital his internist requested that he be seen by a second psychiatrist. After five sessions in the hospital, a decision was made that the patient should be discharged and should begin outpatient psychotherapy with that consultant, starting three days after his discharge. On the night before his first scheduled session, the patient made a serious suicide attempt and was brought to an emergency room. When the second psychiatrist could not be reached, the original examiner was contacted and arrangements were again made for hospitalization, this time in the psychiatric unit of a general hospital. Although the patient still showed some resistance to entering a psychiatric unit, it was made clear to him that under the present circumstances involuntary hospitalization would be used if necessary, and he accepted the plan for inpatient care. It was learned that the patient had agreed to the prior arrangement for outpatient treatment despite severe practical obstacles. When these proved insurmountable the patient felt obligated but trapped and helpless and experienced a resurgence of the self-destructive impulse.

At the patient's request, the psychiatrist who had first seen him undertook to develop a treatment plan. After a 10-day period that included lengthy discussions with both the patient and his family members, it was agreed that outpatient sessions three times weekly would be used. The sessions were arranged to minimize interference with the patient's work schedule, though it was necessary for the therapist to modify his own usual work hours to do so. The focus was initially on day-to-day stresses with special attention to vegetative functions, using whatever time remained to gather a detailed life history.

Amitriptyline (Elavil), up to 300 mg/day, was used for four weeks as a supplement to psychotherapy, but it had no observable benefit and was discontinued. The patient's emotional state stabilized fairly well over the ensuing weeks, and after two months of psychotherapy the sessions were reduced to twice weekly. Diazepam was used, 5 to 10 mg one to three times daily, to reduce tension, especially in the work setting. Six months after treatment began, a series of discouraging personal and work-related developments were associated with a resurgence of intense suicidal impulses. The patient said he had concealed the return of self-destructive impulses over the preceding week as a way of retaining complete control. At one point, a planned suicide attempt, using carbon monoxide from his car exhaust, was interrupted by the unexpected appearance of a neighbor. Erratic sleep and alcohol intake accompanied thoughts of hopelessness about personal goals and discouragement about the outcome of some professional projects. The patient reluctantly agreed to reenter the hospital, but after a 24-hour delay in finding an available bed he indicated he thought he could manage with office visits. The very decision to use the hospital again seemed to exert a stabilizing influence on the patient and to reassure family members that a backup resource was available. The therapist arranged daily therapy sessions and scheduled telephone contact on Saturdays and Sundays. Plans were discussed with the family. The sessions dealt primarily with vegetative functions, especially adequate sleep, with the remaining time being focused on dynamic issues. After two weeks of daily sessions, the patient's emotional state had returned to close to its prior baseline, and the prior therapy schedule was resumed.

Fourteen months after beginning treatment the patient was in a stable emotional state, was doing well on the job, was cautiously optimistic, and was working on long-term issues on a once-a-week schedule. Flurazepam, 30 mg, was used occasionally to help the patient sleep.

Conclusions

How a therapist can best handle a specific clinical problem depends on too many considerations to rely on others' experiences alone, but in the absence of precise guidelines, the points outlined above may provide a starting place. All the situations discussed are derived from clinical practice and represent some of the commonest dilemmas. Some of the suggestions are the results of painful lessons that it is hoped others can avoid.

The focus has been on special characteristics of patients, but therapists also have unique qualities. These are manifested in their treatment philosophy, management style, and temperament and will necessarily modify how they deal with the problem of suicide. One issue that applies to all clinicians, however, is the need to document the basis for management decisions. Whatever approach is taken, prudence suggests that the rationale be recorded in detail for medicolegal reasons.

Other considerations important to all the suicidal cases discussed include the value of collaboration with the patient's own support system, recognition of the patient-therapist relationship as the most significant element in both management and treatment, reliance primarily on intuitive judgments, and, finally, acceptance of the fact that the outcome is often determined to a large extent by forces beyond the therapist's control. Sound management is simply a means by which those forces are influenced in the direction of survival and continued reduced risk.

References

1. Motto J: Suicidal patients in clinical practice. *Weekly Psychiatry Update Series*. 1977; 1:18,.
2. Hendin H. Psychotherapy and suicide. *Am J Psychother.* 1981; 35:469–480,.

3. Jacobs D. Psychotherapy with suicidal patients. In: Jacobs D, Brown H, eds. *Suicide: Understanding and Responding,* Madison, Conn., International Universities Press: 1989.
4. Shneidman E: Psychotherapy with suicidal patients. In: Karasu T, Bellak L *Specialized Techniques in Individual Psychotherapy,* New York: eds. Brunner Mazel: 1980.
5. Motto J. The suicidal patient. In Thase M, Edelstein B, Hersen M, eds. *Handbook of Outpatient Treatment of Adults.* New York Plenum: 1990.
6. Jacobs D. Evaluation and care of suicidal behavior in emergency settings. In Jacobs D, Brown H (Eds.): *Suicide: Understanding and Responding.* Madison, Conn.: International Universities Press, 1989.
7. Motto J. Identifying and treating suicidal patients in a general medical setting. *Resident Staff Physician,* March 1983, 79–87.
8. Mintz R: Basic considerations in the psychotherapy of the depressed suicidal patient. *Am J Psychother.* 1971;25:56–73.
9. Beck A et al. Relationship between hopelessness and ultimate suicide. *Am J Psychiatry.* 1990;147:190–195.
10. Miller D: *Adolescence: Psychology, Psychopathology and Psychotherapy,* New York, Jason Aronson: 1974, pp. 365–376.
11. Pfeffer C. *The Suicidal Child,* Guilford Press, New York, 1986.
12. Sudak H, Ford A, Rushforth N, eds. *Suicide in the Young,* John Wright PSG, Boston, 1984.
13. Peck M, Farberow N, Litman R, eds. *Youth Suicide.* New York, Springer: 1985.
14. Murphy G. Clinical identification of suicide risk. *Arch Gen Psychiatry* 1972;27:356–359.
15. Motto J et al. Communication as a suicide prevention program. In: Soubrier J, Vedrinne J (Eds.). *Depression and Suicide.* Paris: Pergamon Press. 1983.
16. Billings J et al. Observations on long-term group therapy with suicidal and depressed persons. *Life-Threat Behav* 4:160–170, 1974.
17. Kolodny S et al. The working through of patients' suicides by four therapists. *Suicide Life Threat Behav.* 1979;9(1):33–46.
18. Mayer D. A psychotherapeutic approach to the suicidal patient. *Br J Psychiatry* 1971;11 9:629–633.
19. Friedman R. Hospital treatment of the suicidal patient. In: Jacobs D, Brown H, eds. *Suicide: Understanding and Responding.* Madison, Conn. International Universities Press: 1989.
20. Motto J. The right to suicide. *Life-Threat Behav* 1972;2:184–188.
21. Improper commitments lead malpractice claims. *APA Psychiatric News,* Oct. 15, 1976, p. 14.
22. Jones F: Therapists as survivors of suicide. In Dunne E, Mcintosh J, Dunne-Maxim K, eds. *Suicide and Its Aftermath.* New York, Norton: 1987.

13

Liability Potential for Psychiatrists Who Supervise the Care Given by Other Mental Health Professionals

KENNETH DUCKWORTH, M.D., AND THOMAS G. GUTHEIL, M.D.

Editor's Note

More and more psychiatrists find themselves working closely with other psychiatrists and mental health professionals. The relationship between psychiatrists and others may be categorized as follows: (1) Supervisory, wherein the psychiatrist is hierarchically responsible for the overall care of the patient, including the decisions and actions of all professionals under his or her direction; (2) consultative, wherein the psychiatrist offers advice on a "take it or leave it" basis and remains outside the decision-making chain of command; and (3) collaborative, in which there is a mutually shared responsibility for the patient's care.

The legal liability of supervisors is significant; they are responsible for the actions of their staff. The minimal liability of consultants is apparent: they are not directly responsible for the patient. The collaborative setting is the most complicated of the three and requires special attention. A three-way contract with the patient has been suggested,

CME questions for this chapter begin on page 359.

with the role of each professional and his or her responsibilities for and relationship with the patient clearly spelled out for all. The authors also address special aspects of confidentiality in collaborative relationships.

As a final caveat, the authors remind us that "the signature of a physician represents the formal statement that places the physician in a legally and ethically responsible status for the action or consequences of the signed document." As inconvenient as it may seem in some organizational settings, they strongly warn us against such practices as providing prescriptions for or "signing off on" patients whom we have not examined ourselves.

Introduction

Psychiatrists work in a variety of settings and interact in many different ways with other mental health professionals. One relatively unexplored aspect of this interaction is the liability potential that psychiatrists undertake in each of these relationships. Interaction between professionals is likely to increase as market forces promote health maintenance organizations and as pharmacotherapy continues to advance.

The literature currently suggests that the majority of psychiatrists collaborate with other mental health professionals. Two surveys report that approximately two-thirds of psychiatrists prescribe medication for patients in psychotherapy with other clinicians.[1,2] Woodward and colleagues[3] estimate that 10% of patients treated in collaborative relationships are seen by psychiatrists who have only a few medical backup patients; 65% are seen by psychiatrists who have more than 20 such patients. This "medication role" is one of several ways a psychiatrist interacts with other mental health professionals.

Goldberg and coworkers[1] identified concerns psychiatrists have regarding collaborative treatment, including medicolegal responsibility, inappropriate treatment, and possible alienation from nonmedical therapists. Although these concerns are not without merit, there are steps clinicians can take to minimize these risks.

Framework for a Treatment Relationship

The framework for a treatment relationship involving psychiatrists and nonmedical therapists is a crucial but often unexamined aspect of treatment. Fortunately, the American Psychiatric Association (APA) publication "Guidelines for Psychiatrists in Consultative, Supervisory, or Collaborative Relationships with Nonmedical Therapists" outlines these relationships and their corresponding degree of responsibility.[4]

Supervisory relationships are those in which the psychiatrist is hierarchically responsible for the overall care of the patient. The legal doctrine of vicarious responsibility known as *respondeat superior*, which states, "let the master answer for the deeds of his servant," holds true in these situations. The APA guidelines state:

> "In a supervisory relationship, the psychiatrist retains direct responsibility for patient care and gives professional direction and active guidance to the therapist. In this relationship, the nonmedical therapist may be an employee of an organized health care setting or of the psychiatrist. . . . The psychiatrist remains ethically and medically responsible for the patient's care as long as the treatment continues under his or her supervision. The patient should be fully informed of the existence and nature of—and any changes in—the supervisory relationship."[4]

Consultative relationships are different in terms of the level of responsibility and liability. Consultative advice is given on a "take it or leave it" basis. Consultants do not have the ability to hire or fire personnel because they are outside the decision-making chain of command. According to the APA guidelines:

> "In this type of relationship, the psychiatrist does not assume responsibility for the patient's care. The psychiatrist evaluates the information provided by the therapist and offers a medical opinion, which the therapist may or may not accept . . . Consultation is not a one-way process, and psychiatrists do and should seek appropriate consultation from members of other disciplines in order to provide more comprehensive services to patients."[4]

Collaborative relationships lie between these two extremes in terms of the liability potential for psychiatrists. Also, collaborative relationships require a great deal of communication, and the psychiatrist is wise to know with whom he or she is collaborating. Here, the APA guidelines state:

"Implicit in this relationship is mutually shared responsibility for the patient's care in accordance with the qualifications and limitations of each therapist's discipline and abilities. The patient must be informed of the respective responsibilities of each therapist; neither discipline's responsibilities diminish those of the other. Both the psychiatrist and nonmedical therapist are responsible for periodic evaluation of the patient's status to ascertain that the collaboration continues to be appropriate. The therapists must inform the patient, either jointly or separately, if they decide to terminate their collaborative relationship."[4]

Case Vignettes

Dr. A provides medical backup for several patients of a social worker she has never met. She comes into her office to find a patient she has scheduled to see a week from now for a medication evaluation. The patient, who is in obvious distress, states that the social worker is on vacation and told the patient, "Dr. A is covering." Dr. A wonders how to proceed.

Dr. B works as an academic psychiatrist in a university setting. He is the attending physician for an inpatient service team that includes residents, psychology interns, and social work interns. After the suicide of a recently discharged patient, Dr. B wonders whether he is liable for the actions of his resident and social work intern who changed the patient's discharge plan shortly before his release.

Dr. C is surprised to get an angry phone call from a patient referred to him for medication by a psychiatrist with whom he has a consultative relationship. The patient is furious that Dr. C discussed sensitive aspects of the case with the psychologist without telling the patient what he was going to say. Dr. C thinks he is just a consultant in the case and free of liability, even though the patient is threatening legal actions.

Dr. D is disturbed to hear that a patient in her local community health center has harmed a member of his family following a family therapy session. The social worker who conducts the family therapy sessions had Dr. D periodically "sign off" for her treatment plans.

Analysis:
The psychiatrists in these vignettes engaged in treatment relationships with nonmedical mental health professionals, but were unsure of their responsibility. A systematic framework can delineate treatment relationships and clarify responsibilities.

Dr. A is in a collaborative relationship with the social worker but has made the mistake of not clarifying the delineation of responsibility with that clinician (i.e., regarding vacation coverage). The breakdown has led to a situation in which the psychiatrist, who thought she was managing medications only, must perform an emergency evaluation of the patient and, presumably, cover the entire treatment during the social worker's vacation.

Dr. B is in a supervisory relationship and, as such, is responsible for the care of the patient. The actions of his trainees come under the doctrine of *respondeat superior.*

Dr. C believes he is in a purely consultative relationship with the psychologist. However, if he were to decide to treat the patient with medication, it would be difficult for a psychologist to "take the advice or leave it." Dr. C has engaged in a collaborative relationship.

Dr. D, who is unsure of her role, believes she is performing a perfunctory function of being a psychiatrist at the community mental health center; however, she may be liable for the treatment given.

Malpractice Liability
Malpractice occurs when a professional fails to meet the standard of reasonable care and this failure leads to compensable damages. In each of the cases described, the nature of the interaction between psychiatrist and nonmedical therapist probably would define a level of responsibility in the case of a lawsuit.

The Role of Informed Consent and the Treatment Contract:
Dr. A is at little risk of a lawsuit because there has been no harm to the patient. Although she and the social worker arguably breached the standard of care in not communicating their respective roles to the

patient, no harm was done. If Dr. A competently evaluates the patient and prescribes an appropriate treatment, she is at little medicolegal risk. Once the social worker returns, Dr. A would be wise to explore the vacation issue and evaluate the credentials and experience of the social worker before collaborating with her on a regular basis. Moreover, the meaning of their miscommunication and possible blurring of their roles to the patient should be explored actively (perhaps in a three-way meeting). Dr. A should consider consultation from another clinician on how to handle this clinical confusion if she is unable to resolve it. Finally, if Dr. A were to decide to stop working with the social worker, she would have to arrange for other treatment options to avoid abandoning the patient. This is clearly a case where a pound of cure is far more cumbersome than an ounce of prevention in establishing the nature of their collaboration.

With regard to collaborative treatment, some authorities have suggested a three-way contract with the patient, whereby each clinician clearly delineates his or her role and the patient provides informed consent for participation in this process. For instance, the psychotherapist outlines the risks and benefits of psychotherapy, and the prescribing psychiatrist explains the risks and benefits of medication. In addition, this contract would serve to clarify whom the patient should call in case of an emergency, the respective roles of each clinician, and the issues of confidentiality. In this way, there are few surprises because the patient has given informed consent for the collaboration between the psychiatrist and the nonmedical therapist. Vasile and Gutheil[5] have addressed the potential for ambiguity in the delegation of responsibility in the role of medical backup.

Vicarious Liability and Negligent Supervision:

Supervisors are responsible for the acts of their staff. Dr. B, clearly the supervising psychiatrist, is in a different medical liability situation. The responsibility for the actions of his trainees rests with him. Whether he will be held legally responsible (or lose the lawsuit) depends on a variety of factors.

Appelbaum and Gutheil[6] noted that the genesis of lawsuits is most commonly "bad feelings and bad outcome." Suicide is the outcome most often associated with malpractice cases involving psychiatrists. However, not all suicides are the result of negligent care or negligent supervision. There is a limit to the foreseeability of human behavior. For instance, if the patient were clinically unstable, had voiced new suicidal concerns, and had not been reevaluated, any discharge might be considered negligent. However, if the patient had been treated appropriately and assessed as able to seek help, the discharge may have been a "judgment call," as opposed to a negligent decision.

If the treatment team worked with the patient and his family and decided that discharge carried a small risk of suicide but that indefinite hospitalization contained a greater risk of regression or poor quality of life, Dr. B would have been acting from a stance of exercising good clinical judgment. The standard for malpractice is whether the professional standard of care was violated.

In the role of supervisor, Dr. B is charged with tailoring his supervision to the skill and experience of the trainees. Trainees who do not know enough to alert him to their change in plans are his responsibility. In addition to this responsibility, academic psychiatrists have a corresponding advantage in their care of the patient; they may easily access consultation from another clinician on the clinical situation posed to them. Again, consultation does not transfer responsibility for the patient; however, it does illustrate that the psychiatrist was soliciting another opinion, which demonstrates a clinician adhering to a high standard of care, as opposed to making decisions without other input.

Confidentiality Between Psychiatrists and Nonmedical Therapists:

As a collaborating psychiatrist, Dr. C is responsible both for his role in the medication evaluation and in his communication to the clinician with whom he is collaborating. Confidentiality is defined as the clinician's obligation to keep from third parties material that is learned in the professional setting. Psychiatrists must be aware of the issues of confidentiality when speaking to family members, addressing insurance companies, and presenting patients in academic conferences. In a medical backup role, psychiatrists may overlook the fact that the patient may experience confidentiality as compartmentalized and, thus, as something that can be breached between the two clinicians.

The central issue in confidentiality problems is that the patient is now aware that someone has learned information about him or her. The psychotherapist and Dr. C should review with the patient what the communications with the other clinician will be. In other words, before the psychotherapist sends patients to the psychiatrist, he or she should review with the patients that their symptoms will be discussed and that the psychiatrist will attempt to address them. After seeing the patient, the psychiatrist should share his or her findings and concerns with the patient and indicate that the data will be shared with the referral source. Ideally, psychiatrists should give a copy of the evaluation to the patient as well as the psychotherapist so that the patient knows what information has been shared.

At times, patients discuss in psychotherapy matters that are intensely personal and may be surprised to learn that the clinicians take for granted the need to share information. Both clinicians must inform the patient that this information is important to the overall treatment plan. For example, the psychotherapist might say, "I know that your abuse is very personal and shameful to you, but the psychiatrist needs to know about it in order to address symptoms x, y, and z." Conversely, in a consultative report, the psychiatrist may write that he or she elicited a history of postpartum depression with psychosis in the patient; if the patient is ashamed to have this revealed to the therapist, this major clinical issue should be addressed actively by both clinicians. Secrets between an ostensibly collaborating therapist and a psychopharmacologist are fertile grounds for substandard care.

On occasion, an emergency may ensue when confidentiality must be breached. For instance, if a nonmedical psychotherapist learns that the patient has homicidal impulses, he or she may call the psychiatrist because the psychiatrist has the authority to hospitalize the patient. This is a situation in which agreement may be sought but is not required. In emergency settings, the clinician must use his or her judgment and may violate confidentiality to protect the patient's safety or the safety of others. This decision should be made carefully and documented appropriately. Time should be spent with the patient afterward to explain the reasons why the clinician chose to undertake such a decision.

Liability Associated with Physicians' Signatures:

Dr. D did not realize that her signature on the treatment forms had any meaning. Does this mean she is in a supervisory role with the patient? She would do well to establish her responsibility on the part of the clinic, because the plaintiff's attorneys will attempt to define her role in the most active way possible—especially because she probably has greater malpractice coverage than the social worker.

The APA addressed this issue in 1989 in "Guidelines Regarding Psychiatrists' Signatures,"[7] which noted:

> The signature of a physician represents the formal statement that places the physician in a legally and ethically responsible status for the action or consequences of the signed document . . . .The signature of a psychiatrist on a diagnostic formulation or treatment plan signifies that the psychiatrist reviewed it, agreed with the diagnosis, and approved of the plan. This does not necessarily signify that he or she has seen the patient or carried out the evaluation. It may imply only that he or she is head or a member of a multidisciplinary team or supervisor of other professionals or trainees.
>
> The psychiatrist should clarify his or her role in the process of the formulation by writing immediately before his or her signature, "Reviewed by [name]," "Under the supervision of [name]," "Team Leader Approval," or other clarification.

Gutheil's dictum, "If you sign, the case is thine," is a handy guide for questions in this area.[6] To be sure, psychiatrists who sign off on cases are taking responsibility for the contents of the documents they sign.

Preventive Techniques

Medicolegal risk in interaction with other mental health professionals is a necessary part of practice. However, there is a great deal that can be done to minimize this risk. By choosing collaborating clinicians carefully, clearly defining the roles assumed by each of the parties, and establishing open communication, psychiatrists can reduce the problems that stem from the relationship with other clinicians. Psychiatrists should evaluate the credentials of any clinician whom they intend to supervise or with whom they intend to collaborate. Both parties must assess their differing personality styles, perspectives on the value of different therapies, and ability to tolerate the presence of another clinician in what is typically designed as a triad. Commonly, the clinicians will differ in age, gender, attitudes, interpersonal style, and time spent with the patient. The clinician's offices often are starkly contrasting as well. These contextual factors may invite patients to prefer one clinician over the other. In its more serious form, a split can develop.

Clinicians should be wary of the possibility of a therapeutic split; when the psychiatrist hears, "You are so much more helpful" than the nonmedical therapist, this should be a red flag for a split in the relationship. The psychiatrist should communicate this problem to the other mental health professional and ask him or her to do the same, because a therapeutic split defeats the purpose of collaborating in treatment.

One way to decrease splitting is to present a united front. Ideally, this is done as soon as the relationship begins. Who is responsible for what tasks should be outlined clearly. This is part of an informed consent for treatment and will eliminate the pitfall of the mental health professional thinking the psychiatrist is responsible ("he or she has a medical degree") and the psychiatrist thinking the mental health professional is responsible ("he or she sees the patient much more frequently"). Agreement as to these duties must be clear between the clinicians or they will never be clear to the patient. Appelbaum[8] offers recommendations to outline this three-way contract in writing.

The psychiatrist should insist that any medication evaluations be presented properly to the patient. Similarly, the psychiatrist should communicate how he or she will transmit recommendations to the patient and the therapist. Confidentiality concerns also must be reviewed prior to the contact with the second clinician.

Psychiatrists should delineate the medicolegal responsibilities of their duties in clinics and as part of treatment teams. When they are supervisors, they should have the ability to alter treatment *and* clinicians, if necessary. When they are collaborators, they should demarcate the extent of their responsibility and review the qualifications of their partners. Ambiguity in the terms of the relationships serves no one—except the trial attorney!

Conclusion

Psychiatrists currently interact with a variety of mental health professionals in myriad settings. Psychiatrists should formalize the nature of their relationships as supervisory, collaborative, and/or consultative with the mental health professional. Each of these roles involves different responsibilities for the psychiatrist.

Once the relationships are clearly delineated, the psychiatrist must choose mental health professionals with whom he or she feels comfortable, can communicate, and respects as a clinician. Once the psychiatrist has assessed the other mental health professional as competent and communicative, he or she must work to present all appropriate information to the patient in a therapeutic manner.

References

1. Goldberg RS, Riba M, Tasman A. Psychiatrists' attitudes toward prescribing medication for patients treated by nonmedical psychotherapists. *Hosp Community Psychiatry.* 1991;42:276–280.

2. Beitman BD, Chiles J, Carlin A. The pharmacotherapy-psychotherapy triangle: psychiatrist, nonmedical psychotherapist, and patient. *J Clin Psychiatry.* 1984;45:458–459.

3. Woodward B, Duckworth K, Gutheil TG. The pharmacotherapist-psychotherapist collaboration. In: Oldham J, Riba M, Tasman A, eds. *Review of Psychiatry.* Washington, DC: American Psychiatric Press Inc; 1993;12:631—650.

4. American Psychiatric Association. Guidelines for psychiatrists in consultative, supervisory, or collaborative relationships with nonmedical therapists. *Am J Psychiatry.* 1980;137:1489–1491.

5. Vasile RG, Gutheil TG. The psychiatrist as medical backup: ambiguity in the delegation of clinical responsibility. *Am J Psychiatry.* 1979;136:1292–1296.

6. Appelbaum PS, Gutheil TG. *Clinical Handbook of Psychiatry and the Law.* Baltimore, Md: Williams & Wilkins; 1991:chap 4.

7. American Psychiatric Association. Guidelines regarding psychiatrists' signatures. *Am J Psychiatry.* 1989;146:1390.

8. Appelbaum PS. General guidelines for psychiatrists who prescribe medication for patients treated by nonmedical psychotherapists. *Hosp Community Psychiatry.* 1991;42:281–282.

14

Liability Prevention in Psychopharmacology

ROBERT I. SIMON, M.D.

Editor's Note

The standard by which every physician will be judged in a court of law is based on the reasonableness of his or her acts as compared with what an ordinary physician would have done in choosing a particular treatment. The court will look closely at what treatment was chosen and why it was chosen. When treating a patient with medication, a psychiatrist should: conduct a thorough clinical evaluation; see that all appropriate laboratory tests are done; review present and past medication use; obtain a complete background history; be sure the patient has had a recent complete physical examination; consider his or her health in making medication choices; and advise the patient regarding the use of the medication and provide all the information required for informed consent to be obtained.

The author presents certain special cautions, such as the risk of tardive dyskinesia when administering neuroleptics and the need to monitor medication carefully and intervene if and when undesirable side effects occur. In one study, the most common errors made were overdosing, not supplying sufficient information for prescriptions, giving insufficient amounts of a drug, and not taking into account a patient's history of allergic reactions to a family of medications. These errors were committed more often by less experienced physicians.

CME questions for this chapter begin on page 361.

Informed consent has become a cornerstone of current medicolegal policy. The author outlines various dimensions of informed consent, pointing out that one must be familiar with state statutes when obtaining informed consent from someone other than the patient; in some regions, the proxy consent of relatives is not sufficient.

Other specific situations are highlighted, such as prescribing medication for unapproved uses (such as anticonvulsants for mood disorders or antidepressants for phobias), prescribing unapproved drugs (such as clomipramine prior to its FDA approval in the United States), prescribing generic drugs, and prescribing for patients whom the doctor has never seen in person (indeed, a situation to be avoided!).

Introduction

All physicians are judged by a certain standard of care. This standard is based on the reasonableness of their acts compared with what ordinary physicians would have done in choosing a particular treatment. If patients allege that they were treated negligently, the court will look closely at not only what treatment was chosen but also why it was chosen.

Typically, when treating a patient with medication, the exercise of reasonable care involves several factors. The psychiatrist should conduct a thorough clinical evaluation of the patient (including all appropriate laboratory tests), a review of present and past medication use, and a complete background history. Also, the psychiatrist has a duty to advise the patient regarding the use of medication and to provide sufficient information so that informed consent may be obtained.

Medication and Liability

The law recognizes that psychiatric treatment is inexact and, therefore, only reasonable care is required. In administering psychotropic medication, certain pretreatment procedures and posttreatment procedures (i.e., those that occur after treatment has been initiated) are generally considered standard; unless an emergency situation arises, they should be followed. Pretreatment procedures include: a complete clinical history; disclosure of sufficient information to obtain informed consent; and complete documentation of all treatment decisions, particularly when a medication is changed, adjusted, or reinstated. Posttreatment procedures include appropriate supervision of a patient's progress and monitoring the patient's reaction to the medication.

These concerns are greatest when prescribing neuroleptics because of the patient's risk of developing tardive dyskinesia. Several large judgments have been rendered against psychiatrists for failing to obtain a patient's informed consent or failing to monitor a patient's progress properly, which resulted in the development of tardive dyskinesia.[1] Therefore, psychiatrists administering neuroleptic medication *must* be familiar with the suggested tardive dyskinesia management guidelines provided by the American Psychiatric Association (APA) (Table 1). However, no official guideline can substitute for sound clinical judgment in the treatment and management of patients.

In medicine, drug-induced reactions generally are the most common cause of malpractice claims. Of all hospital admissions, it is estimated that 2%—5% are caused by adverse reactions, whereas 5%—30% of hospitalized patients experience an adverse drug reaction during the course of their hospital stay.[2]

One study reported on prescribing errors committed by physicians in a tertiary-care teaching hospital.[3] The authors reviewed 289,411 medication orders written during a 1-year period; 905 prescribing errors were detected and averted. A total of 57.7% of these errors were rated as having potential for adverse consequences. As expected, first-year residents made more errors than experienced physicians. The most common errors were overdosing, writing prescriptions with missing information, and prescribing insufficient amounts of a drug. A total of 6.7% of errors involved giving a drug to a patient who was allergic to the drug. The study concluded that medication errors present a significant risk to patients.

The experience of the APA's professional liability insurance program reveals that improper treatment is the most common complaint.[4] Approximately 35% of cases fall into this broad category. However, this category also includes failure to diagnose, failure to choose or execute proper treatment, and undue familiarity. Most frequently, legal actions are brought against psychiatrists when patients commit suicide.

Some of the most common areas of liability for drug treatment include lack of informed consent, excessive dosage of medication, inappropriate indications for medication, failure to monitor a patient's response to medication properly, failure to intervene properly when undesirable side effects occur, and the development of tardive dyskinesia.

Informed Consent and Liability

Psychiatrists who treat patients without obtaining informed consent are at risk for liability. The patient must have the *mental capacity* to understand *information* presented about the diagnosis, risks (including side effects) and benefits of treatment, alternative forms of therapy that also may be effective, and the consequence of not receiving any treatment. The patient must give his or her *voluntary consent*.[5]

Clinical situations do arise, however, in which the psychiatrist may need to exercise therapeutic privilege and not inform a patient concerning certain aspects of treatment. When patients lack mental capacity to provide competent consent, the consent should be obtained from next of kin or a substitute decision-maker.[6] In some states, "good faith" or the proxy consent of relatives is insufficient; the consent of a legal guardian or the substituted consent of the court is required.[7] Consent may be obtained in written form, but it also should be documented independently that the patient understood the information given and that no coercion was present. Informed consent does not protect a physician who has been negligent in the care of a patient; it only protects against risks that may occur had a "reasonable person been informed of them and rejected the proposed treatment."[8]

The American Medical Association now publishes a Patient Medication Instruction (PMI) form for many classes of psychoactive medications. These forms provide useful information to patients in a format that is easy to read and comprehend. As part of their consent procedures with patients, a number of psychiatrists have found the PMI form useful. In addition, physicians have been advised to inform patients of the following when prescribing a drug: drug name; whether the action of the drug is to treat the disease or to relieve symptoms; how to determine if the medication is effective and what to do if it is not; when and how to take the drug (e.g., before or after meals); how long to take the drug; an explanation of side effects important to the patient and what to do should they occur; possible effects on driving and working around machinery, including the proper precautions to observe; and interactions with other drugs and alcohol.[9]

Obtaining informed consent for the use of investigational drugs is absolutely necessary and rigorous, requiring that the patient be informed of all foreseeable risks associated with taking the medication and the possibility that unforeseeable risks may occur. Malpractice insurance may not cover or may provide only limited coverage for psychiatrists who work with investigational drugs.[10]

Informed Consent Standards:

The traditional professional standard defines the scope of the physician's duty to disclose what a reasonable physician would disclose under similar circumstances.[11] In most jurisdictions, the patient is required to bear the burden of defining the prevailing disclosure standard and proving that the disclosure made to the patient deviated from that practice. In states that have enacted informed consent statutes, a significant number hold to the professional custom standard.[12]

Since the early 1970s, an increasing number of courts have adopted the material risk approach (or "reasonable person" standard). This standard imposes upon the physician a duty to disclose all the information that a reasonable patient would need in order to make an informed decision about a procedure or treatment. This approach is more consistent with the ascendance of patient autonomy.

The major impetus for the reasonable person standard was provided by two 1972 cases, *Canterbury v. Spence*[13] and *Cobbs v. Grant*.[14] The *Canterbury* court rejected a truly patient-oriented standard, the "subjective lay" standard (i.e., what a particular patient would want to know). If the reasonable patient standard prevails, psychiatrists may be able to defend a claim of lack of disclosure on the ground that the patient, had he or she known the information, would have made the same decision.

The psychiatrist is not required to inform the patient of every conceivable risk. A *material risk* is one that "a reasonable person, in what the physician knows or should know to be the patient's position, would be likely to attach significance to in deciding whether or not to forego the proposed therapy."[15] Whether a risk is material depends on the severity and probability of the risk, the likelihood of treatment success, and the availability of alternative, less dangerous treatments. If necessary treatment presents minimal risks, the duty to disclose is not as rigorous as when a treatment presents high risk and is dangerous or intrusive. When less dangerous but equally effective alternative treatments are available, the duty to disclose is heightened when prescribing a riskier treatment. For example, if a neuroleptic is given when a benzodiazepine or buspirone (BuSpar) might be equally effective (such as in the treatment of an anxiety disorder), then detailed disclosure of the risks of neuroleptic treatment is necessary.

Malpractice defense attorneys have recommended the 1% rule as a guideline for physicians.[16] If a particular risk of injury has a chance of occurrence greater than 1%, the risk is considered material and must be disclosed. This rule applies *only* in jurisdictions that have indicated some percentage in specifying what constitutes a material risk. As in all aspects of the informed consent doctrine, uncertainty and inconsistency reign. Courts have been inconsistent in deciding what is a major or minor risk.

Although the general trend of increased physician liability for adverse side effects of prescribed medication continues, a countertrend may be developing, as in the case of *Precourt v. Frederick*[17] in Massachusetts. In this case, an ophthalmologist administered prednisone (Deltasone) to a patient after two separate operations. The patient developed aseptic necrosis of both hips from the steroid. The ophthalmologist gave no warning of side effects. Even though the defendant admitted that aseptic necrosis was a "prominent" complication of steroid use, the court ruled in favor of the physician, stating, "[A] physician is not required to inform a patient of remote risks." The court justified its conclusion by stating, "There must be a reasonable accommodation between the patient's right to know, fairness to physicians' and society's interest that medicine be practiced in this commonwealth without unrealistic and unnecessary burdens on practitioners." The court attempted to treat the interests of individual patients, physicians, and society evenly. *Precourt* hopefully will be the beginning of a countertrend away from holding physicians responsible for the guaranteed health and safety of patients whenever drugs are prescribed.

Physicians should provide patients with individualized information about the diagnosis of the illness, the nature and purpose of the proposed treatment, risks and consequences of the proposed treatment, probability that the proposed treatment will be successful, feasible treatment alternatives (including risks and benefits), and prognosis if the proposed treatment is not given. Psychiatrists may even fulfill a subjective lay standard by informing each of their patients of the risk and benefits of individualized treatment.[18] Furthermore, patients usually are given ample opportunity to ask questions in the give-and-take format of therapy.

All states require informed consent, either by case law or statute.[19] Many states have statutes that require informed consent for treatment.[20] The statutes may specify instances when no consent beyond the patient's understanding the risks of anesthesia and surgery is required. For additional procedures, the state may specify what risks must be told to the patient and in what form (i.e., verbal or written). Under these statutes, only the disclosure of risks specified in the statute are deemed material as a matter of law.[21] Some statutes make compliance to the guidelines voluntary. Most state statutes classify failure to obtain informed consent as negligence rather than battery.[22]

Mental health professionals who inform their patients on the basis of developing and maintaining the treatment alliance will more than likely meet the requirements of the material risk standard. It certainly is not necessary to inform depressed patients about the dopamine hypothesis or the families of patients with dementia about the neuropathology of the nucleus basalis of Meynert in Alzheimer's disease. Providing too much information (overly informed consent) can be distressing and confusing to patients and can itself lead to a malpractice suit.[23] For certain patients with a scientific background, a level of informing in response to questions of causality may be necessary to create the therapeutic alliance. In psychiatry, at least, the professional standard and material risk standard of informing are beginning to move closer together as more psychiatrists appreciate the therapeutic importance of informing the patient as part of the treatment partnership.[24]

Tardive Dyskinesia and Informed Consent:

The vast majority of important litigation regarding tardive dyskinesia has come in the context of equity rather than malpractice cases (e.g., injunction or mandatory relief, such as *Rennie v. Klein*[25]). Nevertheless, a significant number of malpractice suits have been brought against psychiatrists by patients who developed tardive dyskinesia. The allegations of negligence concerning neuroleptic treatment included improper dosages, excessive length of treatment, failure to monitor, inappropriate indications, and failure to obtain informed consent (warning of the risk of tardive dyskinesia).[26]

The greater the risk of any treatment, the greater the obligations to disclose even relatively remote risks. If alternative treatments that present lesser risks or a greater probability of success are available, the duty to disclose increases.

Because the incidence of tardive dyskinesia is quite low within the first 6 months of neuroleptic treatment, some clinicians believe it is not a material risk at the start of treatment and need not be disclosed.[27] Nevertheless, plaintiffs' attorneys are fond of pointing out in court that all psychiatrists have been on notice concerning tardive dyskinesia since 1973. At that time, psychiatrists were first informed of the association between neuroleptic treatment and the possible adverse effect of tardive dyskinesia through the *Food and Drug Administration* [FDA] *Drug Bulletin*, a publication sent to all physicians who have a drug prescription number. Furthermore, informed consent is required by law from the first day of treatment, unless an emergency exists or therapeutic privilege to treat can be asserted legitimately.

When tardive dyskinesia occurs several years after initiation of neuroleptic treatment, the absence of an early informed consent may cause serious legal problems. In addition, many chronic mentally ill patients are mobile and may have been taking neuroleptics for some time that were prescribed by a number of physicians. These patients may not be able to provide an accurate medication history. A delay of 3–6 months in the obtaining of informed consent may further extend the period of cumulative intake of neuroleptics by the patient without valid consent. Apart from legal requirements, full disclosure to patients (with certain exceptions) is the best policy both medically and ethically.

How will a psychotic patient understand information presented about tardive dyskinesia? Because a psychotic patient may have some impaired mental capacity for understanding, only basic information about tardive dyskinesia should be communicated. Psychiatrists sometimes erroneously accept an incompetent patient's consent to treatment as valid because it accords with the psychiatrist's therapeutic intent. In some cases, continued neuroleptic treatment of patients with tardive dyskinesia may represent sound clinical practice consistent with the overall treatment needs of the patient, even though a lawsuit may be filed later. For instance, psychotic patients with tardive dyskinesia who have an acute exacerbation or who require maintenance therapy may need continued neuroleptic therapy. When the mental disorder is severe enough, the psychiatrist and the patient with tardive dyskinesia may be willing to sacrifice long-term outcome for important short-term gains by the continued use of neuroleptics.

When restarting drugs in patients who manifest tardive dyskinesia, informed consent should be obtained *immediately*. When the patient needs to continue neuroleptic pharmacotherapy in the presence of tardive dyskinesia, a confirming second opinion should be obtained.

Prescribing Medication

The *Physicians' Desk Reference* (PDR) is published annually by a private commercial firm. The publisher compiles, organizes, and distributes product descriptions prepared by the manufacturer's medical department or consultants. The FDA requires that products that have official package inserts be reported in the PDR in the identical language appearing on the insert.

The psychiatrist should know that the package insert lists almost all side effects ever reported in drug trials, even if not produced by the specific drug under consideration. In other words, side effects found in similar drugs are reported. The side effects reported in the package insert may not be weighed in terms of probability of occurrence in the course of clinical practice. The legal significance of the package insert or PDR varies with each jurisdiction.

Although the PDR frequently is used by lawyers in court, it would be a professional error for clinicians to regard the PDR as a primary standard of care reference. Psychiatrists are responsible for making informed decisions, taking into account their own clinical training, experience, and the relevant literature. Because the PDR is not a text for psychiatric practice, patient care may be compromised if clinicians view the PDR as their main source of professional guidance, rather than the professional literature and the usual community standards of practice. In essence, the PDR should be considered as one of several sources of information that a psychiatrist may rely upon for making medication decisions. Again, official guidelines cannot take the place of sound clinical judgment.

Prescribing Medication for Unapproved Uses:

Prescribing an approved medication for an unapproved use does not violate federal law. Whenever a psychiatrist prescribes an approved drug that has not yet been approved by the FDA for that particular use (e.g., a tricyclic antidepressant for panic attacks, an anticonvulsant for a mood disorder, or lithium for violent behavior), the decision should be based on reasonable knowledge of the drug and should be supported by firm scientific rationale and valid medical studies. The psychiatrist should have texts or data readily available to substantiate that the decision to prescribe for a nonapproved use was based on sound psychiatric and medical practice.

Nonetheless, the standard for informed consent is correspondingly heightened when medication is prescribed for an unapproved use. The patient or guardian must be informed that he or she will be taking a drug for a use that has not been approved by the FDA and should be warned of all possible, reasonably foreseeable risks. A consent form may provide added protection. The nature of the disclosure should be recorded in the patient's chart. The use of a drug, once marketed, is the responsibility of physicians and is prescribed at their sole discretion.

Prescribing Unapproved Drugs:

The prescription of an unapproved drug technically violates the law. Under 21 USC §355, to "introduce or deliver for introduction into interstate commerce" an unapproved drug is a violation of the law. This issue arose with clomipramine (Anafranil) in the treatment of obsessive-compulsive disorder (OCD) before its official approval. Clomipramine had been approved for use in the treatment of OCD in Canada and Europe but not in the United States. The psychiatric literature supported the treatment of OCD with clomipramine, and the side-effect profile was similar to that of other tricyclic antidepressants.

In general, the FDA's policy is not to prosecute physicians who prescribe legitimate drugs approved in other jurisdictions. However, the risk of malpractice is increased if the patient is harmed by a drug not approved by the FDA for efficacy and safety.

Inappropriate Administration of Psychotropic Medication:

Inappropriate administration of psychotropic medication includes failure to perform an adequate physical examination and failure to obtain a medical history before prescribing psychoactive medication. When psychiatrists decide to prescribe a psychoactive medication for patients, they *must* familiarize themselves with their patients' medical history and physical health. In particular, a history of allergic reactions to medications must be noted. If questions exist about a patient's health, consultation with a medical colleague who can conduct a full medical investigation is in order. Psychiatrists are liable for failing to diagnose organic conditions. They have a firm responsibility to detect organic causes of psychological illness, either by their own examination or by referral to competent specialists.

Prescribing neuroleptics for patients who suffer from neurotic anxiety may be an example of inappropriate administration of medication. However, the clinical needs of the patient are the determining factor. Psychoactive medications that are indicated for one type of psychiatric disorder may be empirically useful for a nonindicated disorder in other patients.

The use of polypharmacy, or multiple medications, often has been disparaged as a "shotgun" approach to treatment that may significantly increase the possibility of serious side effects. Nevertheless, certain patients may benefit from such a regimen.

An attempt to impose social control on mentally ill patients through "chemical straitjackets" represents an inappropriate indication for psychoactive medication if the objectionable behavior is not directly caused by a psychiatric illness. For example, for the severely agitated elderly patient with dementia and psychosis, a neuroleptic may be lifesaving. Neuroleptic medications may be abused if they are prescribed to oversedate a patient in order to squelch objectionable behavior that is a long-standing aspect of the patient's personality and is not reflective of a treatable mental illness. In addition, psychoactive drugs should never be used as a form of punishment. Whenever "chemical restraints" raise deprivation of civil rights issues, malpractice actions are more likely.

The enactment of statutory regulations establishing medication prescribing guidelines influences the standard of care in providing drug therapy. For example, the Omnibus Budget Reconciliation Act of 1987 (OBRA-1987) implemented on October 1, 1990, regulates the use of psychotropic drugs in long-term health care facilities receiving funds from Medicare and Medicaid.[28] The Health Care Financing Administration guidelines for neuroleptic drugs include: (a) documentation of the psychiatric diagnosis or specific condition requiring neuroleptic use; and (b) prohibition of p.r.n. neuroleptic use and gradual dose reductions of neuroleptics combined with attempts at behavioral programming and environmental modification.[29]

Exceeding Recommended Dosages:

Some severely mentally ill patients may require the administration of psychoactive medications that exceed dosage guidelines. The reasons for such a decision must be clearly documented in the patient's record. The patient should be made aware that drug guidelines are being exceeded. Generally, if very high levels of medication are required, the patient may need to be hospitalized until a safer maintenance level of the medication can be achieved.

A patient's failure to renew prescriptions may pose a danger to his or her care. Thus, prescriptions that require frequent renewal may lead to noncompliance. With neuroleptic medication, the prescription of what might appear to be a lethal amount for an ordinary patient may be only a single dose for a chronic patient on long-term maintenance therapy. The psychiatrist should note these differences in the patient's medical record, including the fact that tolerance to the toxic effects of neuroleptic medication develops quickly.

A psychiatrist covering for a colleague should prescribe only enough medication to hold the patient over until the treating psychiatrist returns. If the treating psychiatrist will be away for a long period, the covering psychiatrist may need to evaluate the patient personally. Typically, only a brief history, including diagnosis and treatment, is provided (either orally or in writing) to the covering psychiatrist. Therefore, medications renewed over the telephone must be prescribed with great care. In some instances, renewal of medications may require an appointment with the patient.

Monitoring Side Effects:

Psychiatrists have a duty to use reasonable care in prescribing, dispensing, and administering medication. Monitoring the patient and warning of side effects fall within this duty. As part of the working alliance with their patients, psychiatrists should inform patients of possible side effects of medication, encouraging patients to notify them if any serious side effects arise. Open communication about potential problems with medications enhances the therapeutic process through the establishment of trust and reduces the problem of noncompliance.

Various basic side effects are sometimes overlooked. Patients must be warned about driving or working around dangerous machinery if their medication causes drowsiness or slows reflexes. Similarly, patients must be warned of the dangers of mixing alcohol with psychoactive drugs. Clinicians also must be aware of drug-induced memory impairment, particularly with the use of certain benzodiazepines; any resulting amnesia can be psychologically and socially disabling.

Monitoring the patient's clinical condition rather than placing exclusive reliance upon laboratory test results is imperative. For example, patients undergoing lithium therapy have developed signs and symptoms of toxicity while lithium levels were in the therapeutic range.[30]

Prescribing for Unseen Patients:

Psychiatrists should avoid prescribing medication for patients they have not seen. This problem often arises when psychiatrists who work in clinics are asked to prescribe medications for patients seen by nonmedical therapists. Receiving reports about a patient from nonmedical therapists is not sufficient. Nonmedical therapists are not trained in psychopharmacology, and their reports should not be relied upon to form a clinical opinion about prescribing psychoactive drugs for patients. Psychiatrists who prescribe medication are responsible for such treatment even though another provider is primarily responsible for the overall care of the patient. Under these circumstances, psychiatrists remain highly vulnerable to malpractice actions stemming from improper supervision of patients who develop serious or fatal reactions to medications.

In large hospitals or institutions, the psychiatrist may not be able to see all the patients, and he or she may be required to write a prescription for drugs covering a period of many months that is dispensed by nurses or mental health aides. The only medically acceptable solution to this problem is for the psychiatrist to see the patient each time before a prescription is written; if this cannot be accomplished, the reasons should be documented carefully.

Psychiatrists sometimes authorize a prescription for a person unknown and unseen who lives some distance away and who does not have medical services available nearby. Although this may be done on a one-time basis or as a humanitarian gesture, psychiatrists must understand that should litigation arise, prescribing for unseen patients will likely be viewed as creating a doctor-patient relationship. Patients taking psychoactive medication must be seen as frequently as their clinical needs require. These patients should not be allowed to go unsupervised.

The psychological issues surrounding patient compliance and noncompliance with prescribed medications are complex and need to be explored by the psychiatrist with the patient. For this reason, medications should be dispensed in the context of a therapeutic relationship in which the many psychological meanings involved in the taking of medication can be explored.[26]

Generic Drugs:

Generic drugs that contain the same active ingredients as established proprietary drugs may not possess the same clinical efficacy because of differential dissolution, absorption, and distribution rates in the human body. Therapists may become confused when patients report continued symptoms due to the unrecognized absence of therapeutic efficacy of a generic drug. Whether generic or proprietary, the drug that achieves maximal therapeutic efficacy in the shortest time probably will be cost-effective in the long run.

The psychiatrist is responsible for the selection of the appropriate medication for the patient. Only when the psychiatrist signs the "generic substitution permissible" line may the pharmacist substitute a less-expensive drug with the same active ingredients. In a number of states, drug-product selection laws stipulate that the prescriber must expressly indicate "do not substitute" in some manner when prohibiting generic substitution. To pursue a consistent prescribing and monitoring policy, the psychiatrist should be aware of the legal issues surrounding generic drugs.[26]

Finally, *prescriptions must be written legibly*. If the psychiatrist's cursive penmanship tends to be unreadable, the prescription should be printed. In addition, the amount should be written out so that the number of medications cannot be changed by drug-abusing patients. The pharmacist should be instructed to label all medications, and directions for taking the medication should be specific—rather than "sig: as directed." Unlabeled medications may be difficult to identify by emergency room personnel should the patient require emergency care.

Medications and Motor Vehicles

Felthous[31] cites five major automobile accident cases involving the duty to warn and protect. In one of these cases, *Schuster v. Altenberg*,[32] a manic-depressive patient who was taking alprazolam (Xanax) and phenelzine (Nardil) crashed into a tree at 60 mph within an hour of taking the medications. The patient died, and her 17-year-old daughter was rendered a paraplegic as a result of the accident. The psychiatrist was sued, with the plaintiff alleging negligent care and management of the patient. The trial court granted the defendant's motion for summary judgment. On certification from the court of appeals, the Wisconsin Supreme Court concluded that once negligence is established, the defendants are liable for the unforeseeable consequences of their acts to unforeseeable plaintiffs. Thus, in Wisconsin, one of the broadest *Tarasoff* duties is now the law: there is a duty to protect everyone, identifiable or not.

The Wisconsin Supreme Court ruled that legal sufficiency for the following complaints existed:

• Negligent diagnosis and treatment
• Failure to warn the family of the patient concerning her condition and its dangerousness
• Failure to seek commitment of the patient

On retrial, the psychiatrist was found not guilty. The trial court found the decedent 80% contributorily negligent, the plaintiff 20% negligent, and the defendant psychiatrist not negligent.

Courts collectively are not establishing consistent, coherent law. Relying heavily upon the duty to warn, plaintiffs allege a wide variety of nonclinical duties to disclose, which foster the potential for courts to find "duties and liabilities that are diffuse and unclear." Felthous recommends that if warning or reporting is desired as a matter of public policy, the clarity and consistency of statutory law would be preferable over inconsistent court decisions.

Staying Abreast of Psychopharmacologic Developments

Psychiatrists have an ethical and legal duty to keep abreast of psychopharmacologic developments in psychiatry. Some dynamically trained psychotherapists have avoided acquiring knowledge or skill in administering drug therapy. They, as well as nonmedical therapists, may ask a medical colleague to prescribe medications for their patients. This practice introduces an artificial split into the intimate connection between treating the patient by medication and treating the patient by psychotherapy. Fragmentation of the therapeutic process should be avoided, if possible. Ostow[33] disagrees with fragmented treatment practices because data obtained from psychotherapy are necessary for proper administration of drug therapy. In addition, to understand the patient, drug effects must be distinguished from psychopathologic symptoms. Furthermore, the transference may be split, and the division of treatment is twice as expensive.[34]

Conclusion

As this lesson has emphasized, prescribing clinicians have an ethical and legal duty to remain aware of scientific developments in their specialties, particularly in the burgeoning area of psychopharmacology. Psychiatrists can no longer afford to be therapeutically one dimensional. The psychiatrist who is unfamiliar with a specific treatment modality should avoid its use.

Speaking about the treatment of depression, Lesse[35] states that "those who treat severe depressions should have the broadest possible knowledge of the limitations of various psychotherapeutic techniques. Similarly, they should have an intimate knowledge of the benefits and limitations of the antidepressant drugs." Clinicians' knowledge of developments in psychopharmacology and the law will help avoid inappropriate defensive practices that can lead to substandard care.

References

1. See, e.g., *Clites v State*, 322 NW2d 917 (Iowa Ct App 1982); *Hedin v United States*, #583-3 (D Minn Dec 27th 1984) appeal dsmd #85-5057 MN (8th Cir May 21, 1985); *Barclay v Campbell*, 704 SW2d 8 (Tex 1986); *Faigenbaum v Oakland Medical Center*, 373 NW 2d 161 (Mich Ct App 1985); *American Cyanamid v Frankson*, 732 SW2d 648 (Tex Ct App 1987); *Snider v Harding Hospital* (No 84-CV-06-3582) Franklin Cty Ct Comm Pleas (Columbus Ohio, August 1988).

2. Drug-induced disease called a "double-barreled" liability. *Clin Psychiatr News*. 1984;12(Jan 12):12.

3. Lesar TS, Briceland LL, Delcoure K, et al. Medication-prescribing errors in a teaching hospital. *JAMA*. 1990;263:2329–2334.

4. Risk of malpractice suit for psychiatrists may be rising. *Clin Psychiatr News*. 1984;12(Dec 18):1.

5. King JH. *The Law of Medical Practice in a Nutshell*. 2nd ed. St. Paul, Minn: West; 1986:154–173.

6. *Canterbury v Spence*, 464 F2d 772, 789 (DC Cir), *cert denied*, 409 US 1064 (1972), *citing Fiorentino v Wenger*, 26 App Div 2d 693, 272 NYS2d 557, 559 (1966), *appeal dismissed* 276 NYS2d 639 (1966), *reversed on other grounds*, 280 NYS2d 373, 227 NE2d 296 (App Div 1967)

7. Klein JI, Glover SI. Psychiatric malpractice. *Int J Law Psychiatry*. 1983;6: 131–157.

8. *Cheung v Cunningham*, 214 NJ Super 64a, 520 A2d 832 (1987), *reversed on other grounds*, 111 NJ 573, 546 A2d 501 (1988).

9. Anonymous. What should we tell patients about their medicines? *Drug Ther Bull*. 1981;19:74.

10. Fishalow SE. The tort liability of the psychiatrist. *Bull Am Acad Psychiatry Law*. 1975;3:191–220.

11. *Winkjer v Herr*, 277 NW 2d 579 (ND 1979).

12. Brakel SJ, Parry J, Weiner BA. *The Mentally Disabled and the Law*. Chicago, Ill: American Bar Foundation; 1985:449.

13. *Canterbury v Spence*, 464 F2d 772 (DC Cir), *cert denied, Spence v Canterbury*, 409 US 1064 (1972).

14. *Cobbs v Grant*, 502 P2d 1, 8 Cal 3d 229, 104 Cal Rptr 505 (1972).

15. Miller LJ. Informed consent, I. *JAMA*. 1980;244:2100–2103.

16. Gibbs RF. Informed consent: what it is and how to obtain it. *Leg Aspects Med Pract*. 1987;15(Aug):1–4.

17. *Precourt v Frederick*, 395 Mass 689, 481 NE2d 1144 (1985).

18. Simon RI. *Concise Guide to Psychiatry and Law for Clinicians*. Washington, DC: American Psychiatric Press Inc; 1992:33.

19. Malcolm JG. Informed consent in the practice of psychiatry. In: Simon RI, ed. *American Psychiatric Press Review of Clinical Psychiatry and the Law*. Washington DC: American Psychiatric Press Inc; 1992:3.

20. Solnick PB. Proxy consent for incompetent nonterminally ill adult patients. *J Leg Med (Chicago)*. 1985;6:1–49.

21. Meisel A, Kabnick LD. Informed consent to medical treatment: an analysis of recent legislation. *Univ Pittsburgh Law Rev*. 1980;41:407.

22. Slovenko R. Misadventures of psychiatry with the law. *J Psychiatry Law*. 1989;17(Spring):115–156.

23. *Ferrara v Galluchio*, 5 NY2d 16, 152 NE2d 249, 176 NYS2d 996 (1958).

24. Simon RI, Sadoff RL. *Psychiatric Malpractice: Cases and Comments for Clinicians*. Washington, DC: American Psychiatric Press Inc; 1992.

25. *Rennie v Klein*, 462 F Supp 1131 (D NJ 1978), *remanded*, 476 F Supp 1294 (D NJ 1979) affd in part, *modified in part and remanded*, 653 F2d 836 (3d Cir 1980), *vacated and remanded*, 458 US 1119 (1982), 720 F2d 266 (3rd Cir 1983).

26. Simon RI, ed. *Clinical Psychiatry and the Law*. 2nd ed. Washington, DC: American Psychiatric Press Inc; 1992.

27. Schatzberg AF, Cole JO. *Manual of Clinical Psychopharmacology*. Washington, DC: American Psychiatric Press Inc; 1986:6.

28. Hendrickson RM. New federal regulations, psychotropics, and nursing homes. *Drug Ther*. 1990;Suppl Aug:101–105.

29. Health Care Financing Administration. Medicare and Medicaid requirements for long-term care facilities. Final rule with request for comments. *Federal Register*. 1989;Feb 2.

30. Lewis DA. Unrecognized chronic lithium neurotoxic reactions. *JAMA*. 1983;250:2029–2030.

31. Felthous AR. The duty to warn or protect to prevent automobile accidents. In: Simon RI, ed. *American Psychiatric Press Review of Clinical Psychiatry and the Law*. Washington DC, American Psychiatric Press Inc; 1990;1:221–238.

32. *Schuster v Altenberg*, 144 Wis 2d 223, 424 NW2d 159 (1988), rev'd *Schuster v Altenberg*, 86-CV-1327 (Cir Ct Racine City 1990).

33. Ostow M. Is it useful to combine drug therapy with psychotherapy? *Psychosomatics*. 1979;20:731.

34. Slovenko R. Malpractice in psychiatry and related fields. *J Psychiatry Law*. 1981;9:5–64.

35. Lesse S. Editorial comment. *Am J Psychother*. 1965;19:105.

1 5

Malpractice in Child and Adolescent Psychiatry

EDWARD E. BARTLETT, PH.D.

Editor's Notes

Psychiatrists who specialize in child and adolescent psychiatry are not as likely to be sued for malpractice as those involved with adult care. Nonetheless, certain precautions are in order. The key to malpractice prevention is establishing a good, workable relationship with patients and their parents; trust is the sine qua non *for effective therapy.*

Many of the malpractice prevention principles involved in dealing with children and adolescents are the same as those for adults: explaining practice policies; doing careful assessments; keeping detailed records; wherever possible, involving patient and family in management decisions; and obtaining informed consent. The matter of confidentiality can become somewhat complicated when dealing with adolescents, and the author provides several useful guidelines in this lesson.

Suicide, violence, and medication issues are common sources of legal risk. Special liability responsibilities arise when a psychiatrist is working with other professionals in a group or in clinic/institutional settings. The author advises therapists to refuse to participate in medical systems that reward physicians financially or otherwise for hospitalizing teenage patients.

CME questions for this chapter begin on page 362

Introduction

Psychiatrists are at a relatively low risk of being sued for medical malpractice, and those who specialize in child and adolescent psychiatry enjoy an even lower risk. A review of 711 claims filed with the American Psychiatric Association (APA) professional liability insurance program between 1973 and 1983 revealed that only 36 (5%) involved psychiatrists who specialized in the treatment of children.[1] The 1991 edition of *Physician Characteristics and Distribution,* published by the American Medical Association (AMA), lists 4664 child psychiatrists and 33,603 adult psychiatrists. This suggests that child psychiatrists have a 10-year risk of being sued of only 0.8%, compared with 2% for adult psychiatrists.

A recent survey of 92 child and adolescent residency programs reported details of 18 malpractice actions filed over a 10-year period.[2] Because of the nature of residency training, these lawsuits are weighted toward inpatients. Of the 18 lawsuits, 10 were closed at the time this lesson was published. Of the closed cases, five resulted in a payment to the plaintiff ranging from $7,000 to $500,000, with a mean payment of $167,000.

Establishing the Therapeutic Relationship

The key to malpractice prevention is to establish an effective relationship with the patient and his or her parents. Trust is the *sine qua non* of effective therapy, and psychiatrists who treat children and adolescents must work especially hard to establish a trusting relationship. Countertransference issues further complicate the process. Maintaining a supportive, respectful relationship is particularly important in cases in which: patients or parents are angry or manipulative; the patient was badly abused in childhood; the patient performs self-mutilation; or the therapist experiences a countertransference reaction.

Although the child or adolescent is the primary patient, the relationship with the patient's parents cannot be taken for granted. Frequently, the psychiatrist must negotiate ground rules with the parent to protect the doctor-patient relationship. After the initial evaluation, it is important to set treatment objectives and agree on an initial number of visits. This will reduce the chances of the parent prematurely withdrawing the child from treatment. After the first set of visits, revise treatment objectives and negotiate an additional set of visits, if needed.

At the initial visit, explain in general terms what you hope to accomplish and how. Explain that the therapeutic session is a time for the patient to try new modes of thought and behavior. Ensure that the patient and his or her parents do not place you on a pedestal and that they understand the length and nature of therapy. Explain practice policies regarding telephone calls, medication refills, billing for no-shows, etc. Conduct a thorough medical history to avoid a missed organic diagnosis and obtain a copy of a recent physical examination. Try to obtain a copy of previous psychiatric and medical records.

As therapy progresses, keep the patient informed and involved. Periodically provide information about the progress of therapy, medications, and other options for therapy. Whenever possible, involve the patient and his or her family in management decisions. Provide instructional brochures for the patient to take home.

In the unusual event that you need to terminate the relationship, use caution. Advise the patient verbally and in writing. Send a certified letter. Suggest the names of other qualified psychiatrists. Do not discontinue the relationship abruptly, especially during a crisis.

Managing the Violence-Prone Patient

Psychiatrists often must address the proverbial "half-tamed demons that inhabit the human breast." Sometimes these demons become manifest in violent ways.

A 17-year-old girl had a long-standing diagnosis of psychosis and was taking a psychotropic medication. She voluntarily entered a residential facility that emphasized a psychosocial approach. It was known that the girl was not taking her medication; however, consistent with the facility's philosophy, she was not forced to take it. When she exhibited suicidal tendencies, she was transferred to a nearby hospital. After 2 weeks, she improved and was transferred back to the facility. Three months later, she jumped out of the window of her fourth-story room, landing on a spiked fence. Two spikes pierced her abdomen. An extended course of rehabilitation was necessary.

For most psychiatrists who treat children and adolescents, predicting and preventing suicidal behavior represent the greatest liability challenges. Courts of law recognize that the prediction and management of violence are fraught with difficulties.[3] Nonetheless, the sudden death of a teenager will evoke a remorseful, and possibly vindictive, response from the parents, which may lead to a lawsuit.

The psychiatrist should approach the suicide-prone patient in a systematic and thoughtful manner. The patient's previous history of violence is one of the best predictors.[4] The psychiatrist's assessment of ideation and his or her overall clinical impression can be supplemented with diagnostic tests.

Practice guidelines are being developed to assist psychiatrists. A recent American Academy of Child and Adolescent Psychiatry (AACAP) guideline, *Practice Parameters for the Assessment and Treatment of Conduct Disorders*, provides a number of pertinent recommendations. It includes specific recommendations for managing the violence-prone patient based on whether the patient is deemed to be at moderate or high risk for violence.

Protecting Inpatients from Injury and Violence

Many psychiatrists with a large inpatient practice are unaware of their liability risk that arises from injuries befalling an inpatient.

> A 16-year-old girl presented in the emergency room extremely depressed and anxious. She was admitted to the hospital. During the course of her hospitalization, she was assaulted by another patient. The girl sued, and the hospital and psychiatrist of the assaulting patient were found guilty. The victim received a $500,000 payment.

Psychiatrists must examine the hospital's physical environment, especially the availability of dangerous materials, including call bell cords and medication carts. Access to open windows must be checked. Rights regarding privacy versus protection from violence must be balanced. Procedures pertaining to commitment procedures, assessment of violence potential to others, and roommate assignments must be reviewed. Patients should be advised of unit rules regarding verbal expressions of hostility, fighting, and aggressive behavior. Nursing and other staff should be apprised of the risk and encouraged to be vigilant.

Medication Issues

Many child and adolescent psychiatrists emphasize a psychoanalytic approach and prescribe few medications. Nonetheless, as genetic and neuroscience research expands our understanding of the biologic basis of mental illness, it is likely that medications will come to play a larger role in the therapeutic armamentarium. The most common types of medications leading to lawsuits are major and minor tranquilizers.

The most frequent medication-related allegations in psychiatric practice are:

- Failure to monitor potential side effects of a drug, especially tardive dyskinesia
- Drug dependency
- Lethal overdose of medications
- Discontinuation of medication(s) by a psychotic patient who subsequently commits suicide or homicide
- Lack of informed consent

Confidentiality

Confidentiality refers to the right of a patient to have communications given in confidence and not disclosed to outside parties without implied or expressed authorization. Hippocrates[5] laid the foundation for the modern-day concept of confidentiality: "Whatsoever things I see or hear concerning the life of man, in any attendance on the sick or even apart therefrom, which ought not to be voiced about, I will keep silent thereupon." The legal basis for confidentiality derives from four sources: the constitutional right of privacy, confidentiality provisions in state laws, common law that has evolved from court decisions, and the ethical canons of mental health professionals.

For example, principle VI of the AACAP code of ethics states: "Specific confidences of the patient and the parents or guardians and others involved should be protected unless this course would involve untenable risks or betrayal of care-taking responsibility."[6] Principle X elaborates: "The release of any information regarding a minor unemancipated child or adolescent to persons outside the family (including the noncustodial parent) requires the agreement of parents or guardians." Principle XI addresses the patient's right to know: "It is necessary that the child or adolescent, within his/her capacity for understanding, be clearly apprised of confidentiality in regard both to his/her own communication and to those of parents or guardians."

The psychiatrist should be aware of the various exceptions to confidentiality requirements, as defined by state law, which typically include:

- Court-ordered exams
- Involuntary civil commitment
- Child abuse
- Venereal disease
- Gunshot wounds
- Future violent crimes against an identifiable victim

Be sure that your staff members (especially receptionists and transcriptionists) are familiar with confidentiality requirements. At an initial visit, explain your confidentiality procedures. Outline your confidentiality procedures in a new-patient brochure and/or verbally. Advise the patient that you may wish to discuss his or her problem with other mental health professionals in order to provide the best care.

Provide custodial family members with limited information. With the patient's advance knowledge or permission, advise the custodial family members of the diagnosis, current treatments, medications, prognosis, strategies to manage the patient's illness at home, and community resources. Advise them to report to you any developments or potential danger to self or to others. Obtain consent of the custodial parent before providing information to the noncustodial parent. When caught between conflicting demands of the minor patient, custodial parent, and noncustodial parent, seek to negotiate a middle ground. Remember that your first duty is to the identified patient.

When you receive a request for information from a third party (such as an insurer), use caution. For young minors, the parent's consent is adequate. For mature minors, obtain both the parent's and the child's consent for release of information. Comply with a subpoena only if a judge has ordered it. If in doubt, check with your attorney first.

Custody Issues

No issue poses greater treatment, ethical, and malpractice challenges than the intrusion of a custody conflict into the therapeutic relationship:

> A teenage boy had dysthymia with onset 3 years before, when his parents had divorced. The father retained custody of the boy, and the mother had weekly visitation rights. During these visits, the mother brought the child to a psychiatrist without the knowledge or consent of the father. When the father found out about the therapy sessions, he sued for inflicting emotional injury.

Principle I of the AACAP code of ethics emphasizes: "The primary concerns of the child and adolescent psychiatrist are the welfare and the optimum development of the individual child or adolescent patient or of the population of the children and adolescents being served."[6] With careful foresight and a tenacious focus on doing what is best for the patient, most custody entanglements can be prevented or managed successfully.

Informed Consent

Part of effective malpractice prevention is to provide information via informed consent. Principle VI of the AACAP code of ethics affirms: "The child and adolescent psychiatrist should seek to provide the patients themselves and those involved in their care and/or treatment . . . as thorough an understanding as can usefully be grasped and therapeutically utilized in the care of the child."[6]

Informed consent applies to persons who are legally competent. The law defines competency narrowly in terms of cognitive capacity only. Affective incompetence is not an issue unless it substantially interferes with cognitive capacity. Thus, many, if not most, psychiatric patients are deemed to be legally competent.

Verbal or written consent should be obtained for lithium (Eskalith, Lithane), methylphenidate (Ritalin), neuroleptics, and other medications with major side effects. Written consent affords greater liability protection, assuming the printed form is not used to substitute for a frank discussion of the benefits and risks. Although the parent (or emancipated minor) has the legal right to give consent, the minor patient should be informed, too. Explain the following:

- Diagnosis
- Nature, purpose, and expected outcomes
- Risks and consequences
- Alternative treatments
- Prognosis if no treatment is given

It is not necessary to disclose *every* known risk, only those that are most severe or common, including the possibility of death.

Provide a handout that you have written or one developed by professional organizations such as the AMA, APA, or AACAP. Finally, make a note in the patient's chart that he or she was informed of the benefits and risks of the medication and agreed to its use.

Documentation

Proper documentation of the visit is critical for both therapeutic and malpractice prevention purposes. Detailed documentation can protect the psychiatrist in case of a unfavorable outcome.

A 16-year-old boy with schizophrenia was hospitalized and treated with psychotherapy and neuroleptic medications. After 3 months, he was discharged to the care of his family to continue treatment at an outpatient clinic. Three months later, responding to auditory hallucinations, the patient took several guns available in the house and shot at neighbors, killing several people. At his criminal trial, he was found not guilty by reason of insanity.

The families of the victims sued the hospital and the physician. In its defense, the hospital showed documentation of family conversations made by the social worker who emphasized the need for medication adherence, the role of the family in monitoring the medication, the need to report patient noncompliance to the hospital, the patient's potential for violence, and the need to restrict the patient's access to guns. Based on the documentation, the jury ruled in favor of the hospital and physician.

A defense attorney's worst nightmare is to defend a psychiatrist who has the basis of incomplete, poorly organized, and illegible notes. The psychiatrist should record all important clinical findings and observations, including the treatment plan, consultations, nature of other health problems, and clinical reasoning process. Organize information in a logical manner, such as the problem-oriented medical record.

Document instructions given to the patient and/or parents, especially those that detail therapeutic procedures and risks of medications. If you provide a handout, simply record, for example, "Handout on methylphenidate provided; risks discussed with parent." Document patient noncompliance, missed appointments, and treatment refusals. Then, if a negative outcome occurs, the issue of contributory negligence on the part of the patient can be raised. Record all telephone conversations about major symptoms and medications. Print or legibly write all medication prescriptions and patient instructions.

Do not criticize your colleagues in the chart. Do not write that another physician or therapist made a mistake. If your impression differs, simply state that the information available to you supports a given diagnosis or management course. Be wary of pejorative patient descriptors, such as "secretive," "dishonest," or "uncooperative."

Do not alter your records without clearly indicating "late entry" and the date of the notation. Many defensible cases have been rendered indefensible because the physician penned self-serving notes after a malpractice notice was served. Check with your personal counsel or malpractice insurance carrier regarding the length of time for which you should retain your records.

Working with Other Mental Health Professionals

With the growth of group practices and mental health clinics, psychiatrists have become subject to unique malpractice risks by virtue of their association with other mental health practitioners. Sometimes, the psychiatrist acts solely as a medication consultant, seeing the patient on an infrequent basis. The psychiatrist can become a "deep-pocket" target if the other therapists have no malpractice insurance protection. *Respondeat superior* liability issues arise when the psychiatrist oversees medical students, residents, or fellows.

These problems can be minimized by following certain guidelines. Clarify each therapist's respective responsibilities. For each patient, clarify whether you are the responsible therapist, supervisor, or consultant who gives advice only. Act within the scope of your responsibility. Read the notes of other health professionals involved in the care of the patient consistent with the scope of your relationship. Explain the therapists' responsibilities to the patient; e.g., "Even though we work in a group practice, I still carry the responsibility for your care. In some cases, I may request the advice of one of my colleagues, with your consent." When prescribing medications, you should see the patient often enough to monitor progress, generally every 3 months for a well-stabilized patient.

Obtain a contract that specifies your employer's legal liability for your supervisory and consultative work. For persons you supervise, ensure they are following the proper standard of care. Clarify the nature of your involvement (supervisor versus consultant) in the chart. When you countersign a treatment plan, progress note, or prescription, first indicate "under the supervision of" or "reviewed by." When job requirements preclude you from seeing the patient personally, prudence dictates that you note by your signature, "based on the information provided to me."

Avoiding Undue Familiarity

Although more of a problem in adult psychiatry, sexual involvement of therapists with adolescents does in fact occur.

> A 17-year-old girl exhibited seductive behavior toward her psychiatrist. When she was rebuked, she went to his house one night and threw rocks at his windows. Finally, the psychiatrist let her in, and a sexual encounter ensued. The parents, angered by the absence of professional ethics, filed a lawsuit.

To avoid undue-familiarity lawsuits, promote your personal well-being. Develop strong relationships with persons outside of professional work. Balance work, family, and other commitments. Talk with other mental health professionals about sustaining professional growth. Be aware of life changes that make psychiatrists vulnerable to sexual involvement. These include fatigue, boredom, professional isolation, unhappiness, mid-life crisis, troubled marriage, or troubled children.

Set clear boundaries. Monitor transference-countertransference. Be on the lookout for high-risk situations that might involve: a young, attractive patient or parent; seductive patient behaviors; therapist abuse of alcohol or drugs; or a patient diagnosed with borderline personality disorder.

When temptation strikes, reaffirm your own professional ethics: "I may have sexual thoughts and feelings about the patient, but I will not act on them." Ponder the consequences: "Having sex would be harmful to the patient. I may be sued. I may lose my license to practice medicine. My family will find out." Seek therapy if necessary.

Ethical Considerations and Financial Conflict of Interest

George Pallay, of Boca Raton, FL, and his wife became deadlocked in a bitter custody battle in 1987. During that time, his wife accused him of sexually abusing their three children, then 3, 8, and 9 years old. She succeeded in having the children committed to Fair Oaks Hospital in Boca-Delray. Despite George Pallay's protests, the hospital held the children for 5 weeks, resulting in a hospital bill of $70,000. Then, one day before the insurance benefits ran out, the hospital discharged the children to the parents' joint custody. In the divorce hearing, the judge ruled that the wife's charges of sexual abuse were groundless. George Pallay and the children filed a lawsuit against the hospital for unlawful restraint (*Newsweek*, May 14, 1992).

Reviewing this and other similar cases, Dr. Alan Stone, former president of the APA, noted that the welfare of patients is being eclipsed by marketplace incentives and pressures: "It is *the* major issue in psychiatric care today" (*Newsweek*, May 14, 1992).

In some parts of the United States, psychiatric hospitals are known to pay their high admitters a financial bonus. In Texas, several psychiatric hospitals paid "bounty hunters" (social workers, school counselors, and law enforcement personnel) to recruit children and adolescents, prompting an investigation by the state attorney general.[7] To participate in such practices is unethical and undermines the public's trust in the profession. Psychiatrists should not engage in self-referral or other similar practices.

Conclusion

Psychiatrists engaged in treating children and adolescents enjoy a relatively low malpractice risk. However, when a lawsuit is filed, the emotional impact on the therapist can be devastating. Following the recommendations presented in this lesson will help further reduce liability risk. More important, it will improve the quality of care provided to children and adolescents.

References

1. Slawson P. Psychiatric malpractice: ten years' loss experience. *Med Law.* 1989;8:415–427.
2. Wagner KD, et al. Malpractice litigation against child and adolescent psychiatry residency programs, 1981–1991. *J Am Acad Child Adolesc Psychiatry.* 1993;32:462–465.
3. Brizer DA. Predicting violence: current research and clinical approaches. *Psychiatr Malpract Risk Management.* 1992;2(3).
4. Motto JA. Management of the suicidal patient in clinical practice. *Psychiatr Malpract Risk Management.* 1992;2(2).
5. Hippocrates; Jones EHS, trans. *On Decorum and the Physician.* London, UK: William Heinemann; 1923;2.
6. *Code of Ethics.* Washington, DC: American Academy of Child and Adolescent Psychiatry; 1980.
7. Berry V. Psychiatric facilities. Presented at the 14th Annual Meeting of the American Society for Healthcare Risk Managers; Nov 10, 1992.

1 6

Protecting Others from Violence*

MICHAEL L. PERLIN, ESQ.

Editor's Note

If and when a physician or psychotherapist believes that a patient represents a real threat toward the physical well-being of another person, the courts have determined that he/she has a duty to warn the intended victim or others likely to apprise the potential victim of the danger, including the police. This obligation is not negated by the fact that no one, even the most skilled professional, can predict violence with absolute certainty.

Of course this mandate conflicts with the confidentiality which patients enjoy, also as a right. But the courts have ruled that, "The protective privilege ends where the public peril begins."

The famous Tarasoff decision has been extended to include victims of a class as well as specific victims; e.g., a serious threat to children. Another court has also extended the implications to include property damage, although such damage was related to an act of arson in which life could be endangered.

Another important point has been made. While one would not expect a nonmedical therapist to be held to the same standard of care as

---

*This section by Mr. Perlin is largely adapted from Chapter 13 of Perlin, *Mental Disability Law: Civil and Criminal* (©Kluwer Law Books, 1988).

CME questions for this chapter begin on page 363.

a medically trained one, nonmedical therapists cannot avoid liability if they have failed to make available to themselves medical information relevant to diagnosis and treatment.

Controversy and debate still surrounds this mandate.

Introduction

In addition to those malpractice and other tort cases brought by or on behalf of mentally disabled individuals as plaintiffs,[1] intense attention has recently focused on cases in which the mentally disabled are "third parties." In these instances either therapists or governmental officials are sued for failing to adequately protect individuals against the commission of tortious acts. In other words, although it is the act of the mentally disabled person that precipitated the lawsuit, the defendant is someone else.

By far the most important development in this area has been in the so-called "duty to protect" (often inappropriately labeled the "duty to warn") as first articulated in the important case of *Tarasoff v. Regents of the University of California*.[2] Subsequent cases either adopted, extended, distinguished, limited, or rejected *Tarasoff,* but, in each case, *Tarasoff* has clearly been the benchmark against which all other fact patterns have been assessed. This article will first examine *Tarasoff* in some depth, and will then consider its progeny, in an effort to clarify the current state of the law in this most volatile area.[3]

The Tarasoff Case

Prosenjit Poddar, a graduate student undergoing voluntary outpatient psychotherapy at the University of California hospital, told his therapist (Dr. Moore) that he intended to kill Tatiana Tarasoff, a young woman whom he had known and seen socially for several months a year before, but who did not share his view that the relationship was a serious one.[5] After the therapist (a psychologist) learned that Poddar—whom he viewed as "at times . . . quite rational, at other times . . . quite psychotic"[6]—planned to purchase a gun, he consulted with his supervisor (assistant to the director of the department of psychiatry) and the psychiatrist who had originally examined the patient. He then contacted the campus police (both orally and in writing) to ask for assistance in having Poddar committed.[7]

After the campus police officers took Poddar into custody, they questioned him, extracted a promise that he stay away from Tatiana, and released him without hospitalizing him (when they were satisfied that he was "rational").[8] Subsequently, the director of psychiatry at the university hospital (Dr. Powelson) "asked the police to return Moore's letter, directed that all copies of the letter and notes that Moore had taken as therapist be destroyed, and ∞ordered no action to place Prosenjit Poddar in 72-hour treatment and evaluation facility.∞"[9]

About two months later, Poddar went to Tatiana's home, and killed her.[10] Her parents subsequently filed suit against all relevant parties[11] on four separate tort theories, including the failure to warn of a dangerous patient (alleging that the defendants negligently permitted Poddar to be released from police custody "without notifying the parents . . . that their daughter was in grave danger from . . . Poddar").[12]

After the trial court dismissed the complaint, the plaintiffs appealed.[13] Initially,[14] the California Supreme Court found that a psychotherapist has a duty to warn when, "in the exercise of his professional skill and knowledge, [he or she] determines, or should determine, that a warning is essential to avert danger arising from the medical or psychological condition of his patient."[15] Following a request by the American Psychiatric Association and other professional organizations,[16] however, the Court agreed to rehear the case.

In its second opinion, the Court vacated its earlier decision, holding that a duty existed, but defining it more broadly and "with more latitude for professional judgment by the therapist."[17] Writing for a divided court, Justice Tobriner set out the case's holding:

> When a therapist determines, or pursuant to the standards of his profession should determine, that his patient presents a serious danger of violence to another, he incurs an obligation to use reasonable care to protect the intended victim against such danger. The discharge of this duty may require the therapist to take one or more of various steps, depending upon the nature of the case. Thus it may call for him to warn the intended victim or others likely to apprise the victim of the danger, to notify the policy, or to take whatever other steps are reasonably necessary under the circumstances.[18]

In coming to this conclusion, the Court examined several key factors. First, it asked whether plaintiff's interests were entitled to legal protection against the defendants' conduct, and concluded that the appropriate test was that if one person was placed in a position with regard to the other so that "if he did not use ordinary care and skill in his own conduct . . . he would cause danger of injury to the person or property of the other, a duty arises to use ordinary care and skill to avoid such danger."[19]

Factors to be balanced in assessing cases under this formula included, most importantly, the foreseeability of harm to the plaintiff,[20] the degree of certainty the plaintiff would suffer injury, the closeness of the connection between the defendant's conduct and the plaintiff's injury, the moral blameworthiness attached to defendant's conduct, the burden on the defendant, and the potential consequences to the community.[21]

Second, if avoidance of foreseeable harm requires a defendant to control the behavior of others or to warn, there will only be liability if the defendant bears a "special relationship"[22] to the dangerous person. The therapist-patient relationship satisfies this test, the Court found,[23] and a duty may thus be imposed on a therapist to exercise reasonable care to protect others against the dangers which might stem from a patient's mental illness. By entering into the therapist-patient relationship, the defendant "becomes sufficiently involved to assume some responsibility for the safety, not only of the patient himself, but also of any third person whom the doctor knows to be threatened by the patient."[24]

The Court rejected the defendants' argument that liability should not be allowed because mental health professionals could not accurately predict dangerousness:

> The role of the psychiatrist, who is indeed a practitioner of medicine, and that of the psychologist, who performs an allied function, are like that of the physician who must conform to the standards of the profession and who must often make diagnoses and predictions based upon such evaluations. Thus the judgment of the therapist in diagnosing emotional disorders and in predicting whether a patient presents a serious danger of violence is comparable to the judgment which doctors and professionals must regularly render under accepted rules of responsibility.[25]

Also, in the case before the Court, there was no question as to the failure of defendants to accurately *predict* that Poddar would harm Tatiana; the negligence alleged was in their failure to *warn* as to the ensuing harm.[26]

The adequacy of the therapist's conduct must be measured, the Court reasoned, "against the traditional negligence standard of the rendition of reasonable care under the circumstances,"[27] stressing that the ultimate question of "resolving the tension between the conflicting interests of patient and potential victim is one of social policy, not professional expertise."[28] Professional inaccuracy in predicting violence cannot negate the therapist's duty to protect the victim, the Court continued; the risk that unnecessary warnings would be given "is a reasonable price to pay for the lives of possible victims that may be saved."[29]

Rejecting the defendants' argument that the giving of such warnings would be a breach of trust, the Court countered that it was necessary to balance the patient's right to privacy with the public's interest in safety from violent assaults.[30] The Court noted a statutory exception to the psychotherapist's privilege in cases where the therapist had "reasonable cause to believe that the patient is in such mental or emotional condition as to be dangerous to himself or to the person or property of another and that disclosure of the communication is necessary to prevent the threatened danger":[31]

> We conclude that the public policy favoring protection of the confidential character of patient-psychotherapist communications must yield to the extent to which disclosure is essential to avert dangers to others. *The protective privilege ends where the public peril begins.*[31]

The police defendants, however, could not be held liable, because they had no "special relationship to either Tatiana or Poddar sufficient to impose upon such defendants a duty to warn respecting Poddar's violent intentions."[33]

Justice Mosk issued a separate opinion, concurring in part and dissenting in part, stressing that he concurred in the judgment "only because the complaints allege that defendant therapists *in fact* predict that Poddar would kill and were therefore negligent in failing to warn of that danger."[34] He parted company with the majority, however, regarding that aspect of the Court's holding which allowed for a finding of liability if a therapist failed to predict his patient's tendency to violence "if other practitioners pursuant to the ∞standards of the profession∞ would have done so."[35] Concluded Justice Mosk:

> I would restructure the rule designed by the majority to eliminate all reference to conformity to standards of the profession in predicting violence. If a psychiatrist does in fact predict violence, then a duty to warn arises. The majority's expansion of that rule will take us from the world of reality into the wonderland of clairvoyance.[36]

Justice Clark dissented (for himself and Justice McComb),[37] charging that imposition of the majority's "new duty is certain to result in a net increase in violence."[38] In addition, he read the pertinent statutory provisions[39] to reflect a "clear legislative policy"[40] against disclosure:

> Establishing a duty to warn on the basis of general tort principles imposes a Draconian dilemma on therapists—either violate the act thereby incurring the attendant statutory penalties,[41] or ignore the majority's duty to warn thereby incurring potential civil liability.[42]

The same result must be reached, he concluded, under a common law tort analysis. Confidentiality must be assured for three independent policy reasons: (1) without a "substantial assurance" of confidentiality, those requiring treatment will be deterred from seeking assistance;[43] (2) a guarantee of confidentiality is "essential" in eliciting the "full disclosure necessary for effective treatment";[44] and (3) without trust in a psychotherapist (in which an assurance of confidentiality is a prerequisite), treatment will be frustrated and most likely will not be successful.[45]

Finally, by imposing a duty to warn, the dissent concluded, "the majority contributes to the danger to society of violence by the mentally ill and greatly increases the risk of civil commitment—the total deprivation of liberty—of those who should not be confined."[46]

Because of the "predictive uncertainty"[47] and the concomitant large number of necessary disclosures, treatment will be necessarily impaired: "neither alternative open to the psychiatrist seeking to protect himself"—warn or commit—"is in the public interest."[48]

The Critical Response to Tarasoff[49]

The *Tarasoff* decision immediately unleashed a "torrent"[50] of "profuse academic comment"[51] and analysis, a significant portion of which was severely critical. Psychiatric commentators[52] attacked the opinion as an unwarranted "judicial intrusion [into] private psychotherapeutic practice"[53] for three major reasons:[54] (1) it was premised on the "false view"[55] that valid professional standards enabling psychotherapists to accurately predict future violence did exist; (2) it compromised confidentiality which was essential to successful psychotherapy;[56] and (3) by raising the therapist's obligation to the public over the obligation to the individual patient, it compromised "central professional ethical precepts."[57]

Those legal commentators who took issue with the California Court's decision focused most closely on confidentiality issues, generally predicting that the decision would reduce the success of therapy by (1) decreasing patients' trust in their therapists, (2) discouraging patients from communicating sensitive information because of fear of subsequent disclosure, and (3) causing patients to terminate treatment when they learn that breaches of confidentiality could have occurred or did occur.[58] At least one student note viewed the decision as, perhaps, a therapeutic Armageddon: *Tarasoff* "may have precipitated the decline of effective psychotherapy in California."[59]

Not all legal commentary was so harsh, however. Professor Merton focused on the law/psychiatry role conflicts which appeared to be inevitably "exacerbate[d]"[60] by *Tarasoff,* and noted that the decision "seems to have brought home to many psychiatrists the double-bind quality of their professional obligations," and that it may require psychiatrists to act "collectively, to develop a consensus that simply will not permit certain practices,"[61] such as the common (if discredited) long-term prediction of dangerousness at criminal sentencing hearings. And, in a somewhat different context, Professors Shuman and Weiner have suggested that the need for absolute confidentiality in the context of the physician–patient relationship has been "overstated" by its proponents.[62]

Tarasoff's *Progeny*[63]

Subsequent decisions have been far from unanimous in their construction of *Tarasoff*. Some cases have, with slight modifications, adopted its holding, others have extended its reach (as to the identifiability of victim and forseeability of harm), others have factually distinguished or limited it (on both identifiability and forseeability issues), while several cases have declined to follow it.

Nonetheless, in spite of the fact that, as of 1985, only seven jurisdictions outside of California have explicitly adopted and applied the *Tarasoff* duty in the decade since the case was decided, *Tarasoff*'s symbolic value is so compelling that no one has questioned Dr. Beck's conclusion that the *Tarasoff* duty to protect "is, in effect, at present a national standard of practice."[64]

Adopting *Tarasoff*:

In the case closest to *Tarasoff* on a factual level, a New Jersey trial court substantially adopted the California court's statement of psychotherapeutic duty to third parties in a wrongful death action brought against a psychiatrist (Milano) after one of his patient's (Morgenstein) murdered the plaintiffs' (McIntoshes') daughter (Kimberly).[65]

In denying the defendant's motion for summary judgment at the ensuing civil trial, the Court generally adopted the *Tarasoff* formulation, focusing on the question of the predictivity of dangerousness:

It may be true that there cannot be 100% accurate prediction of dangerousness in all cases. However, a therapist does have a basis for giving an opinion and a prognosis based on the history of the patient and the course of treatment. Where reasonable men might differ and a fact issue exists, the therapist is only held to the standard for a therapist in the particular field in the community. Unless therapists clearly state when called upon to treat patients or to testify that they have no ability to predict or even determine whether their treatment will be efficacious or may even be necessary with any degree of certainty, there is no basis for a legal conclusion negating any and all duty with respect to a particular class of professionals. This is not to say that isolated or vague threats will of necessity give rise in all circumstances and cases to a duty. Whether a duty for a therapist to warn or guard against a criminal or tortious event by a patient to some third party, depends, as with other situations giving rise to a possible legal obligation to exercise due care, ultimately on questions of fairness involving a weighing of the relationship of the parties, the nature of the risk involved, and the public interest in imposing the duty under the circumstances. . . . [66]

The court then summarized its holding:

[A] psychiatrist or therapist may have a duty to take whatever steps are reasonably necessary to protect an intended or potential victim of his patient when he determines, or should determine, in the appropriate factual setting and in accordance with the standards of his profession established at trial, that the patient is or may present a probability of danger to that person. The relationship giving rise to that duty may be found either in that existing between the therapist and the patient, as was alluded to in *Tarasoff* . . . , or in the more broadly-based obligation a practitioner may have to protect the welfare of the community, which is analogous to the obligation a physician has to warn third persons of infectious or contagious disease.[67]

Extending *Tarasoff*:

In other cases, courts have extended the *Tarasoff* duty where the victim was a young child of a threatened victim[68] even where no specific victim has been threatened (on the theories that forseeable violence may involve a "class of persons at risk,"[69] and therapists have a duty "to take reasonable precautions to protect *anyone* who might forseeably be endangered" by the patient in question).[70]

Perhaps most importantly, the Vermont Supreme Court, in *Peck v. Counseling Service of Addison County*,[71] has enlarged the *Tarasoff* duty to include *all* "mental health professionals" in a case involving property, not personal, injury, holding that a "mental health professional who knows or, based upon the standards of the mental health profession, should know that his or her patient poses a serious risk of danger to an identifiable victim has a duty to exercise reasonable care to protect him or her from that danger."[72] Although only property damage was involved, the court noted that arson "is a violent act and represents a lethal threat to human beings, who may be in the vicinity of the conflagration."[73]

Peck is significant for several reasons.[74] First, no other post-*Tarasoff* case has extended its holding to property damage questions.[75] Second, the extension of duty to therapists in addition to psychiatrists and individuals with doctorates in clinical psychology (under state law, a mental health professional includes "a person with professional training, experience and demonstrated competence in the treatment of mental illness, who shall be a physician, psychologist, social worker, nurse or other qualified person designated by the commissioner of mental health"[76]) places the duty to warn on a whole range of therapists, including those not specifically enumerated in the statute in question.

Third, the decision raises important questions as to what professional standard of care[77] is to be used in the case of a "generic *mental health practitioner*."[78] Expert medical testimony was produced at the trial indicating that the patient suffered from temporal lobe epilepsy. While it might be argued that a non-medical counselor should not be held to the same standard of care as a physician in the treatment and management of such a patient, that question became "irrelevant"[79] when testimony showed that the therapist "was not in possession of [the patient's] most recent medical history" because the counseling service had neither a cross-reference system between its therapists and outside physicians nor written policies "concerning formal intra-staff consultation procedures when a patient presented a serious risk of harm to another."[80]

Concludes Stone in his pessimistic analysis of the *Peck* case:

> The smell of the Vermont-expanded *Tarasoff* decision is in the air. Every mental health professional now faces the Tarasoff dilemma: is it in my interest to avoid potential liability by warning potential victims of the potential violence and fire setting of my patient-client?[81]

Distinguishing *Tarasoff:*

Several courts have found that, while there is a general *Tarasoff* duty, it is inapplicable in specific cases where there was either no identified victim,[82] where the therapist lacked control over the patient in question,[83] or where the therapist could have reasonably believed that the patient's fantasies did not pose a danger to an identifiable victim.[84]

Declining to Follow *Tarasoff:*

On the other hand, several jurisdictions[85] have declined to follow the California Supreme Court and impose a *Tarasoff* duty to warn, either—or instead—limiting the scope of *Tarasoff*[86] or rejecting it.[87] The latter decision, however, appears to focus on "failure to confine" rather than "duty to warn."[88] There, where the court declined to find liability in a case where a voluntary outpatient killed someone 14 months after his last date of treatment, it ruled that the plaintiff would have to show "more than a mere possibility that the patient would be very likely to cause harm to himself or to others."[89]

References

1. See generally, Sections 1, 2, & 3, *supra* (this volume).
2. 17 Cal. 3d 425, 131 Cal. Rptr. 14, 551 P. 2d 334 (Sup. Ct. 1976).
3. In addition to the issues raised and discussed here, there have been other important "third party" cases involving questions of premature release, failure to control mentally disabled petitioners or parolees, acts of patients on conditional leave from institutions, and failure to appropriately prosecute involuntary civil commitment applications. These are beyond the scope of this article. See generally, Perlin, *Mental Disability Law: Civil and Criminal* §§13.14 to .19 (©Kluwer Law Books 1988).
4. Although Tatiana was not named by Poddar, she was "readily identifiable" by his description. *Tarasoff,* 131 Cal. Rptr. at 21.
5. *People v. Poddar,* 10 Cal. 3d 750, 111 Cal. Rptr. 910, 912, 518 P. 2d 342 (Sup. Ct. 1974).
6. *Tarasoff v. Regents of the University of California,* 33 Cal. App. 3d 275, 108 Cal. Rptr. 878, 880 (Ct. App. 1973), rev'd 13 Cal. 3d 177. 118 Cal. Rptr. 129. 529 P. 2d 553 (Sup. Ct. 1974), mod. 17 Cal. 3d 425, 131 Cal. Rptr. 14, 551 P. 2d 334 (Sup. Ct. 1976).
7. *Tarasoff,* 131 Cal. Rptr. at 21.
8. *Id.*
9. *Id.*
10. See generally, *Poddar, supra.*
11. Defendants are listed in *Tarasoff,* 131 Cal. Rptr. at 20 n.2.

12. *Id*. at 21. In addition, plaintiffs also sued on three independent tort theories: (1) the failure to detain a dangerous patient; (2) abandonment of dangerous patient (seeking punitive damages only from defendant Powelson on this count); and (3) breach of primary duty to a patient and the public (stating basically the same allegations as the first count, but characterizing defendants' conduct as a breach of duty "to safeguard their patient and the public." *Id*. at 20–21.

13. *Id*. at 20.

14. But see *Tarasoff*, 131 Cal. Rptr. at 22.

15. *Tarasoff*, 118 Cal. Rptr. at 131.

16. See generally, Mills & Beck, "The *Tarasoff* Case," in Beck, ed., *The Potentially Violent Patient and the Tarasoff Decision in Psychiatric Practice* 1, 4–5 (1985) (Beck).

17. *Id*. at 5.

18. *Tarasoff*, 131 Cal. Rptr. at 20.

19. *Id*. at 22, quoting *Rowland v. Christian*, 69 Cal. 2d 108, 70 Cal. Rptr. 97, 443 P. 2d 561 (Sup. Ct. 1968), quoting *Heaven v. Pender*, 11 Q.B.D. 503, 509 (1883).

20. A defendant owes a duty of care "to all persons who are forseeably endangered by his conduct, with respect to all risks which make the conduct unreasonably dangerous." *Tarasoff*, 131 Cal. Rptr. at 22, quoting, *inter alia, Rodriguez v. Bethlehem Steel Corp.*, 12 Cal. 3d 382, 115 Cal. Rptr. 765, 776, 525 P. 2d 669 (Sup. Ct. 1974).

21. *Tarasoff*, 131 Cal. Rptr. at 22.

22. *Id*. at 23: see *Restatement (Second) of Torts* (1965), at §315.

23. *Tarasoff*, 131 Cal. Rptr. at 23-24.

24. *Id*. at 24, quoting Fleming & Maximov, "The Patient or His Victim: The Therapist's Dilemma," 62 *Calif. L. Rev*. 1025, 1030 (1974).

25. *Tarasoff*, 131 Cal. Rptr. at 25.

26. *Id*.

27. *Id*.

28. *Id*., quoting Fleming & Maximov, *supra* note 24, at 1067.

29. *Tarasoff*, 131 Cal. Rptr. at 26.

30. *Tarasoff*, 131 Cal. Rptr. at 26.

31. *Id*. at 27, quoting *Calif. Evid. Code* §1024 (1965).

32. *Tarasoff*, 131 Cal. Rptr. at 27 (emphasis added).

33. *Id*. at 29. Finally, the court rejected defendant therapists' argument that they were statutorily immune, see *Calif. Gov't Code* § 820.2 (1980), declaring that "a public employee is not liable for an injury resulting from his act or omission which was the result of the exercise of the discretion vested in him, whether or not such discretion [was] abuse," construing state law to provide such immunity only in the cases of "basic policy decisions," *Tarasoff*, 131 Cal. Rptr. at 29, quoting *Johnson v. State of California*, 69 Cal. 2d 782, 73 Cal. Rptr. 240, 447 P. 2d 352 (Sup. Ct. 1968), and concluding that its scope "should be no greater than is required to give legislative and executive policymakers sufficient breathing space in which to perform their vital policymaking functions," *Tarasoff*, 131 Cal. Rptr. at 30. This, the court concluded, required of publicly em-

ployed therapists "only that quantum of care which the common law requires of private therapists." *Id.* at 31. On the other hand, the court found (1) defendant therapists statutorily immune—see *Calif. Gov't Code* §856 (1980)—from liability for failure to *confine* Poddar (noting the need to protect therapists "who must undertake this delicate and difficult task"). *id.,* citing Fleming & Maximov, *supra* note 24, at 1064, (2) defendant police officers statutorily immune— see *Calif. Welf. & Instn. Code* §5154(c) (1986 Supp.)—from liability for *their* failure to confine Poddar (nothing that, while campus police were not strictly "peace officers" within the controlling statutory language, they *were* "responsible for [Poddar's] detainment" within the same phrase), *id.* at 33, and (3) no cause of action for punitive damages under state law in a wrongful death action. *Id.,* citing *Pease v. Beech Aircraft Corp.,* 38 Cal. App. 3d 450, 113 Cal.. Rptr. 416 (Ct. App. 1974). The case never went to trial on remand, but settled on terms "within the range for wrongful death of a college girl." Merton, "Confidentiality and the ∞Dangerous, Patient: Implications of *Tarasoff* for Psychiatrists and Lawyers," 31 *Emory L. J.* 263, 295 (1982).

34. *Id.* at 33 (Mosk, J., concurring and dissenting) (emphasis added): Thus, the issue here is very narrow: we are not concerned with whether the therapists, pursuant to the standards of their professions "should have" predicted potential violence; they allegedly did so in actuality.

35. *Id.* at 34. Asked Justice Mosk rhetorically, "The question is, what standards?" *Id.,* relying on *People v. Burnick,* 14 Cal. 3d 306. 121 Cal. Rptr. 488.535 P. 2d 352 (Sup. Ct. 1975), to demonstrate that "psychiatric predictions of violence are inherently unreliable." *Tarasoff,* 131 Cal. Rptr. at 34.

36. *Id.*

37. *Id.* at 34 (Clark, J., dissenting).

38. *Id.* at 35.

39. See id. at 35–38.

40. *Id.*

41. See *Calif. Welf. & Instn. Code* §5330(2) (1984), providing for treble damage recovery for unlawful confidential disclosures. See *Tarasoff,* 131 Cal. Rptr. at 35.

42. *Id.* at 38.

43. *Tarasoff,* 131 Cal . Rptr. at 39, citing, *inter alia,* Fisher, "The Psychotherapeutic Professions and the Law of Privileged Communications," 10 *Wayne L. Rev.* 609 (1974); Rappeport, "Psychiatrist-Patient Privilege," 23 *Md. L. J.* 39 (1963).

44. *Tarasoff,* 131 Cal. Rptr. at 39, citing, *inter alia, In re Lifschutz,* 2 Cal. 3d 415. 85 Cal. Rptr. 829, 467 P. 2d 557 (Sup. Ct. 1970)

45. *Tarasoff,* 131 Cal. Rptr. at 39 40, citing, *inter alia,* Dawidoff, "The Malpractice of Psychiatrists," [1966] *Duke L. J.* 696.

46. *Tarasoff,* 131 Cal. Rptr. at 40.

47. *Id.* at 41.

48. *Id.* at 41. Soon after the *Tarasoff* decision. California legislators drafted a series of bills intended to mitigate the decision's impact, culminating in the 1984 introduction of A.B. 2900, which would have granted statutory immunity to psychotherapists for failing to "warn of and protect from" a patient's actual or

threatened violent behavior except where the patient communicated an "actual threat of physical violence against a reasonably identifiable victim or victims." See Comment, "Psychotherapists' Duty to Warn: Ten Years After *Tarasoff*," 15 *Golden Gate U. L. Rev.* 271. 292 n.160 (1985) ("Golden Gate Comment"). The bill was supported by mental health professional associations, but was opposed by the Citizens' Commission on Human Rights. which characterized it has "an emotional piece of legislation which open[ed] the door to potential violence by removing current protection afforded the public." *Id.* at 293–295. Although the bill was passed by the legislature, it was vetoed by California's governor who feared that it would increase the likelihood of danger to the public and perhaps "excuse conduct which should be actionable." *Id.* In 1985, the bill was reintroduced with two significant changes. In place of the phrase "an actual threat of physical violence," the new bill substituted "a serious threat of physical violence." Also, the duty could be discharged not only by making reasonable efforts to communicate to the victim, but also, in the alternative, "to a law enforcement agency." See *Calif. Civil Code* §43.92 (1986 Supp.). With these changes, the bill was signed and became effective January 1, 1986. See "New California Law Limits Therapists' Liability for Violent Acts Committed By Their Patients," 37 *Hosp. & Commun. Psych.* 87 (1986); there has been no subsequent reported litigation as of yet.

49. On the questions of *Tarasoff*'s empirical impact, of suggested therapeutic approaches in its wake, and of the concomitant rise of "victimology," see Perlin, *supra* note 2, §§13.10 to .13; see generally Wexler, "Patients, Therapists, and Third Parties: The Victimological Virtues of *Tarasoff*," 2 *Int'l J. L. & Psych. I* (1979). See generally, Sadoff, *Commentary on Protecting Others from Violence*, this section.

50. George *et al.*, "The Therapist's Duty to Protect Third Parties: A Guide for the Perplexed." 14 *Rutgers L. J.* 637 (1983) (George).

51. See Note, "Discovery of Psychotherapist-Patient Communications After *Tarasoff*," 15 *San Diego L. Rev.* 265, 266 (1978), and *id.*, 266–267 n.8 (listing articles).

52. At least one review of the literature has noted that criticism of *Tarasoff* was especially strong by psychiatrists who "advocate psychoanalytic therapy." George, *supra* note 50, at 637.

53. Givelber, Bowers & Blitch, "The *Tarasoff* Controversy: A Summary of Findings From an Empirical Study of Legal, Ethical, and Clinical Issues" (Givelber). in Beck, *supra* note 16, at 35, 37.

54. See, *e.g.*, Stone, "The *Tarasoff* Decision: Suing Psychotherapists to Safeguard Security," 90 *Harv. L. Rev.* 358 (1976) (Stone I); Gurevitz, "*Tarasoff*, Protective Privilege Versus Public Peril," 134 *Am. J. Psych.* 289 (1976); Roth & Meisel, "Dangerousness, Confidentiality, and the Duty to Warn," 134 *Am. J. Psych.*, 508 (1977).

55. Givelber, *supra* note 53, at 37.

56. See generally, Dubey, "Confidentiality as a Requirement for the Therapist: Technical Necessities for Absolute Privilege in Psychotherapy," 131 *Am. J. Psych.* 1093 (1974).

57. Givelber, *supra* note 53, at 37.
58. Note, "Where the Public Peril Begins: A Survey of Psychotherapists to Determine the Effects of *Tarasoff*," 31 *Stand. L. Rev.* 165, 166 n.9 (1978); See e.g., sources cited at "Golden Gate Comment," *supra* note 48, at 272 n.7.
59. Note, "*Tarasoff v. Regents of the University of California:* The Duty to Warn: Common Law & Statutory Problems for California Psychotherapists," 14 *Cal. West. L. Rev.* 153 (1978). Concluded the author, "Mental health care and psychotherapy must survive in spite of *Tarasoff.*" *Id.* at 181.
60. Merton, *supra* note 33, at 341.
61. *Id.* at 276.
62. Shuman & Weiner, "The Privilege Study: An Empirical Examination of the Psychotherapist-Patient Privilege" 60 *No. Car. L. Rev.* 893, 927 (1982).
63. For a helpful discussion of the cases discussed below, see Beck, "The Psychotherapist and the Violent Patient: Recent Case Law" (Beck II), in Beck, *supra* note 16, at 9.
64. Beck II, *supra* note 63, at 33. "[M]ost commentators agree that all psychiatrists should practice as if the *Tarasoff* duty to protect is the law." *Id. Cf.* Roth & Levin, "Dilemma of *Tarasoff:* Must Physicians Protect the Public or Their Patients?" 11 *L., Med . & Health Care* 104, 110 (1983) (*Tarasoff* doctrine has been adopted "from coast to coast"). *Tarasoff* issues continue to emerge in "new" jurisdictions. See, *e.g.,* Marcus, "Case Underlines Psychiatric Issue: To Keep Confidences or Report Threats," *N. Y. Times* (May 23, 1986), at A10 (discussing recent Louisiana case).
65. 168 N.J. Super. 466, 403 A. 2d 500 (Law Div. 1979). The *McIntosh* case is discussed extensively in Perlin, *supra* note 2, §13.06.
66. *McIntosh,* 403 A. 2d at 508 (footnotes and citations omitted).
67. *Id.* at 511–512. The *Tarasoff* duty has also been adopted in state and federal cases in Michigan and in the Ninth Circuit. See, *e.g., Davis v. Lhim,* 124 Mich. App. 291, 335 N.W. 2d 481 (Ct. App. 1983), *Chrite v. United States,* 564 F. Supp. 34 1 (E.D. Mich. 1983), *Jablonski v. United States,* 712 F. 2d 391 (9 Cir. 1983). *Davis* and *Chrite* are discussed in Givelber, *supra* note 53, at 14–16, *Jablonski* is discussed in Meyers, "The Legal Perils of Psychotherapeutic Practice (Part 11): Coping with *Hedlund* and *Jablonski,*" 12 *J. Psych. & L.* 39, 40–41 (1984).
68. *Hedlund v. Superior Court of Orange County,* 34 Cal. 3d 695, 194 Cal. Rptr. 805, 669 P. 2d 41 (Sup. Ct. 1983).
69. *Lipari v. Sears, Roebuck & Co.,* 497 F. Supp. 185, 187 (D. Neb. 1980).
70. *Petersen v. Washington,* 100 Wash. 2d 421, 671 P. 2d 230, 237 (Sup. Ct. 1983) (following *Lipari*).
71. *Peck v. Counseling Service of Addison County,* 146 Vt. 61, 499 A. 2d 422 (Sup. Ct. 1985).
72. *Id.* at 427. As Vermont is a comparative negligence case, the trial court had found John's father 50% negligent because he knew his son would be "enraged" if asked to falsify his benefits application. *Id.* This finding was affirmed by the Supreme Court. *Id.*
73. *Id.* at 424 n.3.

74. For a detailed analysis of *Peck*, see Stone, "Vermont Adopts *Tarasoff*: A Real Barn-Burner," 143 *Am. J. Psych.* 352 (1986) (Stone II).

75. See, *e.g.*, Leong, "*Tarasoff* and Property Damage," 143 *Am. J. Psych.* 1488 (1986) (letter to the editor) (*Peck* has "ominous implications for the practice of psychiatry"). *Cf. Bellah v. Greeson*, 73 Cal. App. 3d 911. 141 Cal. Rptr. 92, 94–95 (Ct. App. 1977) (refusing to extend *Tarasoff* to property damage or suicide).

76. *Vt. Stat. Ann.* 18 §7101 (2) (1984 Supp.)

77. See generally, Section 1, *supra* (this volume).

78. Stone II, *supra* note 74, at 354.

79. *Id.*

80. *Peck*, 499 A. 2d at 426.

81. Stone II, *supra* note 74, at 354–355 (emphasis in original).

82. See, *e.g.*, *Thompson v. County of Alameda*, 27 Cal. 3d 741. 167 Cal. Rptr. 70, 614 P. 2d 728 (Sup. Ct. 1980); see also, *Leedy v. Hartnett*, 510 F. Supp. 1125 (M.D. Pa. 1981), aff'd o.b. 676 F. 2d 686 (3 Cir. 1982), *Holmes v. Wampler*, 546 F. Supp. 599 (E.D. Va. 1982); *Furr v. Spring Grove State Hospital*, 53 Md. App. 474, 454 A. 2d 414 (Ct. Spec. App. 1983); *Cairl v. State*, 323 N.W. 2d 20 (Minn. Sup. Ct. 1982).

83. See, *e.g.*, *Hasenei v. United States*, 541 F. Supp. 999 (D. Md. 1982); *Brady v. Hopper*, 570 F. Supp. 1333 (D. Colo. 1983), aff'd 751 F. 2d 329 (10 Cir. 1984).

84. See *White v. United States*, 780 F. 2d 97 (D.C. Cir. 1986).

85. In addition to the cases discussed below, see also, *Hopewell v. Adibempe, Pitt. L. J.* 107, No. G.D. 78–2875 (Pa. Ct. C.P. 181), discussed in Beck II, *supra* note 63, at 30–31, and in Klein & Glover, "Psychiatric Malpractice," 6 *Int'l J. L. & Psych*, 131. 153 n.59 (1983) (premising its holding on a state confidentiality statute), and *Schneider v. Vine Street Clinic*, No. 15344 (111. App. Ct. 1979), discussed in Merton, *supra* note 33. at 328–329.

86. See *Shaw v. Glickman*, 45 Md. App. 718, 415 A. 2d 625 (Ct. Spec. App. 1980), a decision characterized by Professor Menon as "frustratingly opaque." Merton, *supra* note 33, at 326. The *Shaw* case's facts were described floridly by the appellate court:
    This case concerns a new strand to an old yarn, the eternal triangle. It is new in that in addition to the usual cast, *le mari, la femme, et l'amant* (the husband, the wife, and the lover), new characters, the husband's "psychiatric team" have been joined as parties. In fact, the "team" has been sued for injuries inflicted on *l'amant* by *le mari*. *Shaw, supra*.

87. See *Case v. United States*, 523 F. Supp. 317 (S.D. Ohio 1981), aff'd o.b. 709 F. 2d 1500 (6 Cir. 1983).

88. *Case v. United States*, 523 F. Supp. 317 (S.D. Ohio 1981) aff'd o.b. 709 F. 2d 1500 (6 Cir. 1983).

89. *Id.* at 319. In the course of its opinion. the court simply stated that plaintiff's citation to *Tarasoff* was "not controlling," *id.* at 318, and that that case "stands almost alone in its holding," *id.* n.1.

Protecting Others from Violence

ROBERT L. SADOFF, M.D.

Editor's Note

Even though psychiatrists may not be able to predict dangerousness per se, they may be able to predict imminent violent behavior as a part of a clinical pattern of behavior. Hence, as far as possible, they should restrict their willingness to testify as experts to what they can legitimately address.

Patients who are both mentally ill and present a clear and present danger of harm to self or others may be committed. However, when the time for discharge comes, the doctors must face a special challenge. For example, what if the patient is no longer mentally ill, in the strict sense of the term, but still poses a threat of violence? Certainly, a careful assessment of risk should be carried out, as in the case of suicidal patients, and carefully recorded. In most states, persons who have been violent and found "not guilty by reason of insanity" may not be discharged by the psychiatrists alone, but only after a hearing in court.

Introduction

The prediction of violence has been studied, evaluated, assessed, and determined by a number of writers. Perhaps the most important contribution to the prediction of violent behavior is the study by Monahan and colleagues, who ultimately concluded psychiatrists cannot predict dangerousness, per se, but may be able to predict imminent violent behavior or violence as part of a clinical pattern of behavior.[1] Long-range predictions of violent behavior are inadequate, inaccurate, and invalid.

Psychiatrists should not be held to a standard of long-range predictions that courts have imposed upon them in some cases. Because studies have shown psychiatrists cannot successfully predict over the long term, expert psychiatric testimony will be consistent with that lack of expertise. Courts need to learn what psychiatrists can and cannot do. Without supporting expert psychiatric testimony, the courts will not be able to hold psychiatrists liable for long-term predictions.

The confusion in psychiatry and law appears to lie in the definition of dangerousness and violence. The mental health legislation involving commitment states that patients who are both mentally ill and a clear and present danger of harm to self or others may be committed involuntarily. This rule supplanted the previous guideline that a person may be involuntarily committed if he were both mentally ill and in need of hospitalization. The current ruling involves the concept of dangerousness. Psychiatrists cooperate with the law. They frequently testify in commitment cases that a patient is both mentally ill and "dangerous." Many psychiatrists have explained they do not know what "dangerous" means and would prefer not to testify to the concept of dangerousness. However, they complain, the judge, by law, has required such testimony. As a result, psychiatrists have frequently established themselves as experts on dangerousness by testifying that a particular patient is dangerous and, therefore, requires involuntary hospitalization.

The danger of such testimony lies in the concept of dangerousness and its confused definition and interpretation among many judges and courts. The psychiatrist may be in a position to testify that a particular patient at a particular time represents a clear and present danger of harm to self or others because of his mental illness and his verified behavior. That psychiatrist is not, however, an expert on the prediction of dangerousness nor is he able to predict when people who are mentally ill will become violent or dangerous. As a result of the change in mental health law to require the testimony of psychiatrists about dangerous patients, a number of consequences have negatively affected psychiatry and psychiatrists.

Assessing the Potential for Violence in Patients

The first consequence with a negative impact on psychiatry involves the release of patients who had been committed as mentally ill and dangerous. When is the patient no longer dangerous? Is the violent behavior directly related to his mental illness, or are they two separate issues? If the patient's mental illness is not related to his violent behavior, then when he goes into remission of his acute psychotic illness, he may be eligible for discharge. However, he may still present a risk of violent behavior unrelated to his psychotic condition. If the psychiatrist discharges the patient from the hospital, since he can no longer obtain medical benefit in that setting, he is assuming a risk that is unwarranted. The patient may go out and harm someone, and the doctor may well be charged with negligence for prematurely releasing a dangerous patient into the community.

The doctor, then, assumes the mantle as the expert on the prediction of nondangerousness. There are guidelines the psychiatrist may follow that would indicate whether a patient may become violent to others in the near future. This is not to assume that he has guidelines on the "dangerousness" of his patient, however. He may use the same standards and guidelines that he uses in predicting suicidal behavior. At Level One, the patient may be thinking about harming someone else. For the Level Two patient, his thoughts concern harming someone in particular. At Level Three, the patient has the means by which he can harm that particular person, and at Level Four, the patient has attempted to harm or has threatened to harm that person in the past.

Other factors to be considered include the relationship of the patient to the person he wishes to harm; the environment in which the patient will be placed, which may be conducive to further violent behavior; and the presence or absence of mental illness, which may distort the patient's thinking regarding the potential victim.

In several cases, psychiatrists have released patients to the community only to see them commit a violent act. Sometimes, they have killed family members; other times, they have killed strangers in a violent rage. In many cases, the psychiatrist and the hospital were charged with prematurely releasing a violent person into the community. In some of those cases, the court found no liability on the part of the hospital or the doctor because there was no means by which the psychiatrist could determine that the patient was potentially violent. In other cases, the court found the doctor and/or the hospital liable because there were clear indications by the patient that he was going to harm somebody else, and threatened to do so throughout his hospitalization. The standard of care requires that appropriate questions be asked of the patient to determine whether he has the potential for violent behavior in the imminent future. Those questions ought to be recorded in the chart, and the responses noted. They are the essential elements that attorneys who review the chart following a violent act by a former patient will look for in determining whether there is a valid lawsuit. If the record shows the patient had been violent in the past, precautions should be taken at discharge to advise protection against similar conditions or clinical situations that may foster similar violent behavior.

Assessing the Potential for Violence in Outpatients

In the case of *Brady v. Hopper,*[2] the plaintiffs charged that Dr. Hopper was negligent in his care of John W. Hinckley, Jr., in that he knew, or should have known, Hinckley was going to attempt to harm someone in authority in order to impress Jodie Foster. They charged the doctor with responsibility for the damage that resulted from the shooting of President Reagan by Hinckley in 1981. The lower Federal Court and the Court of Appeals did not agree with the complaint, and dismissed the charges. However, some attorneys believe psychiatrists are responsible for the behavior of their outpatients, should have better control over them, and should be aware of a patient's intention to harm someone else. Those are general cases, without specific third parties involved. The issue is raised in order to illustrate the risks that psychiatrists bear in treating potentially violent outpatients. Again, the guidelines include the careful questioning of the patient, who may have a violent history, to determine whether he has current thoughts of harming others, and if he wishes to harm anyone in particular. The questions and responses should be recorded in the patient's chart as bases for the clinical decision making.

The Noncompliant, Potentially Violent Patient

If a patient who has a history of violent behavior is in remission from his acute mental illness, is sent for outpatient treatment, and has a history of noncompliance with his medication or follow-up visits, what is the responsibility of the psychiatrist? Is the psychiatrist to reach out into the community and bring the patient to the clinic for treatment and injection of long-acting psychotropic medication, or is he to leave the patient alone, as many lawyers contend is the patient's right? There have been conflicts in philosophy and in practice about this issue. If the patient harms someone else when he is "written off the books" as noncompliant, is the doctor and/or hospital or mental health clinic responsible for his behavior?

Some attorneys have argued that the psychiatrist has a responsibility to reach into the community and treat the patient when there is a history of previous violent behavior. Others have argued against it, because it violates the patient's right to be left alone if he is not currently violent. No clear cases have been found on this subject yet, but there appears to be a trend that favors the outreach approach. The patient would be deemed incompetent to determine for himself the treatment he needs and would not be in a position to know that if he does not take his medication, he is likely to become violent. The psychiatrist may then be seen as the protector of society, bringing the treatment to the patient if the patient will not come in for his treatment.

It should be noted that despite the studies by psychiatrists, psychologists, and attorneys about the inability of psychiatrists to predict future violent behavior, especially over the long term, the courts have deemed the psychiatrist the expert in such predictions in criminal cases. The leading case is that of *Barefoot v. Estelle*,[5] in which the U.S. Supreme Court, two years after its decision in *Estelle v. Smith*[6] (indicating that a psychiatrist may not testify at the sentencing phase of a criminal case leading to the death penalty if he has not warned the defendant that he may be called to so testify), stated that in a case in which the psychiatrist did not even examine the patient, he may testify at the sentencing phase to the hypothetical question of whether the defendant is dangerous and a psychopath and, therefore, eligible to receive the death penalty. Over the objections of the Amicus Brief of the American Psychiatric Association, the court stated the judicial system was not concerned whether psychiatrists *believed* they could predict such dangerousness; it held the position that the court would tell the psychiatrists what they could do in court. In essence, the U.S. Supreme Court has declared psychiatrists to be experts in the prediction of dangerousness, and they will be held to such a standard.

Therefore, it is strongly suggested that psychiatrists who testify in court do not use the word "dangerous." Psychiatrists may testify on a particular patient's involuntary hospitalization, his mental illness, and his imminent violence or potential violence under specific, enumerated clinical conditions. Thus, the psychiatrist remains a clinician and couches his testimony in clinical terms or in imminent-violence terms, which is part of his expertise. To do other than that, in my opinion, goes beyond psychiatric expertise and should not be allowed in court. The risks of testifying to dangerousness include all of the problems noted above regarding malpractice by psychiatrists. In order to avoid appearing as experts on "dangerousness," which we are not, we should restrict our comments to clinical concepts, such as violent behavior or self-destructive behavior.

Another potentially useful recommendation is to administratively separate, on commitment, those individuals who are mentally ill and suicidal from those who are mentally ill and violent toward others. It is suggested and recommended that all patients who are violent toward others not be discharged from the hospital by the psychiatrist alone, but by a rule of court. In most states, by law, persons found not guilty by reason of insanity may not be discharged by the psychiatrist alone, but only after a hearing in court. We have thus recognized violence is more a community issue than a psychiatric one.

It is essential for psychiatrists to educate others regarding our limitations of expertise as well as what we are able to do. We have no expertise in the prediction of long term violence, and should not be held to a standard of such prediction. We must differentiate between violence to others and self-destructive behavior. We have much more expertise in treating the suicidal patient than we do in treating the homicidal patient. The community has a vested interest in the behavior of the violent person and may prohibit his exposure to the community, even if his mental illness is in remission. Some people who kill are not mentally ill. In fact, most people who kill are not mentally ill. Furthermore, there is no good definition for the word "dangerous." Therefore, psychiatrists who are clinicians should speak only in terms of clinical entities such as violence or self-destructive behavior.

References

1. Monahan J: The prediction of violent behavior; Toward a second generation of theory and policy. *Am J Psychiatry* 141(1):10–15, 1984.
2. *Brady v. Hopper*, 570 F. Supp. 1333 (1983).
3. *Tarasoff v. Regents of the University of California, et al.*, 551 P.2d 334 (1976).
4. *Jablonski, by Pahls v. U.S.*, 712 F.2d 391 (1983).
5. *Barefoot v. Estelle*, 103 S.Ct. 3383 (1983).
6. *Estelle v. Smith*, 451 U.S. 454 (1981).

PART III

Confidentiality and Boundary Issues

1 7

Tarasoff v. Regents
and the Duty to Protect

MICHAEL L. PERLIN, ESQ

Editor's Note

There seems to be a certain degree of confusion with regard to how to interpret the famous Tarasoff *decision, which held that in certain limited circumstances, the psychiatrist who determines (or should have determined) that his or her patient presents a serious danger of violence to another incurs a duty to use "reasonable care to protect the victim." In the* Tarasoff *case itself, the psychiatrist did notify the campus police, but not the parents of the victim; the failure to notify the parents constituted the basis of the suit. Many factors come into play: the foreseeability of harm to the victim, the degree of certainty that he or she would suffer injury, the closeness of the connection between the patient's action and the victim's injury. Confidentiality concerns cannot bar the issuance of warnings.*

A variety of other rulings have followed. For example, one case extended the potential class of defendants to include all mental health professionals. Yet another applied the ruling to property damage.

Three main criticisms have been put forward: no valid standards exist to enable mental health professionals to predict violence accurately; confidentiality may be unnecessarily compromised; and raising

---

CME questions for this chapter begin on page 365.

the therapist's obligations to the public over his or her obligation to the patient may compromise basic professional ethical principles. The Tarasoff *decision may well have led to distorted psychiatric hospital admission and release decisions. On the other hand, it may also have insured proper treatment and rehabilitation for patients in need while saving potential victims from harm.*

As the author points out, oversimplification of the meaning of the Tarasoff *ruling can lead to seriously erroneous decisions, both by clinicians and by courts. Psychiatrists, for example, may misconstrue it to mean that they must render accurate predictions of violence, which they cannot, while others believe the duty to be triggered by the utterance of any threat. Fear of the consequences can lead practitioners to avoid questioning patients about violent impulses, altering record keeping, declining the responsibility for releasing violent patients, and refusing altogether to deal with patients in whom such problems could ever surface.*

Introduction

One of the most controversial aspects of the legal regulation of mental disability practice[1] is the so-called "duty to protect" that stems from case law construing the California Supreme Court's 1976 decision in *Tarasoff v. Regents of the University of California*.[2] *Tarasoff* held that in certain limited circumstances, the psychiatrist who determines (or should have determined) that his or her patient presents a serious danger of violence to another incurs a duty to use "reasonable care to protect the victim."[3] If the psychiatrist fails to do this, he or she may be liable for tort damages.[4]

Over the past 18 years, the legend of the *Tarasoff* case has grown to mythic proportions. The case has spawned a cottage industry of commentary.[5] Mental health professionals have attacked it as a prime example of unwarranted "judicial intrusion" into psychotherapeutic practice;[6] legal commentators have predicted it marked "the decline of effective psychotherapy";[7] and empirical surveyors have found it has had a profound impact on mental health practice even in jurisdictions where it is inapplicable.[8] Widely misunderstood,[9] it remains the benchmark against which all other litigation and statutory reforms in this area are measured, as well as the subject of the most common questions directed to the American Psychiatric Association's legal consultation service.[10] According to the most comprehensive empirical survey conducted on *Tarasoff* awareness among mental health professionals, "it is a fair guess that there is no other legal decision, with the possible exception of controversial cases such as *Brown v. Board of Education*, which could command this level of recognition from laypersons."[11]

Tarasoff has become a shorthand for a large number of situations and issues that transcend both the unique situation faced by the California court 18 years ago and the broader question of how liability should be imposed in cases in which mentally disabled persons are litigational "third parties"; i.e., where they are neither plaintiffs nor defendants but where it is alleged that their violent actions caused the injury that led to the victim's suit against the therapist.[12] Issues of confidentiality, informed consent, scope of insurability, patients' rights, predictability of dangerousness, and limits on governmental intervention in psychotherapeutic practice all have been considered through the *Tarasoff* filter in ways that eventually should help illuminate the underlying core issues: what must a psychiatrist do when he or she believes that a patient is potentially dangerous to a third party, and what implications does the resolution of this issue have for malpractice jurisprudence?

The Tarasoff *Case*

The facts of *Tarasoff* are well known. Prosenjit Poddar, a University of California graduate student, told his therapist (Dr. Moore) that he intended to kill Tatiana Tarasoff, a young woman whom he previously had dated.[13] The therapist consulted with his supervisor and then contacted the campus police, who questioned Poddar and released him once he promised to stay away from Ms. Tarasoff.[14] Two months later, Poddar went to Ms. Tarasoff's home and killed her.[15] Subsequently, her parents filed suit based on a variety of tort theories,[16] including failure on the part of Poddar's therapist to warn Tatiana's parents that Poddar was a grave danger to their daughter.[17]

In its second decision in the case,[18] the California Supreme Court[19] found a "duty to protect" (rather than a "duty to warn") to exist:

> When a therapist determines, or pursuant to the standards of
> his profession should determine, that his patient presents a

serious danger of violence to another, he incurs an obligation to use reasonable care to protect the intended victim against such danger. The discharge of this duty may require the therapist to take one or more of various steps, depending upon the nature of the case. Thus, it may call for him to warn the intended victim or others likely to apprise the victim of the danger, to notify the police, or to take whatever other steps are reasonably necessary under the circumstances.[20]

In answering the question of whether a plaintiff would be entitled to legal protection against a defendant's conduct in such a case, the Court sought to balance the foreseeability of harm to the plaintiff, the degree of certainty that he or she would suffer injury, the closeness of the connection between the defendant's conduct and the plaintiff's injury, the moral blameworthiness attached to the defendant's conduct, and the potential consequences to the community.[21] In such cases, liability will only lie where the defendant bears a "special relationship" to the dangerous person;[22] the therapist-patient relationship satisfies this test.[23]

The Court rejected the argument that mental health professionals' *inability to predict dangerousness accurately* should insulate them from liability[24] and stressed that the alleged failure here was not in the accuracy of prediction (because the therapist did contact the campus police) but in *the failure to warn* once the prediction was made.[25] Although it was possible that unnecessary warnings might be given, that risk was "a reasonable price to pay for the lives of possible victims that might be saved."[26] Finally, the Court rejected the defendant's argument that confidentiality concerns barred the issuance of warnings. Looking both at the patient's right to privacy and the public's interest in safety, the Court concluded that "the public policy favoring protection of the confidential character of patient-psychotherapist communications must yield to the extent to which disclosure is essential to avert danger to others. The protective privilege ends where the public peril begins."[27]

Tarasoff's Progeny

Subsequent decisions from other jurisdictions have been far from unanimous in their interpretation of *Tarasoff*.[28] Some have adopted its holding,[29] some have extended its reach,[30] others have limited it,[31] and others simply have declined to follow it.[32] Courts have extended the *Tarasoff* duty where the victim was the young child of a threatened victim,[33] where the foreseeable violence might involve a "class of persons at risk,"[34] and, in one case, to anyone who might foreseeably be endangered by the patient in question.[35] In the broadest extensions, one case extended the potential class of defendants to include *all* mental health professionals, rather than simply psychiatrists and psychologists, as well as the type of injury involved, to include property damages where the patient burned down his parents' barn.[36] Another court held that a physician might be liable for failing to warn of a medication's side effects if those side effects should have led him or her to caution the patient against driving where it was foreseeable that an accident could result.[37]

Courts have distinguished *Tarasoff* in a variety of cases. Most have involved settings where the victim was neither identified nor identifiable.[38] Similar results were reached in which the therapist lacked sufficient control over the patient in question.[39] Such cases included those in which: (a) The therapist could have reasonably believed that the patient's fantasies did not pose a danger to an identifiable victim;[40] (b) the foreseeable victim had preexisting knowledge of the patient's potential danger;[41] (c) a separate statutorily created privilege protected the therapist from disclosing the patient's actual confidential communication;[42] (d) by the time of the disclosure, the communication was no longer confidential;[43] or (e) it was unsuccessfully alleged by the plaintiffs that a mentally ill adult's parents had undertaken a custodial relationship with their son when they allowed him to live with them after his release from a psychiatric hospital.[44]

In spite of this remarkable common law variation (including cases litigated in several jurisdictions that either severely limit the *Tarasoff* duty or flatly reject its holding),[45] the symbolic value of *Tarasoff* remains compelling. No one has seriously questioned either Dr. James Beck's conclusion that the duty to protect is now "a national standard of practice"[46] or his admonition that mental health professionals should practice "as if the *Tarasoff* duty to protect is the law."[47]

A Critique of Tarasoff and Its Progeny

Both *Tarasoff* and its supportive progeny were greeted initially with a torrent of largely critical academic commentary.[48] Commentators trained in the mental health professions initially criticized it for three main reasons: (1) It was purportedly premised on the false view that valid professional standards exist to enable psychotherapists accurately to predict future violence;[49] (2) it allegedly compromised confidentiality essential to successful psychotherapy;[50] and (3) by raising the psychotherapist's obligation to the public over his or her obligation to the individual patient, it supposedly compromised "central professional ethical precepts."[51] Critical legal commentators looked primarily at confidentiality issues, predicting that the decision would reduce the success of therapy by decreasing patients' trust in their therapists, discouraging patients from communicating sensitive information because of fear of subsequent disclosure, and causing patients to terminate therapy prematurely when they learn of the potential (or actual) breach of confidentiality.[52] Others expressed concern that *Tarasoff* might lead to the overcommitment of patients as a means of attempting to insure the potential victim's safety.[53] Moreover, the warnings themselves might cause the putative victim unnecessary emotional distress[54] or lead to preemptive retaliatory violence on the part of the warned victim,[55] or the requirement of giving warnings might drive therapists away from treating potentially violent patients.[56]

Recent literature has considered the case from a variety of other perspectives. Influential professional associations and commentators have urged state legislatures to adopt statutes to limit potential liability for patients' future violent acts,[57] arguing, in part, that such measures are a necessary step if any order is to be made of the disharmony caused by the incoherent case law.[58] Other commentators have "unpacked" the reasoning supporting *Tarasoff*-esque decisions to focus on the implicit expectations of clairvoyance on the part of mental health professionals.[59]

Commentators are now beginning to explore carefully and sensitively the linkage between *Tarasoff*-type duties, preventive detention, and requirements that the therapist engage in social control[60] (a question that has special troubling implications when the therapist and patient are from different cultural backgrounds).[61] The fear that *Tarasoff* concerns distorted psychiatric hospital admission and release decisions and led to improper use of psychiatric facilities is critical to the underlying inquiries.[62]

On the other hand, others have begun to react positively to the *Tarasoff* duty,[63] reasoning it could result in more proper treatment and rehabilitation for patients who would thus avoid criminal and civil proceedings that might otherwise have resulted from the threatened activity.[64] Others have reported instances in which warnings actually strengthened the therapeutic alliance and contributed to a patient's progress in therapy.[65] It is necessary to assess these findings to determine the ultimate therapeutic (or antitherapeutic) impact of *Tarasoff*-type cases.[66]

Alternative Analysis of Tarasoff

If *Tarasoff* is to be truly understood, it is necessary to consider these issues in light of yet another set of concerns. First, it is necessary to consider recent developments from the perspective of cognitive psychology and to look at the way in which heuristic reasoning shapes both *Tarasoff* decision making as well as mental health professionals' *responses* to *Tarasoff*-type cases. It is thus necessary to turn to therapeutic jurisprudence as a means of identifying and examining the extent of the relationship between legal arrangements and therapeutic outcomes.[67] This analysis should help determine the ultimate impact of *Tarasoff* on malpractice jurisprudence.

Cognitive Psychology:

Interest recently has been kindled in the use of cognitive psychology (focusing primarily on concepts that describe and explain heuristic reasoning and thinking) as a means of explaining judicial, legislative, and lay decision making, and as a vehicle by which to interpret mental disability law developments.[68]

Heuristics refers to the implicit devices that persons use to simplify complex information-processing tasks, leading to distorted and systematically erroneous decisions and causing decision makers to "ignore or misuse items of rationally useful information."[69] The vivid, outrageous case overwhelms reams of abstract data upon which rational choices should be made;[70] mental health professionals are as susceptible to these devices as judges, jurors, legislators, or other lay persons are.[71]

Some empirical research and commentary that have developed around the *Tarasoff* case reflect this phenomenon. Thus, more than three fourths of clinicians surveyed reported that the issuance of warnings was the sole acceptable means of protecting potential victims.[72] Also, commentators have significantly *overstated* the precedential effect of *Tarasoff* and its application in all federal and state jurisdictions.[73] Beyond this, it is not difficult to predict that the distortions inherent in the heuristic reasoning will have an important impact on an area of mental disability jurisprudence as volatile, demanding, and contentious as the duty to warn. The power of heuristic reasoning must be weighed carefully in this inquiry.

Therapeutic Jurisprudence:

It is also necessary to consider the construct of therapeutic jurisprudence as a model by which to assess the ultimate impact of case law and legislation that affects mentally disabled persons. Therapeutic jurisprudence studies the role of the law as a therapeutic agent.[74] This perspective recognizes that substantive rules, legal procedures, and lawyers' roles may have either therapeutic or antitherapeutic consequences and questions whether such rules, procedures, and roles can or should be reshaped to enhance their therapeutic potential but not to subordinate due process principles.[75]

Tarasoff should be the source of a variety of therapeutic jurisprudential inquiries. What impact will the need to comply with *Tarasoff* have on clinical practice? Will courts' construction of empirical evidence that is developed about such impact take into consideration therapeutic jurisprudential values? What impact will *Tarasoff* litigation have on clinical practice?

Much of the first wave of *Tarasoff* commentary addressed the first of these concerns.[76] Thus, after Alan Stone initially assailed *Tarasoff*, warning that it would "destroy the patient's expectation of confidentiality,"[77] the first wave of empirical studies seemed to belie this prediction.[78] Whereas warnings *not* discussed with patients were interpreted to be therapeutically harmful, warnings that *were* discussed were interpreted to have positive therapeutic effects.[79] Other empirical inquiries have focused on ways that clinician awareness of *Tarasoff* has altered the therapeutic relationship, suggesting that the increased awareness of and concern about possible violence may lead to "heightened anxiety . . . in any clinical situation in which the potential violence of a patient becomes an issue, or in which the prospect of a duty to warn arises."[80]

These findings lead to other inquiries. To what extent does *therapist misinformation* about the scope of *Tarasoff* negatively affect therapist-patient relationships? Surveys indicate that therapists have overstated both the *Tarasoff* prescription (as to ways of effectuating the duty) as well as its national precedential applicability; they also frequently simply misstate its holding.[81] *Tarasoff* is misunderstood in other ways: a significant number of therapists have construed it to require accurate predictions;[82] others believe the duty to be triggered by the utterance of *any* threat.[83] Also, it has been argued that professionals have been misled by professional association newsletters that have distorted or misstated the holdings of *Tarasoff*'s progeny and that these misunderstandings serve to further alienate law and psychotherapy.[84]

These inquiries raise yet another set of concerns: have therapists responded to *Tarasoff* by adopting a passive-aggressive style of behavior?[85] Commentators have speculated that the motivations of some clinicians who have responded to *Tarasoff* by overpredicting violence and overissuing warnings[86] may be simply their concern to escape legal liability.[87] Others have reported that some physicians have become reluctant to probe into areas of their patients' lives dealing with violence[88] or have altered their record keeping (either by obscuring information that might suggest violence or by padding a record with information to support a decision not to warn).[89] Still others have argued that clinicians in hospitals should decline to assume final responsibility for releasing violent patients and should require court interventions in all such cases.[90] As Professors Schopp and Wexler[91] have concluded:

> "If the clinician is sufficiently concerned about tort liability to conduct the therapeutic relationship with a wary eye toward protecting his own interests regarding liability, that attitude may be sufficient to dilute the therapist's apparent trustworthiness and concern for the patient's welfare and thus to undermine the therapeutic relationship."

All this must be further weighed in light of yet another body of data that found that doctors sued in malpractice cases reported significantly more emotional and psychological distress than nonsued physicians. Furthermore, this body of data indicates that significantly more of the sued group were likely to stop seeing certain types of patients, to discourage their children from entering medicine, and to think about early retirement.[92]

Others have concluded that it is not simply the reality but the *possibility* of malpractice litigation that is the source of marked anxiety in many mental health professionals.[93] Indeed, Simon[94] claims that "iatrogenic liability neurosis" can capture a therapist's professional judgment. If clinicians believe (accurately or inaccurately) that adopting the sort of behavior described will minimize their malpractice exposure, it is not unreasonable to conclude that more will follow this approach. This conclusion must be read in the context of yet other evidence that suggests that many physicians believe that if they were to release a patient who subsequently commits a violent act, their liability exposure (both as to likelihood of being sued and to the extent of potential monetary damages) would be much greater than in a case in which they were to civilly commit a patient improperly who does not meet statutory commitment criteria.[95]

It is necessary to consider the ways that courts construe empirical evidence in *Tarasoff* cases. The few courts that have considered the issue have not responded in a uniform or coherent way. Two cases—including *Tarasoff* itself—have simply concluded that there was little empirical evidence to support the prediction that imposing a duty would lead to overcommitment.[96] One of the courts that distinguished *Tarasoff* relied on Stone's prediction that the duty would deter treatment.[97] However, one of the most expansive readings of *Tarasoff* buttressed its holding by relying upon survey results in which psychotherapists self-reported they could accurately predict dangerousness,[98] notwithstanding the "overwhelming academic and empirical evidence to the contrary."[99] The fact remains that there is no reliable database of empirical evidence as to the therapeutic value of *Tarasoff* warnings or of the case's ultimate "real life" impact.[100]

Conclusion

There is no dispute as to the controversy or confusion spawned by the *Tarasoff* decision and its progeny. Its very existence has reshaped the configurations of mental health practice and altered the relationship between clinicians and public authorities. It has been responsible for legislative debate and statutory amendment in a significant number of states, including some in which *Tarasoff*-type issues have never been litigated.[100] The extent to which it is both known and materially misunderstood assures maintenance and continuation of its symbolic status. The fact that clinicians self-report changes in their therapeutic approach because of fear (real or imagined) of *Tarasoff*-inspired legal liability attests to the dominance of its image.

References

1. *See generally* 3 ML PERLIN, *MENTAL DISABILITY LAW: CIVIL AND CRIMINAL* §§13.05–13.21 (1989) (hereinafter ML PERLIN). The text in this section is generally adapted from Perlin, Tarasoff *and the Dilemma of the Dangerous Patient: New Directions for the 1990s,* 16 LAW PSYCHOLOGY REV 29 (1992), and from ML PERLIN, THE LAW AND MENTAL DISABILITY §3.19 (1994).
2. 17 Cal 3d 425, 131 Cal Rptr 14, 551 P 2d 334 (1976).
3. *Tarasoff,* 131 Cal Rptr at 20.
4. *Id* at 20–22.
5. *See generally,* 3 ML PERLIN, *supra* note 1, §13.05 at 51 n. 70 (1992 pocket part) (listing articles); Note, *The Psychotherapist's Duty to Warn: Walking a Tightrope of Uncertainty,* 56 CINCINNATI LAW REV 269–70 n. 1 (1987) (same).
6. Givelber, Bowers, & Blitch, *The* Tarasoff *Controversy: A Summary of Findings From an Empirical Study of Legal, Ethical and Clinical Issues* (Givelber) in THE POTENTIALLY VIOLENT PATIENT AND THE *TARASOFF* DECISION IN PSYCHIATRIC PRACTICE 35, 37 (J Beck ed. 1985) (THE *TARASOFF* DECISION).
7. *Note,* Tarasoff v Regents of the University of California: *The Duty to Warn: Common Law and Statutory Problems for California Psychotherapists,* 14 CALIF WEST LAW REVIEW 153 (1978).
8. *See* Givelber, *supra* note 6, at 39–54.
9. *See* Givelber, Bowers & Blitch, Tarasoff, *Myth and Reality: An Empirical Study of Private Law in Action,* 1984 WIS LAW REV 443, 465 (Givelber II).
10. Beck, *The Psychotherapist's Duty to Protect Third Parties From Harm,* 11 MENT PHYS DIS LAW RPTR 141 (1987).
11. Givelber II, *supra* note 9, at 457–458.
12. I explain this use of the term in 3 ML PERLIN, *supra* note 1, §13.05, at 134 n. 70.
13. *Tarasoff,* 131 Cal Rptr at 21. *See also,* People v Poddar, 10 Cal 3d 750, 518 P 2d 342, 111 Cal Rptr 910, 912 (1974).
14. *Tarasoff,* 131 Cal Rptr at 21.
15. *See generally,* Poddar, *supra.*
16. *See Tarasoff,* 131 Cal Rptr at 20–21 (listing causes of action).
17. *Id* at 21.
18. In its initial decision, the California Supreme Court had found that a psychotherapist was under a duty to warn when, "in the exercise of his professional skill and knowledge, [he] determines, or should determine, that a warning is essential to avert danger arising from the medical or psychological condition of his patient." Tarasoff v Regents of Univ of Calif, 13 Cal 3d 177, 529, P 2d 553, 118 Cal Rptr 129, 131 (1974), modified, 17 Cal 3d 425, 551 P

2d 334, 131 Cal Rptr 14 (1976). The Court reheard the case at the request of the American Psychiatric Association and other professional organizations. Mills & Beck, The *Tarasoff* Case, in THE TARASOFF DECISION, *supra* note 6, at 1, 4–5; *see also*, Merton, *Confidentiality and the "Dangerous" Patient: Implications of* Tarasoff *for Psychiatrists and Lawyers,* 31 EMORY LAW J 263, 294 n. 70 (1982).

19.   The decision was a split one. Justice Mosk concurred in part and dissented in part, stressing that his partial concurrence was premised on the fact that the defendant therapist did predict that Poddar would kill Tatiana. *Tarasoff*, 131 Cal Rptr at 33. Justice Clark dissented, warning that the majority's rule "is certain to result in a net increase in violence." *id* at 35.

20.   *Id* at 20.

21.   *Id* at 21–22.

22.   *Id* at 23; see RESTATEMENT (SECOND) OF TORTS, §315 (1965).

23.   *Tarasoff*, 131 Cal Rptr at 23–24.

24.   *Id* at 25.

25.   *Id*.

26.   *Id* at 26.

27.   *Id* at 27.

28.   On the collateral question of the existence of a duty to warn in cases involving persons with AIDS, *see* Bisbing, *Psychiatric Patients and AIDS: Evolving Law and Liability,* 18 PSYCHIATR ANN 582 (1988); Note, *AIDS: Establishing a Physician's Duty to Warn,* 21 RUTGERS LAW J 645 (1990); Weiss, *AIDS: Balancing the Physician's Duty to Warn and Confidentiality Concerns,* 38 EMORY LAW J 299 (1989); Labowitz, *Beyond* Tarasoff: *AIDS and the Obligation to Breach Confidentiality,* 9 ST LOUIS UNIV PUBLIC LAW REV 495 (1990); Zonana, *The AIDS Patient on the Psychiatric Unit: Ethical and Legal Issues,* 18 PSYCHIATR ANN 587 (1988); Weiss, *AIDS: Balancing the Physician's Duty to Warn and Confidentiality Concerns,* 38 EMORY LAW J 299 (1989); Rosmarin, *Legal and Ethical Aspects of HIV Disease,* in A PSYCHIATRIST'S GUIDE TO AIDS AND HIV DISEASES 63–76 (American Psychiatric Association, ed. 1990); Dyer, *AIDS, Ethics, and Psychiatry,* 18 PSYCHIATR ANN 577 (1988); Botello et al., *A Proposed Exception to the AIDS Confidentiality Laws for Psychiatric Patients,* 35 J FORENSIC SCIENCE 653 (1990); *see also* Estate of Behringer v Princeton Medical Center, 249 NJ Sup 597, 592 A2d 1251 (Law Div 1991) (discussing obligation of surgeon to reveal his AIDS condition to patients); Application of Milton S. Hershey Medical Center, 407 Pa Sup. 565, 595 A2d 1290 (1991) (permissible for hospital to disclose physician's AIDS condition to patients and colleagues).

29.   *See generally*, 3 ML PERLIN, *supra* note 1, §§13.10–13.11.

30.   *Id*, §13.12.

31.   *Id*, §§13.13–13.16.

32.   *Id*, §13.17.

33.   Hedlund v Superior Court of Orange County, 34 Cal 3d 695, 669 P 2d 41, 194 Cal Rptr 805 (1983); see 3 ML PERLIN, *supra* note 1, §13.12, at 159–160 n. 269 (discussing *Hedlund*).

34. Lipari v Sears, Roebuck & Co, 497 F Supp 185 (D Neb 1980); see 3 M.L. PERLIN, *supra* note 1, §13.12, at 160 n. 270 (discussing *Lipari*).

35. Petersen v Washington, 100 Wash 2d 421, 671 P 2d 230 (1983); see 3 ML PERLIN, *supra* note 1, §13.12, at 160–161 n. 271 (discussing *Petersen*).

36. Peck v Counseling Service of Addison County, 146 Vt 61, 499 A 2d 422 (1985). Peck is criticized sharply in Stone, *Vermont Adopts* Tarasoff: *A Real Barn-Burner*, 143 AM J PSYCHIATRY 352 (1986). *Compare* Bellah v Greenson, 73 Cal App 3d 911, 141 Cal Rptr 92, 94-95 (1977) (refusing to extend *Tarasoff* to cases involving property damage or suicide).

37. Schuster v Altenburg, 144 Wis 2d 223, 424 NW 2d 159 (1988). Schuster is characterized as "the current apex of *Tarasoff*'s legal manifestation," and as an indication of "expanding liability" following *Tarasoff*, in Note, *The Psychotherapist's Calamity: Emerging Trends in the* Tarasoff *Doctrine*, 1989 BRIGHAM YOUNG UNIV LAW REV 261, 267, 281.

38. *See e.g.*, Thompson v County of Alameda, 27 Cal 3d 741, 614 P 2d 728, 167 Cal Rptr 70 (1980), and see generally, 3 ML PERLIN, *supra* note 1, §13.14, at 164–165 (listing cases).

39. *See e.g.*, Hasenei v United States, 541 F Supp 999, 1009 (D Md 1982); Lindsay v United States, 693 F Supp 1012 (WD Okla 1988).

40. White v United States, 780 F 2d 97, 102 (DC Cir 1986).

41. Moye v United States, 735 F Supp 179 (EDNC 1990); *see also*, Rogers v South Carolina Department of Mental Health, 377 SE 2d 125, 126 (SC Ct App 1989) (family had knowledge of patient's mental illness and its manifestations).

42. *In re* Daniel CH, 220 Cal App 3d 814, 269 Cal Rptr 624, 633—634 (1990) (construing CALIF EVID CODE §1016).

43. People v Clark, 50 Cal 3d 583, 789 P 2d 127, 151, 268 Cal Rptr 399 (1990).

44. Kaminski v Town of Fairfield, 216 Conn 29, 578 A 2d 1048 (1990).

45. *See, e.g.*, Shaw v Glickman, 45 Md App 718, 415 A 2d 625 (1980) (sharply limiting scope); Case v United States, 523 F. Supp 317 (SD Ohio 1981), *aff'd*, 709 F. 2d 1500 (6th Cir 1983) (rejecting *Tarasoff*).

46. Beck, *The Psychotherapist and the Violent Patient*, in THE *TARASOFF* DECISION, *supra* note 6, at 9, 33; *see also*, Menninger, *The Impact of Litigation and Court Decisions on Clinical Practice*, 53 BULL MENNINGER CLINIC 203, 207 (1989) (same); *cf* Givelber II, *supra* note 6, at 474 (*Tarasoff* "potentially the law everywhere").

47. *Id, Cf* Roth & Levin, *Dilemma of* Tarasoff: *Must Physicians Protect the Public or Their Patients?* 11 LAW MED HEALTH CARE 104, 110 (1983) (*Tarasoff* has been adopted "from coast to coast").

48. George, Korin, Quattrone, & Mandel, *The Therapist's Duty to Protect Third Parties: A Guide for the Perplexed*, 14 RUTGERS LAW J 637 (1983) (George); Givelber, *supra* note 6, at 37; McCarty, *Patient Threats Against Third Parties: The Psychotherapist's Duty of Reasonable Care*, 5 J CONTEMP HEALTH LAW POL 119, 120 (1989).

49. Givelber, *supra* note 6, at 37. There is even a question as to whether clinical standards for the prediction of dangerous behavior even exist. *See* Wettstein,

The Prediction of Violent Behavior and the Duty to protect Third Parties, 2 BEHAV SCIENCE LAW 291, 311 (1984); Kaufman, *Post*-Tarasoff *Developments and the Mental Health Literature,* 55 BULL MENNINGER CLIN 308, 311 (1991).

50. *See e.g.,* Dubey, *Confidentiality as a Requirement for the Therapist: Technical Necessities for Absolute Privilege in Psychotherapy,* 131 AM J PSYCHIATRY 1093 (1974); Griffith & Griffith, *Duty to Third Parties, Dangerousness, and the Right to Refuse Treatment: Problematic Concepts for Psychiatrist and Lawyer,* 14 CALIF WEST LAW REV 241, 247 (1978); Stone, *The* Tarasoff *Decisions: Suing Psychotherapists to Safeguard Society,* 90 HARV LAW REV 358 (1976). Stone, whose criticism of *Tarasoff* has been termed "the most elegant," *see* Wexler, *Patients, Therapists, and Third Parties: The Victimological Virtues of* Tarasoff, 2 INT J LAW PSYCHIATRY 1, 2 (1979), has since receded to some extent from this position. *See* A. STONE, LAW, PSYCHIATRY, AND MORALITY 181 (1984) ("the duty to warn is not as unmitigated a disaster for the enterprise of psychotherapy as it once seemed to critics like myself").

51. Givelber, *supra* note 6, at 37.

52. Note, *Where the Public Peril Begins: A Survey of Psychotherapists to Determine the Effects of* Tarasoff, 31 STANFORD LAW REV 165, 166 n. 9 (1978); Comment, *Psychotherapists' Duty to Warn: Ten Years After* Tarasoff, 15 GOLDEN GATE UNIV LAW REV 271, 272 n. 7 (1985) (citing sources).

53. Note, *Imposing a Duty to Warn on Psychiatrists—A Judicial Threat to the Psychiatric Profession,* 48 UNIV COLO LAW REV 283, 297 (1977); McCarty, *supra* note 48, at 133; *Tarasoff,* 131 Cal Rptr at 40—42 (Clark J, dissenting); *cf.* McIntosh v Milano, 168 NJ Sup 466, 403 A 2d 500, 514 (Law Div 1979) ("If psychiatrists now say . . . that therapists are no more accurate than the average layman, serious questions would arise as to the entire present basis for commitment procedures.")

54. Griffith & Griffith, *supra* note 50, at 250–51.

55. Personal communication, Robert L. Sadoff, MD (July 12, 1991).

56. Gurevitz, Tarasoff: *Protective Privilege Versus Public Peril,* 134 AM J PSYCHIATRY 289 (1977).

57. For the most comprehensive overview, *see* Appelbaum, Zonana, Bonnie, & Roth, *Statutory Approaches to Limiting Psychiatrists' Liability for Their Patients' Violent Acts,* 146 AM J PSYCHIATRY 821 (1989); *see also,* Note, *Statutes Limiting Mental Health Professionals' Liability for the Violent Acts of Their Patients,* 64 IND LAW J 391 (1989) (*Indiana Note*); Note, *supra* note 53, at 286–293. On the potential implications of a Colorado statute (COLO REV STAT §13-21-117 [1987]) partially limiting liability in cases involving a mental health worker's failure to warn or protect adequately, *see e.g.,* Note, *A Proposal to Adopt a Professional Judgment Standard of Care in Determining the Duty of a Psychiatrist to Third Persons,* 62 UNIV COLO LAW REV 237, 258–59 (1991) (*Colorado Note*) (statutory exceptions "effectively nullify" immunity grant); Note, 103 HARVARD LAW REV 1192, 197–198 (1990) (immunity laws dilute psychiatrists' incentives to improve monitoring and diagnostic techniques).

58. *See* Felthous, *The Ever Confusing Jurisprudence of the Psychotherapist's Duty to Protect*, 17 J PSYCHIATRY LAW 575, 576, 590 (1989); *see also*, Bloom, *The* Tarasoff *Decision: Dangerousness and Mandated Outpatient Treatment*, 30 INT J OFFENDER THER COMPAR CRIMINOL vii, viii (1986) (statutes reflect "orderly progression in the attempt to define more narrowly the situations in which the *Tarasoff* requirement will apply, and provide clarity in the law"). California is among the states that has adopted such a law. *See* CAL CIV CODE §43.92; *see e.g.*, Note, *Tort Liability for California Public Psychiatric Facilities: Time for a Change*, 29 SANTA CLARA LAW REV 459 (1989); *see generally*, 3 ML PERLIN, *supra* note 1, §13.07 (discussing legislative responses to *Tarasoff*).

59. *See* Rachlin, *Limiting the Dimensions of* Tarasoff, J AM ASSOC PSYCHIATR ADMINS 1, 14 (Winter 1989-90).

60. *See* Appelbaum, *The New Preventive Detention: Psychiatry's Problematic Responsibility for the Control of Violence*, 145 AM J PSYCHIATRY 779 (1988); Leong, *The Expansion of Psychiatric Participation in Social Control*, 40 HOSP COMMUNITY PSYCHIATRY 240 (1989); *compare* Greenberg, *The Psychiatrist's Dilemma*, 17 J PSYCHIATRY LAW 381 (1989) (recommending that psychiatrists use a low threshold of dangerousness as a basis for commitment so as to avoid liability as a vehicle to spur legislative statutory reform).

61. Griffith & Griffith, *supra* note 50, at 258 ("There is a tendency in such situations for aggressive behavior to be misinterpreted as a sign of dangerousness"). On the impact of socioeconomic variables such as status, race, sex, and interpersonal variables such as physical attractiveness and social likability on mental health professionals' attitudes, *see e.g.*, Rogers, *Ethical Dilemmas in Forensic Evaluations*, 5 BEHAV SCIENCE LAW 149, 152 (1987).

62. *See* Appelbaum, *supra* note 60, at 783; *see also*, Appelbaum, *Hospitalization of the Dangerous Patient: Legal Pressures and Clinical Responses*, 12 BULL AM ACAD PSYCHIATRY LAW 323, 325 (1984) ("The natural response on the part of clinicians has been to feel compelled to commit [or admit involuntarily] *all* dangerous patients, regardless of their suitability for hospitalization") (emphasis in original).

63. Note, *Affirmative Duty After* Tarasoff, 11 HOFSTRA LAW REV 1013, 1034 (1983); Note, *Untangling* Tarasoff: Tarasoff v Regents of the University of California, 29 HASTINGS LAW J 179, 180 (1977); George, *supra* note 48, at 650. *Cf.* Shuman & Weiner, *The Privilege Study: An Empirical Examination of the Psychotherapist-Patient Privilege*, 60 NC LAW REV 893, 927 (1982) (need for absolute confidentiality in context of patient-physician relationship has been "overstated").

64. *See e.g.*, McCarty, *supra* note 48, at 121–122.

65. Mills, Sullivan, & Eth, *Protecting Third Parties: A Decade After* Tarasoff, 144 AM J PSYCHIATRY 68, 72 (1987), discussing findings reported in Beck, *When a Patient Threatens Violence: An Empirical Study of Clinical Practice After* Tarasoff, 10 BULL AM ACAD PSYCHIATRY LAW 189 (1982), and Wulsin, Burstzajn, & Gutheil, *Unexpected Clinical Features of the* Tarasoff *Decision: The Therapeutic Alliance and the "Duty to Warn,"* 140 AM J PSYCHIATRY 601 (1983).

66. *See e.g.*, Klotz, *Limiting the Psychotherapist-Patient Privilege: The Therapeutic Potential*, 27 CRIM LAW BULL 416 (1991).

67. Wexler, *Putting Mental Health into Mental Health Law: Therapeutic Jurisprudence*, 16 LAW HUMAN BEHAV 27, 32 (1992).

68. 1 ML PERLIN, *supra* note 1, §1.05A n. 156.1, at 4–5 (1992, pocket part). *See generally*, Saks & Kidd, *Human Information Processing and Adjudication: Trial By Heuristics*, 15 LAW SOCIETY REV 123 (1980-81).

69. Perlin, *Are Courts Competent to Decide Competency Questions? Stripping the Facade from* United States v. Charters, 38 UNIV KAN LAW REV 957, 966 n. 46 (1990), quoting, in part, Carroll & Payne, *The Psychology of the Parole Decision Process: A Joint Application of Attribution Theory and Information-Processing Psychology*, in COG SOCIAL BEHAV 13, 21 (J Carroll & J Payne eds. 1976); *see generally*, Bersoff, *Judicial Deference to Nonlegal Decision Makers: Imposing Simplistic Solutions on Problems of Cognitive Complexity in Mental Disability Law*, 46 SMU LAW REV 329 (1992).

70. Rosenhan, *Psychological Realities and Judicial Policy*, 19 STANFORD LAW REV 10, 13 (1984). Thus, one instance in which an ex-patient (or an individual denied admission to a mental hospital) commits a crime of violence may have the effect of dramatically increasing civil commitment rates in a jurisdiction in spite of whether or not the commitment criteria are amended in response to the violent incident. *See e.g.*, Bagby & Atkinson, *The Effects of Legislative Reform on Civil Commitment Admission Rates*, 6 BEHAV SCIENCE LAW 45, 46 (1988); Fischer, Pierce, & Appelbaum, *How Flexible Are Our Civil Commitment Statutes?* 39 HOSP COMMUNITY PSYCHIATRY 711, 712 (1988).

71. *See e.g.*, Webster, Menzies, & Jackson, *Clinical Assessments Before Trial* 121 (1982); Jackson, *The Clinical Assessment and Prediction of Violent Behavior: Toward a Scientific Analysis*, 16 CRIM JUST BEHAV 114 (1989); Jackson, *Psychiatric Decision Making for the Courts: Judges, Psychiatrists, Lay People?* 9 INT J LAW PSYCHIATRY 507 (1986).

72. *See* Givelber II, *supra* note 9, at 465.

73. *See e.g.*, Roth & Levin, *supra* note 47.

74. See THERAPEUTIC JURISPRUDENCE: THE LAW AS A THERAPEUTIC AGENT (D Wexler ed. 1990); ESSAYS IN THERAPEUTIC JURISPRUDENCE (D Wexler & B Winick eds. 1991); Wexler, *supra* note 67.

75. Wexler, *Health Care Compliance Principles and the Insanity Acquittee Conditional Release Process*, 27 CRIM LAW BULL 18, 19 n. 5 (1991); *see generally*, Wexler, *supra* note 50.

76. Some also spoke to it openly. *See* Wexler, *supra* note 50, at 4 ("*Tarasoff* . . . has the clear-cut potential of prompting and prodding practicing therapists to terminate their continued clinging to an outmoded 'individual pathology' model of violence, and to accept the paradigm of 'interactional' or 'couple' violence already endorsed by the professional literature"); for a consideration of Wexler's insights, *see* 3 ML PERLIN, *supra* note 1, §13.21, at 182–84.

77. Stone, *supra* note 36.

78. *See* Mills, Sullivan, & Eth, *supra* note 65, at 70, discussing findings reported in del Rio, *Ellsberg Psychoanalytic Situation*, 5 INT J PSYCHOANAL PSYCHOTHER 349 (1976); Schmid, Appelbaum, Roth, et al, *Confidentiality in Psychiatry: A Study of the Patient's View*, 34 HOSP COMMUNITY PSYCHIATRY 353 (1983). On Stone's recession from his initial position, see A STONE, *supra* note 50.

79. Carlson, Friedman, & Riggert, *The Duty to Warn/Protect: Issues in Clinical Practice*, 15 BULL AM ACAD PSYCHIATRY LAW 179, 181—184 (1987), discussing, in part, Beck, *supra* note 10; Finney, *Breaking Confidences: An Application of the* Tarasoff *Rule*, 3 AM J FORENS SCIENCE 134 (1982–1983). *See also*, Treadway, Tarasoff *in the Therapeutic Setting*, 41 HOSP COMMUNITY PSYCHIATRY 88, 89 (1990) ("Fulfilling *Tarasoff's* duty encourages patients to make choices, to be involved in decisionmaking, and to accept that they, not the therapist, have the ultimate responsibility for impulse control").

80. Note, *supra* note 52, at 186–188. In response to such concerns, thoughtful commentators have crafted a series of guidelines to therapists to help them deal with the *Tarasoff* "paradox." *See* Roth & Meisel, *Dangerousness, Confidentiality, and the Duty to Warn*, 134 AM J PSYCHIATRY 508, 509–511 (1977); *see also*, Appelbaum, Tarasoff *and the Clinician: Problems in Fulfilling the Duty to Protect*, 142 AM J PSYCHIATRY 425, 426–427 (1985).

81. *See* Givelber II, *supra* note 9, at 466. *See also*, Runck, *Survey Shows Therapists Misunderstand* Tarasoff *Rule*, 38 HOSP COMMUNITY PSYCHIATRY 429 (1984).

82. See Dickens, *Legal Issues in Medical Management of Violent and Threatening Patients*, 31 CAN J PSYCHIATRY 772, 773 (1986). Compare *Tarasoff*, 131 Cal Rptr at 20 (exercise of reasonable care required).

83. Appelbaum, *supra* note 80, at 427.

84. George, Hedlund *Paranoia*, 41 J CLIN PSYCHOL 291, 293—294 (1985).

85. See Perlin, *supra* note 69, at 984–985, 989 (discussing passive-aggressive behavior in the context of right to refuse medication litigation). *Compare e.g.*, Greenberg, *supra* note 60 (recommending the adoption of a lower standard of dangerousness in commitment decision making by clinicians).

86. *See* Runck, *supra* note 81, at 430. *Compare* Roth & Meisel, *supra* note 80, at 509–511 (in *Tarasoff* situations, therapists should avoid being "stampeded" into giving unnecessary warnings, should provide information as to limits of confidentiality prior to entering into the therapeutic relationship, should employ "social and environmental manipulations"—such as bringing third parties into the therapeutic setting—prior to compromising confidentiality; should obtain, wherever possible, permission of patients prior to discussing confidential communications with others; and should assess any such intervention in light of its potential impact on therapy and the likelihood that it will be successful in preventing future violence).

87. Sonkin, *Clairvoyance vs Common Sense: Therapists' Duty to Warn and Protect*, 1 VICTIMS VIOL 7, 19 (1986).

88. *Compare* Perlin, *Psychodynamics and the Insanity Defense: "Ordinary Common Sense" and Heuristic Reasoning*, 69 NEB LAW REV 3, 35–36 (1990) (discussing

reluctance of judges and insanity defense policymakers to "'go deeper' when we unconsciously fear what we may learn at a deeper level of exploration").

89. Note, *supra* note 52, at 188–189.

90. Mills, Sullivan, & Eth, *supra* note 65, at 72.

91. Schopp & Wexler, *Shooting Yourself in the Foot with Due Care: Psychotherapists and Crystallized Standards of Tort Liability*, 17 J PSYCHIATRY LAW 163, 184 (1989).

92. Charles, Wilbert, & Franke, *Sued and Nonsued Physicians' Self-Reported Reactions to Malpractice Litigation,* 142 AM J PSYCHIATRY 437 (1985); *cf* Rosoff, *Physicians as Criminal Defendants: Specialty, Sanctions, and Status Liability,* 13 LAW HUM BEHAV 231, 235 (1989) (questioning whether "status liability"—the positive relationship found between punishment and status when a high-occupational-status defendant commits a serious criminal offense—operates in the context of medical malpractice cases as well).

93. Appelbaum, *supra* note 80, at 429.

94. R Simon, CLINICAL PSYCHIATRY AND THE LAW xxiv (1987).

95. Brown & Rayne, *Some Ethical Considerations in Defense of Psychiatry: A Case Study,* 59 AM J ORTHOPSYCHIATRY 534, 539-40 (1989).

96. *See Colo Note, supra* note 57, at 255-56, discussing, inter alia, *Tarasoff,* 131 Cal Rptr at 26 n. 12; Currie v United States, 644 F Supp 1074, 1082 (MDNC 1986), *aff'd* 836 F 2d 209 (4th Cir 1987); *see also,* Goodman, *From* Tarasoff *to* Hopper: *The Evolution of the Therapist's Duty to Protect Third Parties,* 3 BEHAV SCIENCE LAW 195, 219 (1985) ("there is no credible evidence either that the practice of psychotherapy has suffered or that violence within our society has increased because of the imposition of the duty to protect others upon the mental health professions").

97. *See* Littleton v Good Samaritan Hospital & Health Center, 39 Ohio St 3d 86, 529 NE 2d 449, 459 n. 20 (1988), discussing Stone, *supra* note 50. The patient in Littleton was a voluntary inpatient who did not "manifest violent propensities while being hospitalized." *id* at 460.

98. Schuster v Altenberg, 424 NW 2d 159, 169 (1988).

99. *Colo Note, supra* note 57, at 279.

100. *See e.g.,* Appelbaum, *supra* note 80, at 425; Leong, Eth & Silva, *The* Tarasoff *Dilemma in Criminal Court,* 36 J FORENS SCIENCE 728, 734 (1991).

101. *See Colo Note, supra* note 57, at 289 n. 100 (discussing, inter alia, legislative amendments in New Hampshire (NH REV STAT ANN §330-A:22)), and *Ind Note, supra* note 57, at 407 n. 88 (discussing, inter alia, legislative amendments in Utah (UTAH CODE ANN §78-14a-102(1)). No "duty to protect" case has been litigated in either jurisdiction.

1 8

Boundary Issues in Psychiatric Treatment

KATHLEEN MERO MOGUL, M.D.

Editor's Note

In the relationship between psychiatrist and patient, boundary violations apply to those transgressions that are damaging to the therapeutic process and, most importantly, to the patient. Sexual involvement is the ultimate boundary violation and is clearly unethical. But other violations occur as well, such as exploiting information gained from the patient; in one notable case, a psychiatrist was found guilty of using inside information secured from the wife of a noted business figure to profit in stock trading.

It's important to keep in mind that many patients are themselves not clear regarding boundaries; most boundary violations are initiated by patients; but for the therapist, this is no excuse. Certain patients are more prone to this, including those who were not respected by parents and early caregivers, those with strong dependency needs, and those who may have experienced sexual and/or emotional abuse as well as various physical intrusions. Many patients "test" therapists by demanding that the boundaries of the therapeutic relationship be crossed. And therapists themselves, as they experience empathy, may momentarily identify with a patient's feelings and be subject to blurring of boundaries.

CME questions for this chapter begin on page 366.

Certainly, some psychiatrists have antisocial personalities and take serious advantage of patients' vulnerability. Most do not. It would be a mistake to assume that boundary violations can only occur with other professionals and not oneself. To be on guard, be prepared to recognize patients in whom boundary violations are more likely to be encouraged, as well as issues and problems in therapy that may increase the risk. Also, be aware of one's own susceptibility, as during times of stress, loneliness, or other personal conflict.

A particularly complex issue involves socializing with patients. In general, it is best to avoid contact with patients outside the consulting room. This rule may apply to patients' families, too. In smaller communities and other special circumstances, this may be difficult to implement. The author feels that one should be quite firm in handling even minor boundary infractions. Although the author's admonitions seem, at times, rather stringent, the basic principle of preserving the integrity of the therapeutic relationship is vital to successful practice.

Introduction

The subject of boundary violation has received considerable attention in the psychiatric literature over the past few years as a result of the recognition that such transgression is the general precursor of sexual involvement between patient and therapist.[1–4] The term *boundary* has two meanings in the clinical literature. In the more important—although perhaps less often specified—sense, it refers to the boundary between patient and therapist as two separate people. The other meaning refers to the usual structures or rules of therapy that form the framework within which therapy can take place safely. These include the place of therapy, the established therapy schedule, the expected fee, and, more generally, the expectation that the therapist will offer needed treatment (and only that) and the patient will pay a specific fee (and only that).

A useful distinction can be made between boundary violations and boundary crossings.[4] A boundary crossing is any change or variation from the established boundaries: a value-neutral term that includes harmful instances as well as those that prove valuable to the therapeutic process. Boundary violations apply to those transgressions that are damaging to the therapeutic process, and most especially to the patient.

The Standards of the Profession

It is universally accepted among mental health professionals that sexual involvement with patients is the ultimate boundary violation and unethical. The ethics principles of the American Psychiatric Association (APA) state that "sexual activity with a current or former patient is unethical."[5] It has been observed repeatedly that the sexual involvement of therapists with patients is usually preceded by a series of other boundary infractions of escalating character.

The ethics code of the APA recognizes that boundary crossings, even those that do not entail sexual violation, *may* be violations of the patient and of the therapeutic relationship; thus, they *may* be unethical.[5] Section 6, annotation 1, of the ethics principles of the APA reads,

> Physicians generally agree that the doctor–patient relationship is such a vital factor in effective treatment of the patient that preservation of optimal conditions for development of a sound working relationship between a doctor and his/her patient should take precedence over all other considerations.[5]

This clearly makes it an overarching principle to structure the relationship so that psychiatric treatment can proceed in an optimal fashion. Section 3, annotation 2, which states, "A psychiatrist who regularly practices outside his/her area of professional competence should be considered unethical,"[5] places an obligation on psychiatrists to recognize the importance and difficulty of protecting this working relationship with certain difficult-to-treat patients whose wishes for more intense personal relationships could endanger the therapeutic relationship. Exploitative relationships are addressed specifically in section 1, annotation 1:

> The patient may place his/her trust in his/her psychiatrist knowing that the psychiatrist's ethics and professional responsibilities preclude him/her from gratifying his/her own needs by exploiting the patient. This becomes particularly important because of the essentially private, highly personal, and sometimes intensely emotional nature of the relationship established with the psychiatrist.[5]

Such exploitation of the patient or of the therapeutic relationship may not be recognized consciously by inexperienced or incompetent therapists, or may involve more intentional or careless behavior.

Section 2, annotation 2, enjoins against exploitation of information gained from the patient and against exerting undue influence on the patient by stating that "the psychiatrist should diligently guard against exploiting information furnished by the patient and should not use the unique position of power afforded him/her by the psychotherapeutic situation to influence the patient in any way not directly relevant to the treatment goals."[5]

Boundary Between Psychiatrist and Patient

Patients (particularly those who are sicker and at the less-differentiated end of the developmental spectrum) frequently are not clear regarding the boundary between the therapist and themselves. Others may lose the distinction transiently, especially in certain phases of the transference. For example, projection and projective identification are known mechanisms by which this confusion expresses itself. Thus, it is not uncommon for a patient to provide the first indication of feeling angry or sad by greeting his or her psychiatrist with, "You look angry (sad), Doctor," and it is only somewhat less common for the psychiatrist to recognize that his or her feeling of anger or hopelessness during a therapeutic session reflects how the patient feels. Therapy should help such patients attain a clearer sense of themselves, their own feelings, and, thus, their boundaries. For therapists, empathic attunement to the patient, necessary for effective therapy, involves temporary, almost momentary, identification with the patient's feelings involving a blurring of boundaries. However, it is essential that the therapist quickly return from this state to one that includes cognitive validation so that his or her countertransference does not mistake projections and identification for empathy.[6]

Boundaries of the Therapeutic Structure

There is general agreement that the framework for psychotherapy must be defined and clear to both psychiatrist and patient. The psychotherapeutic encounter should occur at regular intervals, at specific times, and for a fixed duration in a habitual and professionally appropriate setting. Within this "space," the patient is free to confide in the psychiatrist with assurance of confidentiality, except under unusual circumstances (usually legally prescribed) involving imminent danger to the patient or another person. The psychiatrist's attention and interventions are addressed to the therapeutic needs of the patient, with care that these interventions are not the expressions of the therapist's needs. The therapist must set a mutually acceptable fee and expect it to be paid promptly and regularly. This structuring seems elementary, but negotiations around these boundaries and their meanings regularly occur and profit the therapy. Breaches of this structure may, however, also be precursors of damaging boundary violations and the substance of ethical complaints brought against psychiatrists.

General adherence to structure and its continued presence as a point of secure reference is good psychiatric practice. Rigid adherence is safe for risk management and protects patients against exploitation. On the other hand, it also can be used to subject patients to a sometimes cold and sadistic assertion of the psychiatrist's power. Even under more benign circumstances, it may make for rather sterile therapy, in which many opportunities for useful explorations of patients' wishes in relationships are lost.[7,8] Nowhere is this more directly and movingly expressed than in the letter from "Ann, a patient."[9]

Boundary Crossings
Patients as Initiators:

Most often, boundary crossings are initiated by patients. Such crossings may be manifestations of unconscious wishes or expressed consciously and insistently. Frequently, the importance of having a request or wish gratified can be rationalized persuasively.

Because of developmental failure in self-object differentiation, there may be a lack of appreciation of boundaries and the need for them on both an emotional and cognitive level. To such patients, the very idea of boundaries makes no sense. They may have experienced object closeness and emotional gratification only in early infancy and in later repetitions of merged states. They seek these in all relationships, and thus also in the relationship with their therapist. Similar predispositions exist in patients whose personal boundaries were not respected by parents and early caregivers. At the extreme, this may be due to sexual abuse, but also to physical intrusions and violations (such as frequent enemas or rigid control of food intake), or to parental attempts to ascribe their own feelings to the children.

Dependency wishes and needs for approval frequently are expressed in wishes or demands to extend or change the treatment boundaries. For some patients, no amount of attention, work at understanding, and willingness to tolerate painful affects or rage (even directed at the therapist) constitute caring; they insist that only something perceived as different (outside of the therapeutic agreement), special, or extra would constitute caring.

Other patients may have a need, often unconscious, to test their therapist to ascertain whether this person cares enough to withstand the patient's persuasive or threatening demands. There is often an underlying conviction that no one can pass the test. The profoundly ambivalent position of wishing for a trustworthy object (necessary for successful therapy and recovery) combined with the wish to maintain the view of people as untrustworthy and corruptible, which then requires no change in the defensive and maladaptive make-up of the patient, may leave the therapist feeling helpless and trapped for long periods. At times, the patient's rage and wish for vengeance toward old objects can, in their transference manifestation, lead to a relentless effort (disguised as neediness, dependency, and "real" love) to defeat the therapist in his or her attempt to be a trustworthy person.

Therapists as Initiators:

There are psychiatrists with antisocial character pathology who willfully and repeatedly exploit patients in various ways, including sexually. These therapists gratify their own wishes consciously and without concern for their patients, although they may have glib and blatantly unconvincing rationalizations that these activities do not harm or may even benefit their patients. These therapists usually do not benefit from educational or therapeutic endeavors and constitute a continued hazard to the patients they treat.

Various authors have noted that it is hazardous for psychiatrists to think of boundary violations (even sexual ones) as something that happens only to others, emphasizing that intensive therapeutic involvement presents such risks for everyone.[10] This is particularly true in cases in which the exploitation is not blatant. In these cases, various factors, either separately or together, may place the therapist at risk of misjudging the patient's needs in considering the appropriateness and meaning of certain boundaries.

A therapist's training, experience, and skills may not be adequate for treating patients who repeatedly strain boundaries. It in no way shifts the blame for boundary violations from psychiatrists to patients to recognize that there are certain patients with early developmental arrests, personality organizations, childhood abusive and other traumatic experiences, or diagnoses (such as borderline personality disorder) who manifest feelings or behavior in therapy that may place them at particular risk for blurring or transgressing boundaries.[1]

Psychiatrists should be trained cognitively and have supervised experience to recognize such patients, be able to diagnose them, and be alert to issues and problems that may arise in treatment. Such intellectual awareness is accompanied by knowledge of countertransference pitfalls that frequently develop with such patients. Experienced therapists often recognize that certain wishes or needs of patients are particularly difficult and taxing for them to work with and, thus, likely to lead to nontherapeutic interventions; they wisely avoid working with such patients. Fortunately, each therapist is different; therefore, the therapist who cannot work well with clinging, dependent patients may work well with belligerent ones and vice versa.

Intellectual knowledge can be defeated by pressures that occur in the therapist's life or from his or her personality make-up. Therapists, too, are more vulnerable at times of loss and, therefore, under more pressure from their own needs. Illness, divorce, or death in the family may exacerbate personality characteristics and put some therapists at risk of using their patients to gratify their own needs.

In discussing the different types of sexually exploitative therapists, Twemlow and Gabbard[9] describe the "lovesick therapist," an otherwise competent therapist who falls in love with one particular patient and limits the acting out based on complex dynamics involving losses of boundaries vis-à-vis this patient. They state "one prophylactic measure—one that therapists must enforce themselves—is the avoidance of nonsexual dual roles with patients."[10]

All therapists find that certain patients are better liked, touch a chord in a particularly poignant way, arouse rescue or other fantasies, or preoccupy the therapist more than others. When such feelings are recognized, monitored, and taken as a signal for particular care, they may enrich understanding and need not interfere with the maintenance of therapeutic boundaries or with therapy. If, however, such feelings are truly preoccupying or appear to drive the therapist toward action he or she would not take with other patients, a consultation—and perhaps even a shift of the patient's care to another therapist (with total termination of the relationship with the patient)—is urgently indicated.

Therapists, too, may have an excessive need to be loved and/or may fear abandonment, which may lead to excessive needs to gratify patients' expressed wishes and an inability to set or insist on needed limits lest patients feel angry or decide to discontinue therapy. Current circumstances may play into and combine with these needs of therapists. For example, sometimes therapists have open hours and wish to fill them; when patients interview several potential therapists before selecting one, it is difficult at such times not to try to be "best loved" by the patient by offering to meet the patient's wishes in ways that set the tone for boundary transgressions and problematic therapy. At this early stage, as well as throughout therapy, psychiatrists must be willing to risk losing patients.

Insufficiently curbed narcissistic needs in the therapist also contribute to boundary violations. A therapist may act out a wish to play the role of the "all-good" object, the rescuer, or the only one to be really trusted in a patient's life, thus encouraging greater dependency and more pressing demands for a special relationship. A therapist also may feel so specially skilled or perceptive that he or she feels permitted to say or do things that would not be deemed by that therapist to be acceptable in treatment by others. Related is the problem of the overconfident therapist who does not recognize the need for restraint and self-questioning, and who does not recognize therapeutic problems or impasses and the need for consultation.

The Continuum of Boundary Crossings
Dual Relationships:

Although a sexual relationship with a patient is the most blatant and universally damaging perversion of the relationship between therapist and patient, there are other behaviors that breach therapeutic boundaries. These behaviors are exploitative—if not of the patient, of the doctor-patient relationship—because the relationship (and thus the opportunity for the behavior) would not exist otherwise. However psychiatrists rationalize that entering a dual relationship is for the patient's benefit, they should not engage in dual relationships with patients. For example, therapists have employed patients in their offices, as baby-sitters, or as caretakers for invalid family members and have rationalized that they were providing patients with needed jobs or an opportunity to see a healthy family function, or that they were doing something altruistic and caring to improve those patients' sense of self. Aside from blurring and interfering in the therapeutic relationship, such arrangements are based on and involve the power a therapist has over his or her patients. Therefore, such dual relationships are exploitative, regardless of the apparent benefit. Similarly, psychiatrists should provide only the agreed-upon professional services to patients. Regardless of what other area of expertise the doctor may have, it does not belong in the treatment relationship.

Socializing with patients constitutes a dual relationship. Both the patient and therapist may think that an outside relationship can be kept separate from the therapeutic relationship. Expectations in a social relationship are different, however, for both parties from those that should exist in a treatment relationship; it is impossible to isolate and confine such emotional expectations to certain settings and times. For this reason, therapists also should avoid blurring relationship boundaries that would arise if a social acquaintance, friend, or relative were to seek treatment from them. Social or other outside encounters with patients sometimes are not avoidable but should be handled professionally.

A therapist's personal life should be kept separate from his or her practice and from the relationship with the patient. No matter how lonely a patient is, it is not the therapist's task to remedy the loneliness by including the patient in his or her family life. This not only destroys the possibility of further therapy—the reason for which the patient sought out the therapist—it also generally leads ultimately to feelings of envy, exploitation, and anger on the part of the patient.

Psychiatrists who talk too much about themselves, their activities and experiences, and their families also forget what the patient has come for. In doing so, they intrude themselves into the therapy. Once again, even though self-revelations often are rationalized as being good for the patient by bringing equality into the relationship or educating the patient, they generally serve to satisfy the therapist's needs. Extensive self-revelations, particularly those of an emotional or sexual nature, are intrusive and seductive for patients, deflecting them from their own problems and issues into preoccupation and fantasies about the therapist.

Deviations as Warning Signals:

There are also instances of boundary blurring that may complicate or interfere with therapy but do not necessarily lead to clear-cut exploitative violations. Such minor breaches, however, regularly precede more serious ones. Effective therapy probably has ceased—and a turn toward harmful boundary violations has begun—when: a patient seems special or to have special needs that cause the therapist to make exceptions with any regularity, such as increases in the frequency or length of sessions or sessions at unusual times (e.g., late evening); there are frequent lengthy phone calls, particularly outside of working hours; and nonpayment of fees is accepted without careful consideration and necessity. When such a pattern is recognized, consultation may get treatment back within the proper frame and allow it to proceed; at the very least, however, it may save both patient and therapist from a calamitous course.

A family member seen in conjunction with a patient—to obtain history, provide help in the relationship, or give information—is essentially a patient in the sense that only a professional relationship can exist. Personal or business involvement with that person may violate the patient's treatment boundaries, even if that person was never seen professionally.

Gray Areas/Treatment Dilemmas:

It is relatively easy to identify behaviors that are almost always problematic and best avoided. In almost every therapy, however, questions of appropriate boundaries arise in which the course of action is best decided by understanding the patient, the patient's wishes and needs, the issues in the treatment relationship at that particular time, and the meaning of the action in question.

Very often, it is easier for a therapist to answer questions or grant a minor request than to hold fast to thorough exploration. Indeed, when a patient is in treatment around ongoing troublesome symptoms or major life problems and when treatment is not primarily insight-directed, it may be gratuitous to explore minutely around minor boundary issues; e.g., requests for appointment changes, occasional lateness, or minimally intrusive questions ("Are you going on vacation or to a professional meeting?" or, "What's the flower on your desk?"). In general, however, it is beneficial to adhere to the basic framework of therapy, which imposes abstinence on both patient and therapist. Frequently, when exploration brings understanding, patients have less need to have requests gratified.[11]

Names

A frequent dilemma revolves around the way patients and psychiatrists address each other; i.e., by first or last names. Although first-name relationships predominate in current culture, and there are therapists who work comfortably on a mutual first-name basis, the maintenance of last names is an often useful affirmation and reminder of the professional, adult, and basically mutually respectful nature of the relationship. Patients' wishes to call their doctor by his or her first name often constitute wanting to make the relationship more personal; or they may want to use the first name to express disdain or envy. Wishes by patients to be called by their first names without a wish for reciprocity may signify the wish to mimic an earlier, more dependent relationship. There are cases, however, in which flexibility and acquiescence to the patient may be necessary for therapy to continue, ultimately to include the productive exploration of this insistence.

Although it is difficult to identify exactly the right transition age, it is generally inappropriate to call a late adolescent or very young adult other than by first name, unless one wants specifically to underline the transition to adulthood. A young person may never have been called by anything but his or her first name; the last name may signify the mother or father to the patient. The therapist's insistence, then, may be perceived as phony and rejecting of the patient.

Gifts from Patients

Accepting gifts of significant value from patients is a boundary violation and likely to be exploitative. Patients pay a fee for the psychiatrist's service, and the psychiatrist should not expect or accept anything of value beyond that. The rejection of gifts, however, must be executed in a way that does not result in patients feeling criticized or diminished. Small gifts, sometimes homemade and sometimes expressing some particular feeling, are not uncommonly presented on special occasions (such as at Christmas or at termination of treatment) when gifts conventionally are accepted. To accept such a present is a boundary crossing but generally is minor and harmless, whereas its rejection would be baffling or a narcissistic injury to many patients. Patients who frequently suffer and complain of the inequality in the relationship rectify this feeling by being able to offer something that the therapist appreciates. Exploration of the patient's sense of inadequacy and inequality should be pursued, but generally not in immediate conjunction with the gift.

There are instances in which rejection of a gift has positive therapeutic value. For example, a patient discussed her insecurity in relationships and mentioned somewhat in passing that this caused her to shower people with gifts. At her next appointment, she offered her therapist a bouquet of flowers. The therapist asked her to put down the bouquet and talk about it. She spent much of the session elaborating on her insecurities, her need always to give, and the resentment that went with this. At the end of the hour, she picked up the flowers and said, "I guess I shouldn't leave these," and took them with her without having had her gift rejected. She subsequently made considerable progress in working on self-esteem issues in relatively brief therapy.

Requests

Patients sometimes express rather imperative, urgent demands, and the therapist realizes that there is insufficient motivation and not enough time for full exploration before an answer must be given. For example, an emotional, frequently incensed patient arrived at a session on a snowy winter day and announced that her car had broken down on the way and the therapist would have to lend her money for the way home. She immediately went on to describe angrily a variety of other mishaps and urgent problem situations. The therapist recognized that lending the patient money would constitute an unacceptable transgression of the therapeutic boundaries. The therapist was apprehensive about the patient's rage, and knew that the refusal should not come at the end of the hour when the full expression of the patient's rage could be avoided but the patient would be left alone with it. With some trepidation, the therapist interrupted the patient and announced very simply that he would not lend the patient the money. To the therapist's surprise, the patient stopped her angry outpourings and said, "Oh." After a brief silence, she looked in her wallet and announced, "I guess I can take care of it myself." After this, she appeared much calmer and began to explore productively some of the issues facing her. It appeared that, in this case, the therapist's refusal helped her to take a developmental step.

At other times, the refusal of requests (such as for borrowing a book or a waiting-room magazine or even a questioning of the need for a requested extra appointment) has led to productive exploration of both the expressed wish and the meaning of the refusal or hesitation, thereby exposing issues and conflict that might not have been uncovered otherwise. This sometimes leaves the patient with long-term feelings of pain from the rejection constituted by the refusal. In such instances, it may remain unclear whether the therapy was better served by the strict preservation of boundaries or would have been better served by a well-explored breach. Generally, it is more conducive to the productive exploration of fantasies and wishes if a request is not granted. Personal questions about family, when they are explored, sometimes reveal that patients are actually more content not knowing the answers, because almost any answer may in some way shatter a fantasy or displease them.

It must be apparent that in these gray areas, it is not so much what is done that is correct or incorrect but that the process of arriving at the course of action and dealing with its consequences is productive and crucial for therapy. The willingness of the therapist to give careful thought to the issue, discuss and explore it with the patient, and explore the meanings of the chosen course and of the alternatives is what affords safety from boundary violation and makes the boundary issue a lively part of meaningful therapy. An additional safeguard is that whatever the course of action is, it should not have to be secret. The therapist should not consider a course of action that cannot be disclosed comfortably or discussed with a colleague or consultant, nor should the psychiatrist admonish a patient to keep an event in therapy a secret.

Gender of the Psychiatrist

All evidence indicates that sexual boundary violations are more common between male therapists and female patients than in other gender combinations.[12,13] Some evidence indicates this is also true of nonsexual boundary violations.[14] Experience, mostly clinical and anecdotal, suggests that the motivation for boundary violations differs between genders. With male therapists, the risk stems more frequently from underestimation or abuse of the power factor; with female therapists, the risk comes more often from misguided caretaking impulses, gratifying dependency wishes, or attempting rescue from painful life situations.[15]

Special Circumstances
Occasions for Self-Disclosure:

Although it is important for therapists to limit self-disclosure, there are instances in which self-disclosure is inevitable and others in which it may be appropriate.[16] An example of inevitable self-disclosure is if the therapist is pregnant (a subject on which a substantial body of literature exists) or has a serious illness that may affect the patient and therapy.[17–19] The death of a spouse or a child also is likely to fall into this category.[20] It is more debatable whether, for example, a therapist's divorce, the death or serious illness of someone close but more removed, or the nature of an illness that does not substantially affect therapy should be disclosed. Useful criteria are that therapists should avoid burdening patients with their own problems so that patients are not made to feel that they must spare or take care of the therapist. On the other hand, patients need to know and be helped to deal with aspects of the therapist's life that affect them and therapy. Once again, openness to discussion and understanding is essential if such issues do arise.

Small Communities:

The maintenance of strict boundaries between therapy and personal life is fraught with difficulty in small communities, whether they be small towns, academic communities, or even within larger geographic areas, such as minority communities where the therapist and patient belong to the same ethnic group or sexual minority group. In these settings, it is difficult for patients and psychiatrists to avoid extratherapeutic encounters without severely limiting the life and scope of either or both. Although somewhat greater latitude is necessary when this situation prevails, it is nevertheless the psychiatrist's obligation either not to treat certain patients or ensure that boundaries are defined clearly and that they can be maintained in such a manner that therapy can proceed. At times, this may impose some real privation on the psychiatrist. When necessary, some overlap of professional and personal life can be handled with discretion and awareness of the transference and countertransference hazards.[14,21] Safeguards would be to define clearly the overlap and its extent; i.e., to redefine the boundaries, be vigilant about erosion and extension of the overlap beyond what has been defined, and openly discuss the realities as well as the emotional implications for the patient within the context of therapy.

Conclusion

Boundary crossings must never occur when they entail exploitation of the patient or the therapeutic situation. Psychiatrists must guard against rationalizing boundary crossings when their own needs or wishes are actually being gratified. Under these circumstances, boundary crossings become violations of the patient's trust and of the ethics code of the profession. Both good patient care and good risk management dictate their avoidance.

Regular, more minor boundary transgressions that take place with the same patient, or begin to characterize a psychiatrist's practice, can be signals of possible problems. If recognized as such, they may help to identify the nature of these problems and/or the need for consultation to avoid more serious treatment impasses or difficulties.

Occasional boundary issues arise in most therapies, and are best addressed on an individual basis, with full consideration of the psychodynamics of the patient, the transference issues, and the understanding of what would best further therapeutic movement and understanding. Full exploration with the patient about the meaning to the patient of actions to be taken—or not taken—generally ensures respect for the patient and allows the therapeutic process to proceed effectively.

References

1. Gutheil TG. Borderline personality disorder, boundary violations, and patient-therapist sex: medicolegal pitfalls. *Am J Psychiatry*. 1989;146:597–602.
2. Stone MH. Boundary violations between therapist and patient. *Psychiatr Ann*. 1976;6:670–677.

3. Epstein RS, Simon RI. The exploitation index: an early warning indicator of boundary violations in psychotherapy. *Bull Menninger Clin.* 1990;54:450–465.

4. Gutheil TG, Gabbard GO. The concept of boundaries in clinical practice: theoretical and risk management dimensions. *Am J Psychiatry.* 1993;150:188–196.

5. American Psychiatric Association. *The Principles of Medical Ethics with Annotations Especially Applicable to Psychiatry.* Washington, DC: American Psychiatric Press Inc; 1993.

6. Buie DH. Empathy: its nature and limitations. *J Am Psychoanal Assoc.* 1981;29:261–307.

7. Michels R. Sex, ethics, and psychotherapy. American Psychiatric Association Scientific Meeting; New York, NY; May 14, 1990.

8. Altshul VA, Sledge WH. *Countertransference Problems: Review of Psychiatry.* Washington, DC: APPI Inc; 1989;8:518–530.

9. Ann, a patient. A patient's view of doctor-patient boundaries. [Letter to the editor.] *Am J Psychiatry.* 1990;147:1391.

10. Twemlow SW, Gabbard GO. The lovesick therapist. In: Gabbard GO, ed. *Sexual Exploitation in Professional Relationships.* Washington, DC: APPI Inc; 1989.

11. Goz R. On knowing the therapist as a person. *Int J Psychoanal Psychother.* 1975;4:437–459.

12. Gartrell N, Herman J, Olarte S, et al. Prevalence of psychiatrist-patient sexual contact. In: Gabbard GO, ed. *Sexual Exploitation in Professional Relationships.* Washington, DC: APPI Inc;1989.

13. Gartrell N, Herman J, Olarte S, et al. Psychiatrist-patient sexual contact: results of a national survey, I: prevalance. *Am J Psychiatry.* 1986;143:1126–1131.

14. Mogul KM. Ethics complaints against female psychiatrists. *Am J Psychiatry.* 1992;149:651–653.

15. Gilligan C, Pollak S. The vulnerable and invulnerable physician. In: Gilligan C, Ward J, Taylor J, eds. *Mapping the Moral Domain.* Cambridge, Mass: Harvard University Press; 1988.

16. Gold JH, Nemiah JC, eds. *Beyond Transference: When the Therapist's Real Life Intrudes.* Washington, DC: APPI Inc; 1993.

17. Schwartz HS, Silver AL, Madison CT, eds. *Illness in the Analyst.* New York, NY: International Universities Press; 1990.

18. Dewald P. Serious illness in the analyst: transference, countertransference, and reality responses. *J Am Psychoanal Assoc.* 1982;30:347–363.

19. Gruenbaum H. The vulnerable therapist: on being ill or injured. In: Gold JH, Nemiah JC, eds. *Beyond Transference: When the Therapist's Real Life Intrudes.* Washington, DC: APPI Inc; 1993.

20. Givelber F, Simon B. A death in the life of a therapist and its impact on the therapy. *Psychiatry.* 1981;44:141–149.

21. Beskind H, Bartels SJ, Brooks M. Practical and theoretical dilemmas of dynamic psychotherapy in a small community. In: Gold JH, Nemiah JC, eds. *Beyond Transference: When the Therapist's Real Life Intrudes.* Washington, DC: APPI Inc; 1993.

19

Sexual Boundary Violations

SILVIA W. OLARTE, M.D.

Editor's Note

The deleterious effects of sexual intimacy between psychiatrist and patient are obvious: distrust for psychotherapy and psychotherapists; distrust for the opposite sex in general; shame, guilt, self-blame, depression, suicidal ideation and a number of other adverse emotional and behavioral complications. Such intimacy is clearly unethical and can be the basis of a malpractice suit. Whether a therapist can have an intimate relationship with a patient after treatment has ended remains an area of controversy, but the general opinion is that it should be avoided.

Surveys report that while 96% of men therapists and 76% of women therapists acknowledge attraction to one or more of their patients, only 9.4% of the men and 2.5% of the women report having actual sexual relations with them. Most sexual—but obviously not all—boundary violations occur between male therapists and female patients.

- *The characteristics of therapists who become involved with patients have been studied. The most common offender appears to be a middle-aged man undergoing personal distress, professionally isolated, who overvalues his healing capacities and tends to use unorthodox methods in treatment. Offenders have been described as uninformed and naïve, mildly neurotic, severely neurotic and socially isolated, suffering with impulsive character disorder, narcissistic character*

CME questions for this chapter begin on page 367.

disorder, or with a psychotic or borderline personality. The less patho-
logical the therapist's condition, the more successful the rehabilitation.
• *Patients can be especially erotic at times and use eroticism in a vari-*
ety of ways and for a variety of psychological purposes. Every psy-
chiatrist must be on guard lest he or she becomes emotionally and/or
sexually involved, taking whatever measures are required to mini-
mize such risk.

Introduction

Sexual intimacy with clients during treatment is clearly prohibited in
most mental health professionals' codes of ethics. In spite of this undoubted proscription, sexual boundary violations during treatment
have been documented in various groups of health professionals.[1-4] Its
undoubted deleterious effect on the client includes: distrust for the
opposite sex; distrust for psychotherapy and psychotherapists, with
subsequent difficulty in reinstating treatment; guilt, shame, and self-
blame; impaired sexual relationships; depression, loss of self-esteem,
and suicidal ideation; and feelings of anger, rejection, abandonment,
and reenactment of pathogenic childhood situations, because patients
who were sexually abused as children are more vulnerable to being
sexually abused by therapists.[5-7] Sexual intimacy with a former client
remains an area of controversy. Some argue that it becomes a consenting act between two mature adults after a specific time has passed following termination.[8] The majority adheres to the belief that such
behavior continues to be harmful to the client, no matter how much
time has elapsed since termination of treatment.[9,10]

Sexual attraction between psychiatrist and patient cannot always
be described as part of transference or countertransference feelings.
Among surveyed psychotherapists, 96% of men and 76% of women
acknowledged attraction to one or more of their clients. Of these psychotherapists, only 9.4% of the men and 2.5% of the women reported
having had sexual relations with their patients.[11] Among surveyed
trainees, 86% of men and 52% of women acknowledged sexual attraction to one or more patients.[12] Both the psychotherapists and the
trainees reported that having been attracted to their patients evoked
guilt, confusion, and anxiety. Moreover, they cited their lack of adequate training to contend with their sexual attraction for their patients.
The majority reported insufficient training on the recognition and res-

olution of erotic transference phenomena and minimal discussion during supervision of countertransference feelings pertaining to the development of patients' erotic transference onto therapists.

Most sexual boundary violations occur between male therapists and female patients. Various survey studies found 8%–12% of male therapists and 1.7%–3% of female therapists acknowledged sexual contact with their clients.[1-4]

Phenomena inherent to the psychotherapeutic relationship, such as transference and countertransference, reflect both culturally bound sex-role related factors and intrapsychic factors of the patient and the therapist independent of the gender composition of the dyad. Understanding the role played by such factors fosters appropriate resolution of such inherent therapeutic phenomena and avoidance of its misuse. Neither socio-cultural nor intrapsychic factors alone can explain such a preponderance of sexual boundary violations among the male therapist-female patient dyad. Still, our exploration of the possible influence of culturally bound and intrapsychially bound factors on the psychotherapeutic relationship can help us understand such a preponderance and focus our educational efforts on trying to minimize the occurrence of such boundary violations within the therapeutic relationship.

Sex-Role Related Issues

Kaplan,[13] following Kagan's description of the process of socialization for each sex, describes the therapist's role as a combination of two components, the structural and the functional.

The structural component addresses the therapist's responsibility to define for the patient the specific characteristics of the contractual therapeutic relationship. Frequency, length, and location of meetings; appropriate subjects of discussion; and type of interactive pattern to be developed are examples of contractual characteristics. The patient can attempt to influence part of this structure, but its definition lies primarily with the therapist. This expected structural role is what confers authority on the therapist. The therapists' personality traits that are most conducive to successful accomplishment of the structural task are independence, assertiveness, and emotional distance—traits most consistent with masculine, rather than feminine, patterns of sex-role socialization. On the other hand, the functional component addresses

the therapist's ability to be empathic and intuitive, to be a good lis-
tener, and be capable of showing compassion for others while post-
poning gratification of personal needs in favor of the patient's. These
traits are emphasized in the female socialization process. Men and
women therapists need to possess both sets of characteristics to perform both the structural and functional roles.

The presence of such characteristics in both men and women therapists will depend on their socialization patterns, which in turn depend
on their intimate interpersonal world and their particular sociocultural
context. Men and women therapists need to be aware of the effect of
their sex-related socialization patterns and recognize possible countertransference reactions that stem from such patterns. A therapist who is
a man and not aware of his socially acceptable authority role can be inappropriately accepting of his female patients' tendency to be compliant, to be nonconfrontational, and to idealize his authority by
fostering dependency, not growth. A man therapist unable to recognize a patient's need for an empathic, nurturing stance might deny this
patient's dependency components on an erotic transference, address
only the sexualized aspect of the transference, and mishandle such a
phenomenon, facilitating sexual acting out inside or outside of the
therapeutic situation.[14]

A woman therapist who may feel that her professional authority
role is not congruent with her sex-role socialization patterns, might
overvalue her empathic stance, exaggerating the development of a
nurturing-symbiotic transference. The patient might be inhibited
from expressing any transferred erotic longings to the therapist. This
might interfere with the patient's ability to integrate dependency and
erotic longings for the love object.

Intrapsychic Process

The development of an erotic transference within a psychodynamic
therapeutic relationship is considered a universal phenomenon; still, it
most frequently develops within a woman-patient/man-therapist
dyad. The child's development of his or her sense of gender and psychological self will depend upon integration of both the different socialization patterns for the boy and girl and the different interpersonal
developmental paths followed while relating to the nurturing authority figures of both sexes. Pearson[15] maintains that to understand the

difference in the development of the erotic transference in relation to the gender of the patient and therapist, the cultural conceptualization of femininity and masculinity, patients' early object relations, and the asymmetric structures of the oedipal complex must be considered.

Women develop their female self-identity in terms of their affiliation to others: the establishment and continuation of relationships is crucial to their self development, and emotional interdependence fosters growth. By contrast, men define their male self-identity through achievement and autonomy.[16–18] Both sexes might be equally fearful of psychological engulfment by an image of a powerful, omnipotent, primitive, symbiotic nurturing figure—feelings belonging to an earlier developmental stage—but men and women might react differently to the awakened feelings of dependency and longing for the recognized separate love object. That in turn will affect their development and expression of the erotic transference. In a man-patient/woman-therapist dyad, the patient seems to develop a mild, transient—if at all—erotic transference toward his therapist. The patient tends to separate his dependency needs on the nurturing figure from his erotic desires, experiencing the therapist as a nurturing maternal ally or as a threatening, intrusive authority. He then projects the transferred erotic wishes *outside* the therapeutic relationship. The woman patient, on the other hand, is more comfortable with her awareness of her dependency needs and might tend to eroticize her dependency needs *within* the therapeutic relationship.[16]

The Sexually Abusive Therapist

Prevalence surveys on the existence of sexual boundary violations have been easier to construct and complete than surveys addressing the psychodynamic characteristics of the abusive therapist. Throughout the now-voluminous literature on the subject, three main methodologies have been used to describe the characteristics of the sexually abusive therapist: composite descriptions, profile descriptions, and descriptions based on voluntary evaluations of offenders.

Composite descriptions are derived from the treatment of a few offenders.[19,20] Profile descriptions are based on common characteristics found in anonymous research surveys of responders who acknowledged sexual contact with their clients.[2,3] An alternative source is methodic review of personnel files and medical records for known cases of staff-patient sexual relationships in given institutions.[21] The third methodology is examination of the description of offenders. It is contingent on voluntary evaluations of such offenders by centers that specialize in treating victims of physical and/or sexual abuse.[22]

Composite Descriptions:

The composite profile that most frequently emerges from the treatment and/or consultation with offenders is that the therapist is a middle-aged man who is undergoing some type of personal distress, is isolated professionally, and overvalues his healing capacities. His therapeutic methods tend to be unorthodox; he frequently particularizes the therapeutic relationship by disclosing personal information not pertinent to the treatment, which fosters confusion of the therapeutic boundaries. He is generally well trained, having completed at least an approved training program and at times formal psychoanalytic training.

Twemlow and Gabbard[23] based their observations on their treatment and consultation with offending therapists. They described those who fall in love with their patients as the "lovesick therapist." Lovesickness is a reaction separate from any specific underlying pathology, as it can be experienced by therapists who, upon evaluation, can be considered normal, neurotic, or suffering from assorted personality disorders. Lovesickness is characterized by the following features:

- Emotional dependence
- Intrusive thinking, whereby the thought of the other is almost a constant phenomenon
- Physical sensations like buoyancy or pounding pulse
- A sense of incompleteness, of feeling less than whole, when away from the loved one
- An awareness of the social proscription for such love that seems to intensify the couple's longing for each other
- An altered state of consciousness that fosters impaired judgment on the part of the therapist when in the presence of the loved one

This impaired judgment is not displayed in front of other clients. As a result, the therapist can adequately carry out other clinical functions.

Profile Descriptions:

The most common offender profile extrapolated from anonymous surveys is similar to that derived from treatment of specific offenders: a man who has completed an accredited residency training program and who has undergone some personal psychotherapy or psychoanalysis. A survey by Gartrell and associates[3] found that of the 6.4% of psychiatrists who acknowledged sexual relationships with their patients, 89% were men. Of all the psychiatrist-patient sexual contacts reported, 88% involved a man therapist and a woman patient. Of the offenders, 65% reported they had been "in love" with the patient. The survey did not clarify this state, but it alerts us to the possible frequency of the above-described lovesick state of the therapist, with its subsequent clouding of judgment and possible fostering of sexual boundary violations. Moreover, 33% of the offenders had been involved with more than one patient. All offenders who admitted contact with more than one patient were men. Still, 40% of the offenders regretted the contact, and 41% of the offenders consulted colleagues because of their sexual involvement with patients; women offenders consulted more frequently than men offenders, and repeat offenders were the least likely to seek such consultation.

Sexual exploitation of psychiatric patients admitted to varied institutions is an ongoing problem that is difficult to address. Still, when addressed, two profiles of possible vulnerable staff emerge.[21] One is a young, exploitative staff member, who acts out his/her exploitative tendencies outside as much as within the hospital setting. This would correspond with the antisocial therapist described by Twemlow and Gabbard[23] or one of the severely character-disordered abusive therapists described by Schoener and Gonsiorek.[22] The second group (as with the profile from composite sources) encompasses middle-aged, isolated individuals, undergoing personal difficulties that trigger longing for nurturing. Men in the second group tend to be disillusioned with the workplace and feel slighted or hurt by the institution. Their sexual acting out might express their anger and disappointment with the organization and might well resonate with similar feelings within the patient. Women staff members who abuse patients sexually most often are actualizing rescue fantasies, trying to restore the patient's health through love.

Voluntary Evaluation of Offenders:

Schoener and Gonsiorek[22] have developed a classification of sexually exploitative therapists who have voluntarily agreed to a complete psychological and psychiatric evaluation. They have grouped the offenders into clinical clusters correlated with the offenders' potential for rehabilitation and treatment. These categories have been developed through their extended clinical experience rather than a systematic research approach.

Uninformed/naïve:

These professionals lack knowledge of their expected ethical standards or lack understanding of professional boundaries and confuse personal with professional relationships. If the professional who lacked the appropriate information possesses a mature personality, appropriate supervision and education can correct this lack of knowledge and the vulnerability to transgress professional boundaries disappears. Such is not the case with those therapists whose lack of information is accompanied by different levels of personal pathology. There, the underlying pathology determines the prognosis for rehabilitation.

Healthy or mildly neurotic:

These professionals for the most part know their professional standards. Their sexual contact with a patient is usually an isolated and/or limited incident. Frequently at the time of the boundary violation, these therapists are suffering from personal and/or situational stresses that foster a slow erosion of their professional boundaries. They most often show remorse for their unethical behavior, frequently stop such violations on their own, and/or seek consultation with peers. With appropriate treatment and supervision, the majority can be rehabilitated.

Severely neurotic and socially isolated:

Therapists in this cluster show long-standing and serious emotional problems. They can suffer from depression, low self-esteem, feelings of inadequacy, and social isolation. They frequently confuse personal and professional boundaries and foster inappropriate closeness with their patients in and out of the therapeutic relationship. They share personal information not pertinent to the therapeutic process. When erotic transferences develop, they fail to recognize them because of unresolved countertransference feelings, such as their need for self-gratification.[14] When they transgress the professional boundaries and their behavior becomes unethical, they tend to deny it or justify such transgression as a therapeutic maneuver to enhance the patient's self-esteem, as a restitutive emotional experience, or as a consequence of the patient's existing pathology. These therapists can experience guilt and/or remorse, but seldom do they discontinue their unethical sexual relationship with their patient. They frequently are repeat offenders. Because of their more serious personality pathology, rehabilitation through treatment and supervision is difficult; their prognosis is guarded.

Impulsive character disorder:

These therapists show difficulty with impulse control in most areas of their lives. Their problem is generally long-standing. Most have received adequate training and are aware of their professional standards, but regulations do not work as a deterrent to their impulsivity in or out of their professional lives. Their judgment is poor. They tend to abuse more than one victim, show minimal remorse for their unethical behavior, and are oblivious to the possible harm inflicted on the patient by their impulsive behavior. These therapists are poor candidates for rehabilitation.

Sociopathic or narcissistic character disorder:

These therapists also suffer from long-standing serious pathology in most areas of their lives. They tend to be more calculating and deliberate in their abuse of their clients. They successfully manipulate the treatment situation by fostering erotic transference, by blurring the professional boundaries with inappropriate personal disclosure that enhances and idealizes transference, and by manipulating the length or the time of the sessions as to facilitate the development of a sexual relationship with a given patient. They can successfully manipulate the victim or the system to protect themselves from the consequence(s) of their unethical behavior. If caught, they might express remorse and agree to rehabilitation to protect themselves and/or their professional standard, but they will show minimal or no character change through treatment. Their prognosis is poor.

Psychotic or borderline personality disorders:

The severity of such professionals' psychopathology will directly interfere with their reality testing and/or critical judgment. They generally possess the appropriate knowledge of ethical standards and of clinical aspects of professional boundaries; however, their impaired reality testing or poor judgment impedes them in applying such knowledge. Their capacity for rationalization of their unethical behavior—compared with the neurotic individual—is idiosyncratic and simplistic. Rehabilitation is determined by the seriousness of the underlying pathology, and their prognosis is guarded.

Conclusions

Ethical behavior during a professional relationship is always the responsibility of the professional, independent of the patient's pathology or the intensity of any given therapeutic processes inherent to the therapeutic relationship. Still, even though a patient's given pathology and/or the intensity of inherent therapeutic phenomena such as the development of an erotic transference can tax the therapeutic relationship, it may enhance the therapist's vulnerability to blur professional boundaries.[24]

To ensure ethical performance, professional organizations must assume the responsibility of educating their membership not only on accepted ethical standards but on all other sociocultural, personal, and clinical factors that can influence their ethical behavior. For the recognized offenders, professionals are responsible for developing effective evaluatory methods to determine the possibility for treatment and rehabilitation of the offenders in order to avoid a repeat of their unethical behavior. Only a serious commitment to the education of professionals on ethical matters and a candid, systematic, thorough, nonpunitive evaluation—along with an appropriate treatment and rehabilitative approach for the offenders—can secure professional ethical behavior, protecting the patient from the harm such behavior motivates.

References

1.   Kardener SH, Fuller M, Mensh IN. A survey of physicians' attitudes and practices regarding erotic and nonerotic contact with patients. *Am J Psychiatry.* 1973;130:1077–1081.

2. Bouhoutsos J, Holroyd J, Lerman H, Forer BR, Greenberg M. Sexual intimacy between psychotherapists and patients. *Prof Psychol Res Pract.* 1983;14:185–196.

3. Gartrell N, Herman J, Olarte S, Feldstein M, Localio R. Psychiatrist-patient sexual contact: results of a national survey, I: prevalence. *Am J Psychiatry.* 1986;143:1126–1131.

4. Gartrell N, Milliken N, Goodson WH III, Theimann S, Lo B. Physician-patient sexual contact—prevalence and problems. *West J Med.* 1992;157 (August):139–143.

5. Feldman-Summers S, Jones G. Psychological impact of sexual contact between therapists or other health care practitioners and their clients. *J Consult Clin Psychol.* 1984;52:1054–1061.

6. Apfel R, Simon B. Patient-therapist sexual contact, I: psychodynamic perspectives on the causes and results. *Psychother Psychosom.* 1985;43:57–62.

7. Schoener GR, Milgrom JH, Gonsiorek JC. Therapeutic responses to clients who have been sexually abused by psychotherapists. In: Schoener GR, Milgrom JH, Gonsiorek JC, Luepker ET, Conroe RM, eds. *Psycho-therapists' Sexual Involvement with Clients: Intervention and Prevention.* Minneapolis, Minn: Walk-In Counseling Center; 1990.

8. Appelbaum PS, Jorgenson L. Psychotherapist-patient sexual contact after termination of treatment: an analysis and a proposal. *Am J Psychiatry.* 1991;148: 1466–1473.

9. Vasquez MJT. Sexual intimacies with clients after termination: should a prohibition be explicit? *Ethics Behav.* 1991;1:45–61.

10. Shopland SN, VandeCreek L. Sex with ex-clients: theoretical rationales for prohibition. *Ethics Behav.* 1991;1:35–44.

11. Pope KS, Keith-Spiegel P, Tabachnick BG. Sexual attraction to clients. *Am Psychol.* 1986;41:147–156.

12. Gartrell N, Herman J, Olarte S, Localio R, Felstein M. Psychiatric residents' sexual contact with educators and patients: results of a national survey. *Am J Psychiatry.* 1988;145:691–694.

13. Kaplan AG. Toward an analysis of sex-role related issues in the therapeutic relationship. In: Perry Reiker P, Carmen EH, eds. *The Gender Gap in Psychotherapy.* New York, NY: Plenum Press; 1984:349–360.

14. Gabbard GO. Therapeutic approaches to erotic transference. *Dir Psychiatry.* 1990;10(4).

15. Pearson ES. The erotic transference in women and in men: differences and consequences. *J Am Acad Psychoanal.* 1985;13:159–180.

16. Chodorow NJ. *Feminism and Psychoanalytic Theory.* New Haven, Conn: Yale University Press; 1988.

17. Miller JB. The development of women's sense of self (Work in Progress #12). Wellesley, Mass: Stone Center Working Papers; 1984.

18. Gilligan C. *In a Different Voice: Psychological Theory and Women's Development.* Cambridge, Mass: Harvard University Press; 1982.

19. Dalberg C. Sexual contact between patient and therapist. *Contemp Psychoanal.* 1970;6:107–124.
20. Davidson V. Psychiatry's problem with no name: therapist-patient sex. *Am J Psychoanal.* 1977;37:43–50.
21. Averill SC, Beale D, Benfer B, et al. Preventing staff-patient sexual relationships. *Bull Menninger Clin.* 1989;53:384–393.
22. Schoener GR, Gonsiorek JC. Assessment and development of rehabilitation plans for the therapist. In: Schoener GR, Milgrom JH, Gonsiorek JC, Luepker ET, Conroe RM, eds. *Psychotherapists' Sexual Involvement with Clients: Intervention and Prevention.* Minneapolis, Minn: Walk-In Counseling Center; 1990.
23. Twemlow SW, Gabbard GO. The lovesick therapist. In: Gabbard GO, ed. *Sexual Exploitation in Professional Relationships.* Washington, DC: American Psychiatric Press Inc; 1989:71–87.
24. Gutheil TG. Borderline personality disorder, boundary violations and patient-therapist sex: medicolegal pitfalls. *Am J Psychiatry.* 1989;146:597–602.

20

Are You Liable for Your Patients' Sexual Behavior?

DOUGLAS MOSSMAN, PHD

Editor's Note

The extent to which psychiatrists can be held legally accountable for damage or harm caused by their patients' sexual behavior has not been determined with any degree of unanimity in the U.S. court system. In cases involving matters of consensual sex, the courts' criteria for a person's competence to consent to sexual activity are not uniform. Nevertheless, psychiatrists can reduce their vulnerability to malpractice claims by conducting careful assessments of each patient's competence to make decisions regarding his or her psychiatric care and to consent to sexual behavior. In doing so, psychiatrists will position themselves to make the most informed and legally responsible decisions about treatment planning, patient supervision, and placement of the patient in the hospital.

Psychiatric management of patients infected with HIV is laden with malpractice vulnerability as well. Although no state mandates that a physician notify loved ones, significant others, or contacts of patients who have developed AIDS, some states do permit such notification. In other words, the physician's duty to warn is both variable and nebulous. Official guidelines of the American Psychiatric Association

CME questions for this chapter begin on page 368.

make it "ethically permissible" to inform third parties of their risk of HIV infection if an HIV-positive patient under the psychiatrist's care refuses to cease risk-creating behavior or to inform the parties themselves. Moreover, psychiatrists can hospitalize HIV-positive patients on an involuntary basis if they threaten to endanger others and if they have a mental illness for which hospitalization is indicated. The duties to warn and to protect (i.e., the Tarasoff duties) have been applied legally to physician care of patients with infectious disease as far back as the late 19th century, and physicians should be as familiar as possible with the precedents governing the law in their jurisdictions.

However, as the author of this lesson notes, expert knowledge of the case law regarding psychiatric care is not sufficient to shield oneself from malpractice action over cases involving sexually transmitted diseases and patients' sexual behavior. After all, the law can be subjective; a judge may render a decision based more on personal belief and/or emotional interest than on objective fact and then locate the necessary legal citations to support his or her rationale.

Introduction

In the past two decades, since the California Supreme Court's Tarasoff decisions,[1] U.S. psychiatrists have become acutely aware of their potential liability for the harmful actions of their patients. Most lawsuits that have invoked the Tarasoff duty to protect have dealt with injuries caused by patients' violence toward third parties. However, the arrival of the HIV epidemic in the 1980s led physicians and legal commentators to question the legal responsibility of clinicians and their employing agen-cies for third-party injuries caused by sexual contact with patients. Although Tarasoff duties and malpractice liability are familiar topics for most psychiatrists, the principles that underlie these legal matters are confusing, counterintuitive,[2] and frequently misunderstood.[3]

Suing Psychiatrists: What Makes a Case?

When prosecuting an accused criminal, the state alleges that the defendant has violated the public peace by breaking a law enacted by the legislature. Written laws specify that certain kinds of conduct are illegal and punishable.

Theoretically, a caregiver whose patient knowingly participated with a nonconsenting patient in illegal sexual activity might be charged criminally for facilitating that sexual activity.[4] However, the sexual activities of patients are far more likely to result in civil tort actions against psychiatrists. In a tort action, a citizen (i.e., the plaintiff) seeks compensation from another individual (i.e., the defendant) for an injury caused by conduct that breached a legally recognized interpersonal duty.[5] Occasionally, this duty is one created by or codified in legislation. However, for the most part, the duties that potentially generate civil liability have been established over centuries as courts have heard cases and made decisions about personal compensation for an injury.

Courts are supposed to make judgments about liability in particular cases by applying past decisions (i.e., legal precedent) and any applicable statutes to the new situations before them. The relevant decisions and statutes are those of each court's particular jurisdiction. An Iowa court that is deciding a case might take note of other states' decisions about similar cases; however, it could reach a very different finding based on Iowa statutes, previous Iowa cases, or the court's unique view of what the law should be.

For many areas of conduct, experience, abundant precedent, and consistency across jurisdictions allow a clear statement of the "law of torts," and legal texts[5,6] outline the circumstances that courts would recognize as legitimate causes for lawsuits. However, psychiatrists' liability for harm caused by patients' sexual behavior is not one of these areas. To define this form of potential liability, one must extrapolate from a smattering of existing cases to the many possible scenarios under which patients' sexual behavior could harm a third party. Lawsuits against psychiatrists seeking compensation for patients' sexual activities have asserted either that the psychiatrist committed medical malpractice or that the psychiatrist's actions violated the injured party's civil rights.

Malpractice:

In a psychiatric malpractice suit, the plaintiff seeks compensation for injuries alleged to have resulted from professional negligence (i.e., from a failure to apply the knowledge and skills ordinarily possessed and exercised by other psychiatrists working in similar circumstances). If damages (financial, physical, or emotional) result from the negligence and if the negligence was the "proximate" cause of the damage, the psychiatrist must compensate the injured party. A negligent act is a proximate cause when the result is a foreseeable outcome of the act. "Foreseeability" is a central issue in assessing liability for harm caused by psychiatric patients to third parties.

Typically, physicians owe professional duties only to their patients; however, under certain circumstances, physicians also incur duties to the public. Psychiatrists' potential liability for their patients' harmful actions expanded greatly in the wake of California's Tarasoff rulings[1] and decisions in several other states (the so-called "Tarasoff progeny"[7]) that reached similar conclusions. The Tarasoff decisions concerned a lawsuit filed by the parents of a young woman who was killed by Prosenjit Poddar. Poddar, a graduate student in psychotherapy at the University of California Health Services, told his therapist that he intended to kill Tatiana Tarasoff, who was vacationing outside the country at the time. The therapist notified campus police; they interviewed Poddar, found him to be rational, and released him. Poddar subsequently terminated therapy, and the therapist took no further action. Two months later, Tarasoff returned and Poddar killed her. Following Poddar's criminal conviction, Tarasoff's parents civilly sued the treating practition-ers and their employer, claiming that the clinicians were negligent in not detaining Poddar and in not warning Tarasoff's parents of Poddar's intention. The defendants countered that failure to commit or provide warning was not grounds for a malpractice suit.

In 1974, the California Supreme Court issued the first of two decisions on Tarasoff's parents' claim, holding that the practitioners had statutory immunity from lawsuits concerning commitment decisions; however, failure to warn was a sufficient legal basis for a suit. Mental health professionals' organizations strenuously protested, arguing that issuing warnings violated the professional obligation to maintain confidentiality, that this potential breach of confidentiality might inhibit patients from seeking or being open in psychotherapy, and that warnings would not protect third parties anyway.

In 1976, the California Supreme Court took the unusual step of rehearing the case and issuing a second ruling. The Court drew an analogy between the dangers posed by violent psychiatric patients and the risks to the public from the potential spread of infectious diseases. Invoking older decisions that held physicians responsible for failing to notify potential contacts of infectious patients, the Court declared that confidentiality ends "where the public peril begins." The Court acknowledged that warnings could be inadequate to protect others and revised its earlier decision to state that a therapist "bears a duty to exercise reasonable care to protect the foreseeable victim of" a patient and to "take whatever . . . steps are reasonably necessary under the circumstances."

Most courts that have reviewed cases of violence to third parties have embraced the Tarasoff doctrine. Courts also have extended the doctrine to situations involving persons accompanying an identified victim,[8] damage to property,[9] unidentified victims,[10] and victims injured in automobile accidents.[11] When state courts have chosen not to invoke the Tarasoff duty, they generally have not rejected the duty in principle but have said that particular circumstances distinguished Tarasoff from the specific case under consideration.

Several state legislatures have passed laws specifying how clinicians can fulfill their duty to protect,[12] and legal and medical authorities regard this duty as a national standard of practice.[3,13,14] Commentators also have reasoned that the Tarasoff obligation need not be limited to patients' violent acts, arguing that a psychiatrist's knowledge of a patient's potential to engage in injury-causing sexual activity (e.g., transmission of HIV by a patient to a third party) might generate a lawsuit alleging failure to protect.[15–18]

Civil Rights Actions:

A malpractice suit is not the only legal means for seeking compensation for professional wrongdoing. When psychiatrists act under color of state law, plaintiffs can file tort claims and seek compensation for damages on the grounds that the psychiatrists' behavior violated their civil rights (so-called "1983 actions" for the section of the U.S. legal code[19] describing this type of violation) or other constitutional rights. Plaintiffs have claimed rights violations in suits alleging imposition of unwanted treatment, inadequate supervision of a patient, failure to prevent suicide or death at the hands of another, failure to provide appropriate medical treatment, and failure to prevent sexual assault by another patient.[20] However, psychiatrists often are protected from such lawsuits by statutory-defined immunity from liability or by the additional immunity granted by the U.S. Supreme Court in Youngberg v Romeo. This decision established the professional judgment rule: a professional can be held liable only when damages stem from a decision that was "such a substantial departure from accepted professional judgment, practice, or standards as to demonstrate that the person responsible actually did not base the decision on such a judgment."[21] Mental health professionals also can claim good-faith immunity from liability if inadequate funding of their facility prevents them from satisfying normal professional standards.[20]

HIV Transmission and Psychiatrist Liability

Recent studies have shown that psychiatric patients have higher rates of HIV seropositivity than the general population (7% in one study[22]) and that they frequently engage in behavior that places them at risk of transmitting or becoming infected with HIV.[23] Many patients who receive inpatient psychiatric care—particularly minors and adults suffering from chemical dependency, chronic severe mental illness, or developmental disability—are vulnerable to unwanted sexual advances or cannot make thoughtful decisions about sexual activity.[24] The risk of HIV transmission in any single act of needle sharing or intercourse with an infected person is less than 1%[25]; however, if such behavior occurs repeatedly, the cumulative risk of transmission quickly becomes substantial.[26]

The implications of these statistics were quickly appreciated by mental health professionals. By the late 1980s, many commentators established positions concerning ethical obligations and potential for malpractice liability in situations where HIV-positive psychiatric patients were either unable or unwilling to cease risk behavior or inform sexual contacts about their HIV status.[15,26,27] Psychiatrists have three main sources of guidance in anticipating and dealing with the ethical problems and liability risks associated with potential HIV infection: professional ethical guidelines, statutes, and case law.

Ethical Guidelines:

The American Psychiatric Association's (APA) policies on AIDS have been revised over the past decade in ways that reflect psychiatrists' experience in dealing with HIV infection, treatment advances, and changing perspectives on balancing confidentiality and the duty to protect. The 1993 APA guidelines[28] make it "ethically permissible" for psychiatrists to inform third parties at risk of infection if HIV-positive patients will not cease risk-creating behavior or inform contacts themselves.[29] Informing third parties (either directly or through public health authorities) should be a last resort only after careful consideration of the "profound impact of such a notification." Psychiatrists may hospitalize HIV-positive patients involuntarily because of dangerousness toward others only if the patients have a mental illness for which hospital treatment is appropriate.[28] APA guidelines regard counseling about HIV risk reduction a part of standard inpatient care. The vulnerability and impaired decision-making capacity of many inpatients place a responsibility on caregivers to protect patients in the hospital and to prepare them to protect themselves after discharge. In an inpatient setting, clinicians should respond to behavior that poses a risk of HIV transmission with verbal and pharmacologic treatments; if these measures fail, the patient should be isolated and/or restrained.[24] Commentators who concur with these policies believe that they provide a judicious approach to fulfilling the overriding duty of psychiatrists to protect while limiting breaches of confidentiality.[15,16] (The APA has established a separate policy for dealing with HIV infection in children and adolescents.[30])

Other organizations' policies on AIDS take different views of confidentiality obligations and the duty to warn. The American Medical Association's (AMA) Council on Ethical and Judicial Affairs[31] believes that a physician should inform a third party if the patient will not stop risk-creating behavior and public health authorities take no protective action. The position of the American College of Physicians and the Infectious Disease Society of America[32] is ambiguous, urging that the confidentiality of HIV-infected patients be respected "to the greatest extent possible, consistent with the duty to protect others." The American Bar Association's Model Policy emphasizes concern about potential liability over ethical considerations; it suggests that when clinical efforts to induce infected patients to inform contacts or cease risk behavior have failed, caregivers should consult a lawyer or seek a judicial ruling before breaching confidentiality.[33]

Some commentators have criticized policies that allow or recommend third-party disclosure of HIV status under any circumstances. They argue that making known a patient's seropositivity can have devastating personal consequences. They also believe that by not granting absolute assurance of confidentiality to HIV-positive patients, physicians may deter infected patients from being tested and from discussing their status or behavior with caregivers.[25,27]

Statutes:

All the cited policies recognize that the behavior of clinicians must be guided by applicable laws in their jurisdiction. In the 1980s, several states enacted laws dealing with the physician's duty to warn third parties of the risk of HIV infection; these laws take precedence over any common law principles concerning liability.[34] All states require that physicians report AIDS cases to public health authorities, but most states do not require reporting positive test results of persons who do not have AIDS.[28] No state requires a physician to notify contacts, but laws in several states allow notification[34] and often shield physicians from liability whatever their decision may be.[28] In some states, the physician's duty to protect is satisfied by reporting HIV-positive results to the health department, which bears the burden of notifying contacts.[28,34] Statutes vary greatly in delineating the circumstances requiring warnings and the persons who should or may be warned. States variously allow warnings to spouses, current sexual partners, past sexual partners, needle-sharing partners, jail or prison personnel, emergency medical personnel, persons who handle corpses, and/or guardians; some statutes allow third-party warnings only with the patient's consent.[16,25,28] Physicians must be aware of the statutes in their jurisdiction when making a decision about warning a third party.[34]

Case Law:

No U.S. decision specifically addresses the liability of mental health professionals for HIV transmission to a third party. However, should future cases raise this issue, courts may draw on several existing precedents.

The Tarasoff decisions drew inspiration from statutes that require physicians to report cases of contagious diseases and from decades-old cases involving transmission of infections to third parties. A standard interpretation of these cases (and similar decisions not cited in Tarasoff) is that they establish a physician's duty to warn family members or close contacts of the danger posed by an infectious patient.[35] However, as Table 1 shows, the actual holdings were quite narrow.

Decisions reached after Tarasoff have found physicians liable for third-party injuries caused by infectious disease transmission in three cases as of late 1995:

1. A 1976 Florida court found that a man who shared a hospital room with a surgeon's infected patient had a cause of action against the surgeon who failed to carry out appropriate infection-control precautions.[43]

2. In the 1990 DiMarco v Lynch Homes—Chester County decision,[44] the Pennsylvania Supreme Court found that a man who contracted hepatitis had a cause of action against his sexual partner's physicians for failure to give proper advice. The partner was a blood technician who had stuck herself with a needle while drawing blood from a patient with hepatitis. Her physicians erroneously advised her that if she did not contract hepatitis by 8 weeks, she was not infected. Acting on this information, she refrained from sexual relations for 8 weeks. She developed hepatitis (type B) 3 months after the needle stick, and 3 months later, her partner also was diagnosed with hepatitis (type B).

3. The January 1995 California district court ruling in Reisner v Regents of University of California[45] directly addressed a physician's duty to a third party who contracted HIV through sexual contact. In 1985, one day after performing an operation at the UCLA Medical Center, the surgeon learned that the patient, Jennifer Lawson (then 12 years old), had received HIV-tainted blood. No one told her or her parents. Three years later, Lawson began dating—and became intimate with—Daniel Reisner. Two years after this, Jennifer was diagnosed with AIDS; she told Reisner, who found that, by then, he was HIV-positive. Reisner successfully sued his girlfriend's surgeon and associated defendants. The questions before the appellate court were whether the defendants owed a duty to Reisner and whether Reisner had legal grounds for a suit. Relying heavily on Tarasoff and DiMarco, the court ruled that the caregivers could be liable for Reisner's injury even though his identity was unknown to them. However, the breach of duty was the defendants' failure to issue a warning to the "second party" (i.e., Lawson and/or her parents). "Once the physician warns the patient of the risk to others and advises the patient how

to prevent the spread of the disease, the physician has fulfilled his duty—and no more (but no less) is re-quired."[11] (Emphasis added.)

A common thread running through these cases is that the physicians failed to perform basic medical tasks: make a diagnosis, inform a patient about a condition, and provide accurate medical advice to persons requesting it. Table 2[46–49] summarizes some recent decisions that did not involve such blatant errors and that found no liability.

Using previous cases to predict how courts will decide cases involving HIV transmission by mental patients is tricky. One might opine from Reisner that physicians run a limited risk of liability for patient behavior that transmits HIV if they accurately inform patients about their diagnosis and its implications. However, courts (and the public) often take a unique view of psychiatric patients and their caregivers' responsibilities, believing that mental illnesses impair judgment and self-control and that mental health professionals who accept psychiatric patients for treatment therefore assume a duty to control patients who cannot be responsible for themselves. This view is implicitly endorsed by the APA's guidelines that acknowledge the vulnerability of many inpatients and sanction physical restraint to prevent HIV transmission when other measures fail.[24] Courts may not limit the obligation to control psychiatric patients only to patients ill enough to require hospital care. For example, it has been argued that persistent refusal by an HIV-positive patient to cease risk behavior or to inform contacts would be evidence that the patient's mental condition endangers the public and justifies warning a third party.[15,28] Although this reasoning is circular (i.e., bad judgment proves that a person has a judgment-impairing mental illness), it might sound convincing to a court or a jury.

Liability for Other Consequences of Patients' Sexual Behavior
Sexual Assaults in Hospitals:

Several persons have sued psychiatrists for sexual assaults committed in hospitals. These suits have yielded mixed and sometimes conflicting opinions.

Decisions Favoring Plaintiffs

A former inpatient sued the Ohio Department of Mental Health (ODMH) for exacerbation of her mental condition after she was raped by Michael Preston, another inpatient on her ward.[50] Preston previously had been convicted of sexually assaulting a nurse at another hospital, and prior ODMH "records indicated that he was excitable and violent." The court concluded that "it was foreseeable that Preston would attack and rape not only patients but members of the staff," that ODMH "knew it was assigning the plaintiff to a place of danger," and "that Preston's presence on the same ward . . . presented a dangerous condition and, thus, constituted negligence and the proximate cause of the plaintiff's rape and injury."[50] The court reached this conclusion even though Preston was convicted for the assault, which implies that he was responsible for the act. (Given the histories of many ODMH inpatients, almost any coed ward would be "a place of danger" in the court's eyes; as an ODMH-employed psychiatrist, I am struck by the court's confidence in my ability to "forsee" events.)

Colorado law provides immunity from Tarasoff-type liability unless a patient has expressed a specific threat against a particular person. However, a patient was allowed to sue a hospital after she was sexually assaulted by another patient because the patient alleged that the treatment staff knew of the assailant's "dangerous proclivities and his prior aggressive behavior toward" the victim.[51] Such findings, if true, would constitute specific communication of a threat; therefore, an appeals court overturned the lower court's dismissal of the lawsuit.

A 1983 action was brought on behalf of a profoundly retarded patient against hospital employees (including his primary physician) after an unidentified assailant sexually abused the patient twice in a 12-day period.[52] The defendants sought to have the case dismissed. The court believed that the first incident might have been an "isolated mishap," but failure to institute—or even consider—additional protections before the second incident amounted to "deliberate indifference" and was therefore potentially actionable.

A psychiatrist who was a psychiatric resident's analyst sought dismissal of a suit brought by a boy and his parents who alleged that the resident sexually assaulted the boy while he was hospitalized. During psychoanalytic treatment, the resident revealed that he was a pedophiliac. The analyst also was a residency faculty member and knew that the resident planned to specialize in child psychiatry. The court reasoned that the analyst's faculty status gave him "official control and authority over" the resident (a condition for vicarious liability). The court also said that the analyst could have redirected the resident's career without compromising confidentiality. Finding that "a self-confessed pedophiliac who intends to practice child psychiatry presents a foreseeable risk of harm to future minor patients," the court concluded that the boy had grounds for a suit.[53]

Decisions Finding No Psychiatrist Liability

A female patient brought a civil rights action against Colorado state hospital officials alleging that a male patient attacked, kissed, and fondled her. Both patients were fully clothed. The district court dismissed the suit, finding that the man's act was an isolated incident and thus not an unconstitutional deprivation of rights.[54]

A Pennsylvania woman was admitted following an acute exacerbation of schizophrenia and was judged not in need of special observation in the hospital. Three days after admission, she claimed that another patient had raped her on the day of admission. Her condition worsened and required antipsychotic medication; concern about possible effects of the medication led her to undergo a therapeutic abortion later. She sued, alleging negligent supervision. The trial court entered a verdict for the hospital. The appellate court and state Supreme Court affirmed: the decision to forego special observation conformed to state law requiring the "least restrictive" treatment, and such treatment decisions were immune from suit.[55]

A psychiatrist who provided care to a plastic surgery patient was found immune from legal action after the patient attempted to sexually assault a hospital staff member. Under California statutory law (passed after Tarasoff), psychotherapists are immune from liability stemming from their patients' violent behavior unless a patient has communicated a specific threat of physical violence toward a specific third party. Before the attempted assault, the patient had followed, grabbed, and tried to fondle nurses on the floor where he was hospitalized, but the court said that this behavior did not constitute a "serious threat" of violence.[56]

An inpatient who alleged that another inpatient raped her sued several hospital staff members, including her psychiatrist, claiming violation of her civil rights and negligent supervision. The court dismissed the claim against the psychiatrist, who was not responsible for the training or supervision of the persons who were supposed to have been monitoring the patients. However, because previous incidents at the hospital had potentially placed the supervisors "on notice" about problems with patient supervision, the 1983 action against the persons was allowed to go forward.[57]

Consensual Sex in a Hospital

Just one case has dealt with damages alleged to have resulted from a hospitalized patient engaging in consensual intercourse.[58] Virgie Foy and her son sued her guardian, her physicians, and the mental health facility where she had resided, alleging that the boy's birth resulted from negligence. A California appeals court held that a hospital need not prevent a patient from procreating simply because of the patient's incompetence and that failing to prevent the apparently voluntary act of intercourse, which led to a "wrongful birth," was not grounds for a suit. Failure to provide reproductive counseling and contraceptives might be actionable if Foy could demonstrate that she would have used such assistance. The court noted that case law and statutes express a policy preference for maximizing patient autonomy and reproductive choice. "The threat of liability for insufficient vigilance in policing patients' sexual conduct . . . would effectively reverse these incentives and encourage mental hospitals to accord mental patients only their minimum legal rights."[58]

Discussion

Many scenarios besides those discussed herein might generate a lawsuit (e.g., failure to monitor an inpatient who, while suffering illness-induced confusion or hypersexuality, has sex and becomes infected with HIV; or failure to monitor a disturbed inpatient who commits adultery and becomes pregnant).

Administrators and professionals who care for mentally disabled patients (especially in hospitals and institutions for the mentally retarded) commonly avoid explicit discussions of the sexual behavior of patients and often do not provide adequate guidance for staff members. This can lead to confusion about, and mishandling of, issues arising from sexual interaction. As a result, hospital personnel may respond to incidents of consensual sex in ways that violate rights to liberty and reasonable interaction yet fail to investigate and/or report incidents that might warrant criminal proceedings (e.g., rapes and sexual assaults). They also may not develop institutional practices and procedures to reduce sex-related risks.[4]

A key legal issue in determining a hospital care-giver's responsibility for a patient's sexual behavior is the involved patient's ability to consent to sexual interaction. Mental health care providers have a constitutional responsibility to assess the competence of a person who applies for voluntary psychiatric hospitalization because the need for such hospitalization automatically raises questions about the person's ability to make sound treatment decisions.[59] Protecting patients with impaired decision-making abilities is a primary function of a psychiatric hospital. Courts have taken different positions as to what constitutes competence to consent to sexual activity: some require only that the participant understand the nature of the activity; some require understanding of the nature and factual consequences of the activity; and some require understanding of the nature, factual consequences, and moral or social significance of the activity.[4]

The traditional approach to sex in the hospital simply has been to discourage it.[60] Although clinicians may have good reasons to take this position, the reality is that inpatients engage in sexual activity (usually surreptitiously), probably more often than the clinical staff realize. Policies, practices, and treatment planning that do not recognize this fact are unrealistic.

Consideration of a patient's capacity to consent to appropriate sexual behavior and to refrain from inappropriate sexual behavior should influence decisions about therapy, supervision, and ward placement. Of course, potential sexual activity is just one of many matters to consider in making treatment decisions. Its significance will be a function in part of the anticipated duration of hospitalization. On a short-stay ward, it may be reasonable to ask patients to refrain from sexual interaction and to plan treatment with this expectation. In a long-stay hospital (e.g., one where patients spend years confined), this expectation is not reasonable. Staff who work in long-stay settings must develop policies and procedures that address sexuality and privacy consistent with applicable local laws concerning consent. To carry out such policies, staff members need training in helping patients handle sexual issues, in recognizing and responding to patients' sexual problems, and in reporting incidents of possible criminal behavior.[4]

Institutional policies that address patients' sexual behavior and their capacity to consent to sexual activity provide (at least in theory) some protection against liability. Evidence that a clinician or hospital followed a policy suggests that it was acting with forethought, which is a powerful argument against a claim of negligence. Similarly, following a sensible policy and documenting the exercise of professional judgment should be a barrier to claims of "deliberate indifference" to patients' civil rights. Finally, training and supervision of staff suggest that the hospital has taken precautionary measures to make sure that "isolated mishaps" do not evolve into a pattern of neglect.

Conclusion

Although psychiatrists may be sued for their patients' sexual behavior, it is not clear what circumstances will produce successful lawsuits (i.e., verdicts holding psychiatrists liable for damages). Only a few jurisdictions have established precedents in this area; many of these precedents contradict each other, and courts in other jurisdictions may interpret them selectively or ignore them. Although the tort law doctrine of foreseeability is well established, an individual court's view about whether prior behavior made a particular outcome foreseeable may hinge upon that court's seemingly arbitrary interpretations of facts.

In deciding cases, judges are supposed to apply existing law. However, when asked to decide cases involving sexually transmitted diseases and psychiatric patients' sexual behavior—emotion-laden topics where precedents are ambiguous—there is no reason to suspect that judges will respond differently from other humans: they will make up their minds about cases in ways that inevitably reflect their personal beliefs, political positions, and emotional reactions to the facts before them and then will find legal citations to support their conclusions.

Mental health professionals and legal scholars have attempted to fashion practical approaches for responding to patients' sexual behavior and accompanying fears of liability.4,61 Although these approaches appear sensible on clinical grounds, their usefulness as liability-prevention measures remains uncertain.

References

1. Tarasoff v Regents of University of California, 33 Cal App 3d 275, 108 Cal Rptr 878 (1973), rev'd, 13 Cal 3d 177, 529 P 2d 553, 118 Cal Rptr 129 (1974), modified, 17 Cal 3d 425, 551 P 2d 334, 131 Cal Rptr 14 (1976).

2. Goldman MJ, Gutheil TG. The misperceived duty to report patients' past crimes. Bull Am Acad Psychiatry Law. 1994;22:407–410.

3. Perlin ML. Tarasoff and the dilemma of the dangerous patient: new directions for the 1990s. Law Psychol Rev. 1992;16:29–63.

4. Sundram CJ, Stavis PF. Sexual behavior and mental retardation. Ment Phys Disab Law Reporter. 1993;17: 448–457.

5. Keeton WP. Prosser and Keeton on Torts. 5th ed. St. Paul, MN: West Publishing, 1984.

6. American Law Institute. Restatement of the Law, Second, Torts. St. Paul, MN: American Law Institute Publishers; 1965.

7. Stone AA. Law, Psychiatry, and Morality. Washington, DC: American Psychiatric Press; 1984.

8. Hedlund v Superior Court of Orange County, 34 Cal 3d 695, 669 P 2d 41, Cal Rptr 805 (1983).

9. Peck v Counseling Service of Addison County, 146 Vt 61, 499 A 2d 422 (1985).

10. Lipari v Sears, Roebuck & Co, 497 F Supp 185 (D Neb 1980).

11. Petersen v State Washington, 100 Wash 2d 421, 671 P 2d 230 (1983).

12. Appelbaum PS, Zonana H, Bonnie R, Roth LH. Statutory approaches to limiting psychiatrists' liability for their patients' violent acts. Am J Psychiatry. 1989;146: 821–828.

13. Beck JC, ed. The Potentially Violent Patient and the Tarasoff Decision in Psychiatric Practice. Washington, DC: American Psychiatric Press; 1985.

14. Menninger WW. The impact of litigation and court decisions on clinical practice. Bull Menninger Clin. 1989;53:203–214.

15. Zonana H. Warning third parties at risk of AIDS: APA's policy is a reasonable approach. Hosp Community Psychiatry. 1989;40:162–164.

16. Appelbaum K, Appelbaum PS. The HIV antibody-positive patient. In: Beck JC, ed. Confidentiality Versus the Duty to Protect: Foreseeable Harm in the Practice of Psychiatry. Washington, DC: American Psychiatric Press; 1990:121–140.

17. Lott CM. The case for mandatory HIV testing of active duty sex offenders. Mil Med. 1994;159:386–389.

18. Searight HR, Patricia P. The HIV-positive psychiatric patient and the duty to protect: ethical and legal issues. Int J Psychiatry Med. 1994;24:259–270.

19. 42 USC 1983.

20. Perlin ML. Mental Disability Law—Civil and Criminal. Charlottesville, VA: Michie Press; 1989.

21. Youngberg v Romeo, 457 US 307 (1982).

22. Sacks M, Dermatis H, Looser-Ott S, Burton, Perry S. Undetected HIV infection among acutely ill psychiatric inpatients. Am J Psychiatry. 1992;149:544–545.

23.   Cournos F, Guido JR, Coomaraswamy S, et al. Sexual activity and risk of HIV infection among patients with schizophrenia. Am J Psychiatry. 1994;151:228–232.

24.   Commission on AIDS. AIDS policy: guidelines for inpatient psychiatric units. Am J Psychiatry. 1993;150: 853.

25.   Wiseman M. Hey doc, can you keep a secret? An Ohio physician's right to warn third parties that they may be at risk of contracting HIV. J Law Health. 1991–1992;6:199–221.

26.   Simon RI. Clinical Psychiatry and the Law. 2nd ed. Washington, DC: American Psychiatric Press; 1992.

27.   Perry S. Warning third parties at risk of AIDS: APA's policy is a barrier to treatment. Hosp Community Psychiatry. 1989;40:158–161.

28.   American Psychiatric Association Commission on AIDS. AIDS policy: position statement on confidentiality, disclosure, and protection of others. Am J Psychiatry. 1993;150:852.

29.   Hermann DHJ, Gagliano RD. AIDS, therapeutic confidentiality, and warning third parties. Maryland Law Rev. 1989;48:55–76.

30.   American Psychiatric Association Commission on AIDS. Position statement on HIV infection and psychiatric hospitalization of children and adolescents. Am J Psychiatry. 1994;151:631.

31.   American Medical Association Council on Ethical and Judicial Affairs. Ethical issues involved in the growing AIDS crisis. JAMA. 1988;259:1360–1361.

32.   American College of Physicians Health and Public Policy Committee, Infectious Diseases Society of America. The acquired immunodeficiency syndrome (AIDS) and infection with the human immunodeficiency virus (HIV). Ann Intern Med. 1988;108:460–469.

33.   Rennert S. AIDS/HIV and confidentiality: model policy and procedures. Kansas Law Rev. 1991;39:653–737.

34.   Taub S. Doctors, AIDS, and confidentiality in the 1990s. John Marshall Law Rev. 1994;27:331–346.

35.   Bateman TA. Liability of doctor or other health practitioner to third party contracting contagious disease from doctor's patient. In: American Law Reports, 5th Series. Rochester, NY: Lawyers Cooperative Publishing; 1992:370–393.

36.   Span v Ely, 8 Hun 255 (N Y 1876).

37.   Edwards v Lamb, 69 N H 599, 45 A 480 (1899).

38.   Skilllings v Allen, 173 N W 663 (Minn 1919).

39.   Davis v Rodman, 227 S W 612, 147 Ark 385 (1921).

40.   Jones v Stanko, 160 N E 456, 118 Ohio St. 147 (1928).

41.   Wojcik v Aluminum Company of America, 183 N Y S 2d 351 (1959).

42.   Hofmann v Blackmon, 241 So 2d 752 (Fla App 1970), cert. denied, 245 So 2d 257 (Fla 1971).

43.   Gill v Hartford Accident & Indemnity Company, 337 So 2d 420 (Fla App D2 1976).

44.   DiMarco v Lynch Homes-Chester County, 583 A 2d 422 (Pa 1990).

45. Reisner v Regents of University of California, 31 Cal App 4th 1195, 37 Cal Rptr 2d 518 (Jan 1995).

46. Gammill v United States, 727 F 2d 950 (C A 10 Colo 1984).

47. Knier v Albany Medical Center Hospital, 500 N Y S 2d 490 (Sup 1986).

48. Britton v Soltes, 205 Ill App 3d 943, 563 N E 2d 910 (1st Dist 1990).

49. Heigert v Reidel, 206 Ill App 3d 556, 565 N E 2d 60 (5th Dist 1990).

50. Knoll v Ohio Department of Mental Health, 577 N E 2d 135 (Ohio Ct Cl 1987).

51. Halverson v Pikes Peak Family Counseling, 795 P 2d 1352 (Colo App 1990), rehearing denied, 851 P 2d 233 (Colo App 1992).

52. Shaw by Strain v Stackhouse, 920 F 2d 1135 (3rd Cir 1990).

53. Almonte v New York Medical College, 851 F Supp 34 (D Conn 1994).

54. Knight v People of State of Colorado, 496 F Supp 799 (1980).

55. Farago v Sacred Heart General Hospital, 562 A 2d 300 (Pa 1989).

56. Barry v Turek, 267 Cal Rptr 553 (Cal App 1 Dist 1990).

57. Rogers v State of Alabama Department of Mental Health, 825 F Supp 986 (M D Ala 1993).

58. Foy v Greenblott, 141 Cal App 3d 1, 190 Cal Rptr 84 (App 1983).

59. Zinermon v Burch, 494 U S 113 (1990).

60. Binder RL. Sex between psychiatric patients. Psychiatr Q. 1985;57:121–126.

61. Perlin ML. Hospitalized patients and the right to sexual interaction: beyond the last frontier. NYU Rev Law Soc Change. 1993–1994;20:302–327.

D. The courts have been unanimous in deciding what exactly constitutes competence to consent to sexual activity.

PART IV

New Areas of Liability

21

Guidelines to Avoid Liability in Managed Care

LAWRENCE L. KERNS, M.D. AND
CAROL GERNER, J.D.

Editor's Note

The changing scene in health care delivery has posed the physician with an incredibly vast array of new opportunities to be at risk for malpractice. The best safety strategy is to practice medicine within the boundaries of the generally accepted "standard of care" regardless of financial, bureaucratic, or political pressures that may be placed on you.

Managed care, in particular, contains a number of new risk areas, many of which have yet to be extensively defined by the court system. A new wave of litigation arising from the growth of managed care will, however, provide more legal risks and more clarifications.

• For example, the doctor must adhere to standards of care even if a utilization review decision takes a different stance, and if such a physician complies with such a review and the patient suffers damage as a result, trying to place the responsibility on the review process or the reviewer is little protection.

•Other sources of legal peril exist as well. For example, when groups of physicians contract with a managed care operation, all members may be held liable for the mistakes of one doctor in the group. Although not yet tested, physician reviewers may find themselves involved in suits that deal with issues such as breach of contract, breach of warranty, and breach of the implied covenant of good faith and fair dealing.

CME questions for this chapter begin on page 370.

Introduction

Until recently, the health care delivery system in the United States was primarily a fee-for-service one with a focus on the one-to-one relationship between physician and patient. A physician's relationship to a health care institution was usually limited to an affiliation with a hospital as a member of the medical staff. In such cases the physician was generally considered an independent contractor, not an employee of the hospital. Under those conditions, neither party was generally liable for the actions of the other, as neither controlled the activities of the other.

Under this traditional system of health care delivery, the liability issues confronting a physician were fairly well defined. As a practicing physician, one could be held liable for deviating from what is known as "the standard of care" in the rendering of medical treatment to a particular patient.

But patterns of traditional health care delivery have changed, in large part due to the dramatic rise in health care costs. The traditional fee-for-service practice has given way to a group of strategies collectively known as "managed care."

Regardless of their formats, managed care programs share several common features that may complicate liability issues for physicians. Within each program the physician may be confronted with one or more of the following:

- Preadmission and admission review
- Concurrent review processes
- Discharge planning protocols
- Individual case management
- Second-opinion requirements
- Appeal procedures

The increasing visibility of managed care programs has triggered a new wave of litigation. In recent years, there has been a decided increase in liability claims involving managed care programs. Although the role of the physician in the context of managed care has not always been addressed, legal principles from the days of fee-for-service practice can be utilized to limit potential liability.

This lesson will review liability issues for physicians who fit one of the following major categories in managed care: physicians who practice independently, physicians who provide care under contract to a managed care entity, and physicians who serve as reviewers. The lesson will then analyze potential areas of liability and provide recommendations to minimize liability in the event of an adverse outcome.

Independent Physicians

The independently practicing physician cannot escape the constraints and cost controls imposed by third-party payers and fourth-party managed care or utilization review companies. The vast majority of inpatient cases and a growing number of outpatient cases are now subject to external utilization review. Precertification and second-opinion requirements necessitate scrutiny of the medical necessity of each admission, and physicians who conduct concurrent (as well as retrospective) reviews determine the necessity of each day of inpatient care. Benefit limitations may restrict access to the level of care deemed necessary by the treating physician. Pressures to limit the number of treatment days, the use of specialist consultants, and costly testing may all influence the physician's management of a particular case. In short, various cost-containment measures affect the clinical decision making of the independently practicing physician and potentially increase exposure to malpractice liability.

No physician should forget that medicine must be practiced according to the standard of care. It is beyond the scope of this lesson to review the principles of common law known as medical malpractice, but suffice it to say that a physician cannot escape liability for failure to comply with the standard of care simply because of the influences of external cost-containment measures.

Under existing case law, when a managed care entity becomes involved in medical treatment, numerous questions arise about the distribution of liability or responsibility for patient care. Although the leading cases of *Wickline v. State of California*[1] and *Wilson v. Blue Cross of Southern California*[2] address the liability issues of third-party payers, both cases suggest that the treating physician bears responsibility for clinical decisions, including the appropriate time for discharge. Neither case suggests that a physician can avoid liability by acquiescing to a utilization review decision not in accord with the standard of care. Although others, such as a negligent utilization review entity, may share in the responsibility for harm to a patient, their conduct will not relieve the physician of liability.

Wickline addressed the liability of a third-party payer in the context of medical treatment rendered to a patient, and this case also illustrated how a physician's judgment may be influenced by a cost-containment mechanism, potentially increasing his liability. In *Wickline*, the patient was admitted and approved for a ten-day hospitalization. After the patient's surgery, the physician requested an eight-day extension of the hospital stay. The physician cooperated with the utilization review process and was advised that only a four-day extension was authorized. The physician did not appeal or challenge this decision but instead discharged the patient in 14 days, as dictated by the third-party payer. The patient was eventually readmitted and suffered vascular complications that resulted in the amputation of her leg.

The physician in *Wickline* was not held liable primarily because the decision to discharge the patient earlier than originally contemplated still fell within the standard of care. The physician's medical treatment plan was influenced by the cost-containment restrictions of a third-party payer, but the plan was not influenced to the point that the physician deviated from the accepted standard of care.

Should a physician acquiesce to the decision of the utilization review process if it is against good medical judgment? Clearly, the case law would suggest not. If the physician in *Wickline* had disagreed with the recommendation of the utilization reviewer, several options were available to challenge the decision. First, the physician could have contacted the reviewer to discuss the reasons for the decision. In *Wickline*, the facts suggest that the physician reviewer was not adequately informed about the severity of the patient's condition. Furthermore, the reviewer did not know the reasons for the initial admission. Second, the physician could also have renewed the request for an extension of the admission after a few days.

In *Wilson*, the utilization review decision to limit the inpatient stay resulted in the premature discharge of a patient who eventually committed suicide. Although the issue of physician liability was not addressed in *Wilson*, the third-party payer's determination resulted in the patient's refusal to remain in the hospital because the third-party payer would not guarantee payment. Even under conditions of denial and probability of nonpayment for services, the physician-patient relationship cannot be terminated without risk of medical abandonment.

In such instances the physician should document any action the patient takes to end the relationship or terminate treatment, including making a note that the patient is acting against medical advice. On the other hand, continuing treatment in spite of possible nonpayment may be preferable, and the retrospective utilization review or appeal will often result in recovery of a portion of the payment.

Recommendations for Independently Practicing Physicians

- Vigorously challenge or appeal any utilization review denial that conflicts with your medical judgment, treatment, or discharge planning.
- Personally contact the physician involved in the utilization review and discuss the reasons for the requested treatment and why they were not honored. Demand a written explanation of any utilization review decision, on the grounds that you need it to respond adequately in the appeals process.
- Document all contacts with utilization reviewers and any efforts to challenge the utilization review process, but remember that ultimate responsibility remains with the treating physician. Pursue all available appeals offered by the managed care organization.
- Practice according to the standards of care applicable to your specialty and community.
- Cooperate with external reviews by responding in a timely manner and providing all pertinent information after obtaining the patient's consent to its release.
- Document your treatment, including pertinent findings, the rationale behind clinical decisions, and discussions with the patient (including obtaining informed consent).
- Maintain adequate professional liability insurance to protect against malpractice claims.

Managed Care Physicians

Whereas the independent physician's practice can be influenced by external cost-containment mechanisms, the managed care physician usually practices under the same or even more constraints. Depending on the contractual arrangements between the physician and the managed care organization, financial incentives may further influence the physician to reduce costs by limiting treatment.

Before serving as a managed care physician, it is important that the physician review any pertinent contract to ensure that complying with its terms does not conflict with exercising good medical judgment. Failure to do so can result in the physician's being bound by a contract that may foster imposition of liability. In *Varol v. Blue Cross and Blue Shield*,[3] the court rejected the psychiatrists' challenge that the preauthorization and other managed care requirements of a pilot program for the provision of mental health services violated Michigan laws. The psychiatrists had argued that requiring preauthorization interfered with their "right" to determine methods of diagnosis and treatment, and would result in the unauthorized practice of medicine by the insurer. Although the court concluded that state law claims were preempted by the federal statute known as the Employee Retirement Income Security Act (ERISA), it noted that the physicians had voluntarily agreed to the terms. The court warned that neither the cost-containment nor reimbursement features of the contract superseded the psychiatrists' ethical and legal obligation to provide appropriate patient care.

Courts, however, may not uphold provisions of provider agreements that unduly restrict the physician–patient relationship. In *Humana Medical Plan v. Jacobson*,[4] the court concluded that a liquidated damages clause in an affiliated provider agreement was unenforceable because it was against public policy. The offending clause was included to act as a deterrent— to prevent the physician from changing health maintenance organization (HMO) affiliations, thereby causing the physician's patients to change HMOs along with him. The court found that the clause "needlessly" hindered the continuation of existing physician–patient relationships by "driving a financial wedge" between the doctor and his patients.

The provider agreement in *Humana* also contained a not-to-compete covenant. The enforceability of the clause was waived by the HMO. In *dicta*, the court noted that there was nothing to indicate that the noncompete clause would not run afoul of the same public policy that rendered the liquidated damages clause unenforceable.

When insufficient care results in harm to the patient or it can be demonstrated that financial incentives to the physician limit or reduce care, the physician may face potential liability not only for negligence but also for fraud and breach of fiduciary duty.

In *Bush v. Dake*,[5] the plaintiff alleged that the managed health care plan's system of financial incentive, risk sharing, and utilization review was contrary to public policy and medical ethics. The plaintiff further alleged that the use of such cost-containment systems constituted negligence, fraud, breach of trust, and tortious breach of the relationship with her physician. The court rejected the allegations that such a system was contrary to public policy. It found, however, that a question existed whether the financial incentive system was the proximate cause of the alleged malpractice. Bush was eventually settled, but a "gag order" prohibited disclosure of the settlement terms.

In *Teti v. U.S. Healthcare, Inc.*,[6] the plaintiffs, members, and former members of an HMO, filed a class action complaint against the HMO, alleging that they were not informed of the risk-shifting provisions and other financial incentives. They further alleged that they were denied access to care that they were entitled to by virtue of the premium payments made by them or on their behalf. Since the court dismissed the case on jurisdictional grounds, it did not address the merits of the plaintiffs' allegations.

To date, plaintiffs have been unsuccessful in their attempts to impose liability based on financial incentives. No decision has been rendered imposing liability for financial incentives or other aspects of a cost-containment system. Similarly, no decision has been rendered concluding that such incentives legally cause injuries.

A managed care physician who is a member of a group under contract to a managed care entity may be liable for the malpractice of other physicians in the group if it can be proved that the medical group's contract with the HMO to provide quality medical services that meet a certain standard of care was breached.

In *Stelmach v. Physicians Multispecialty Group, Inc.*,[7] the court upheld liability against the medical group for the negligent care provided by one of its physicians. The court concluded that the medical group had breached its contract with the HMO and that the plaintiff-physician member was a third-party beneficiary of the contract and entitled to damages. The court rejected the group's arguments that the physician was an independent contractor and thus established the legal basis for imposition of liability on a physician group for the action of its individual physicians.

Additionally, third parties may employ antitrust theories to support claims against health plans and providers that are founded on price-fixing, group boycotts, fee or compensation arrangements, or monopolization. (Section 1 of the Sherman Act generally prohibits all contracts, combinations, and conspiracies that constitute unreasonable restraints of trade. Section 2 of the Sherman Act addresses monopolization.) The risks of antitrust liability are increased when the health plan is controlled by the provider by ownership or board makeup, and when the plan and provider control a significant portion of the market in a given service area. However, the full implications of antitrust liability are beyond the scope of this lesson.

To the extent that the managed care physician has a role in the hiring of physicians, liability may arise for failing to make reasonable efforts to verify the credentials of the physician. One court has suggested that the managed care organization could be held liable on a theory of negligent selection if it designates the members of its panel. In *Harrell v. Total Health Care, Inc.*,[8] the court noted that the IPA-model HMO owed a duty to its members to investigate panel members and exclude those who posed a "foreseeable risk of harm." The court in Harrell, however, never addressed the merits of the claim since it dismissed the action for other reasons.

Recommendations for Managed Care Physicians

- Carefully review and negotiate any contract that imposes managed care techniques upon the patient treatment process.
- Consider what disclosure, if any, is warranted for any referral restrictions or financial incentives.
- Review all practice protocols and determine the degree to which they conform to the standard of care.
- Establish a corporate policy for credentialing that includes a check of the following:
     Licensure
     Education, training, and experience
     Board certification
     Competence and ethical character
     Hospital privileges and status
     Malpractice history
     Health
- Exhaust sources of information for credentialing information:
     The applicant
     Licensing agencies

  Hospitals
  Malpractice insurers
  Medical societies
  The National Practitioner Data Bank

- Review all written materials provided to patient members to ensure that they do not refer to "guarantees" or contain false representation. Careful language should be used in all plan summaries, contracts, benefit books, and marketing materials.
- Maintain a level of practice that is consistent with the accepted standard of care.
- Make sure that liability insurance protects the physician against the negligent acts of other member physicians.

Physician Reviewers

The most likely source of physician liability in managed care is the utilization review process. Most lawsuits have been filed as a result of the decision of the review entity or physician reviewer. Although many of the reported cases address the issues of liability of the review entity, the same principles can be applied to address the yet unexplored area of liability for the physician reviewer.

Arguably, when a reviewer denies authorization for treatment, it is foreseeable that the patient may forego that treatment and harm may result. This area of potential liability has yet to be fully tested in the legal system. One possible argument that can be raised by the physician to limit any liability is to establish that the role of a reviewer does not entail a physician-patient relationship that would give rise to a duty of care for that patient. The existence of a professional physician-patient relationship is a legal prerequisite for a cause of action alleging professional malpractice against a physician.

Whether the physician reviewer has the requisite physician-patient relationship with the party whose treatment is the subject of review has not been specifically addressed in the reported decisions. Assuming that the review organization has established certain procedures and protocols for the physician reviewers to follow, the physician should be satisfied that the decisions about medical care and medical necessity meet the standard of care. If liability for the physician reviewer exists, it is likely that the liability will be measured against the same standard of care governing physicians generally. In fact, legislative initiatives now exist in some states that would define utilization review as the practice of medicine.

Other possible theories of liability yet to be tested against the physician reviewer include breach of contract, breach of warranty, and breach of the implied covenant of good faith and fair dealing. In a breach of contract action, the plaintiff alleges that the physician or organization failed to provide comprehensive health services according to the terms of the agreement. If a certain assurance of representation is given to the patient or if the parties contract for a specific result, failure to achieve that result may give rise to a cause of action for breach of warranty. In many jurisdictions, courts imply a covenant of good faith and fair dealing in every contract; that is, they imply that neither party to a contract will do anything to interfere with the rights of the other party to receive the benefits of the contract. The physician's liability in these situations would depend on the nature of the contractual relationship between the payer, the utilization review entity, and the physician.

To the extent that a managed care organization advertises or qualifies its treatment services, it may be held to the standards it describes in written brochures or materials. Some decisions have held advertisements to be puffery and not actionable, but at least one court has indicated that liability may be imposed under breach of warranty if a physician clearly promises a particular result that is not attained (*Pulvers v. Kaiser Foundation Health Plan*).[9]

Regardless of the theory, the plaintiff-patient must establish that the denial of coverage or other action by the reviewers proximately caused the injury. In other words, the plaintiff must establish that the action by the reviewer, in the natural or probable sequence, caused the injury. It need not be the only cause. It is sufficient if the cause coincides with some other cause acting at the same time that, in combination, caused the injury. This issue of proximate cause has not been affirmatively addressed in the case law.

Another potential theory against the physician reviewer could involve an action brought by the physician or other providers against the reviewer for interfering with the physician's prospective economic relationship with a patient (*Slaughter v. Friedman*).[10]

Notwithstanding the numerous legal theories that can be raised over improper utilization reviews, the Employee Retirement Income Security Act (ERISA) may provide a preemptive barrier to such claims. ERISA creates a comprehensive regulatory scheme for employee pension and welfare plans. Accordingly, it can preempt state common-law claims involving the denial of benefits. Thus, the statute severely restricts the damages a participant can recover from a managed care program for improper denial of payment. In *Corcoran v. United Healthcare, Inc.*,[11] the parents of an unborn child, who died after an employee plan determined that hospitalization of the mother was unnecessary, filed a wrongful death action. In granting the defendants' motion for summary judgment, the court concluded that the action against the reviewer was preempted under ERISA. The medical decision was incidental to a benefit determination under the plan.

Recommendations for Physician Reviewers

- Utilize nurse triage personnel (as appropriate) in review processes, but review all decisions that in any way limit the treatment sought.
- Be sure that you have the factual knowledge to recognize the clinical factors that can affect the outcome of treatment.
- Consult with specialist physicians (as appropriate) or review cases only within your own areas of expertise.
- Obtain all necessary information; for example, review the initial treatment authorization, review the patient's chart, and consult with the treating physicians, as appropriate.
- Clearly document the reasons for your decisions.
- Establish well-publicized and readily available appeal mechanisms.
- Make decisions on appeals in a timely manner, as required by the exigencies of the situation.
- Follow internal policies and procedures.
- Seek indemnification from the organization for any claims arising from review activities.
- Do not deny treatment without advising the physician and the patient of the rights-of-review process.

Conclusion

Regardless of the format chosen for practicing medicine, a physician must never forget that the practice of medicine must be performed within the standard of care. No physician will be able to avoid liability by attempting to shift the blame for alleged malpractice to the managed care system. Cost-consciousness and cost-containment measures have become a permanent feature of the health care delivery system in this country. Nevertheless, cost limitation programs cannot be permitted to corrupt medical judgment.

Although many of the reported decisions have addressed some of the potential liability issues, they have not resolved many of the legal questions of responsibility facing physicians in this new era of health care.

The existing case law is very fact-specific and, consequently, of limited precedential value, but it does offer practitioners guidelines on how to minimize liability in these uncharted legal waters.

Generally, the courts have recognized the distinction between retrospective and prospective utilization review processes. The liability risks will be greater for prospective action than for retrospective conduct. The practical consequences of prospective utilization review processes can develop into the withholding of necessary care, with resulting malpractice. Thus, theories of liability will be more likely to develop in this area. The consequences of retrospective denial of payment may not be as severe and may not serve as the basis for as much physician liability.

References

1. *Wickline v. State of California*, 192 Cal. App. 3d 1630, 228 Cal. Rptr. 661 (2d Dist. 1986), *decertified*, 741 P. 2d 613, 239 Cal. Rptr. 805 (Cal. 1987).
2. *Wilson v. Blue Cross of Southern California*, 222 Cal. App. 3d 660, 271 Cal. Rptr. 876 (2d Dist.), *review denied*, Oct. 11, 1990.
3. *Varol v. Blue Cross and Blue Shield*, 708 F. Supp. 826 (E.D. Mich. 1989).
4. *Humana Medical Plan v. Jacobson*, Case No. 91-1396, Ct. App., 3d Dist., 1992.
5. *Bush v. Dake*, No. 86-25767-NM (Saginaw, MI, Cir. Ct., filed June 1, 1987).
6. *Teti v. U.S. Healthcare, Inc.*, 904 F. 2d 694 (1989).
7. *Stelmach v. Physicians Multispecialty Group, Inc.*, No. 53906 (Mo. Ct. App. 1989) (unpub).
8. *Harrell v. Total Health Care, Inc.*, No. W.D. 39809, slip op (Mo. Ct. App. W. Dist., Apr. 25, 1989), *affirmed*, 781 S.W. 2d 58 (1989).
9. *Pulvers v. Kaiser Foundation Health Plan*, 99 Cal. App. 3d 560, 160 Cal. Rptr. 392 (1979).
10. *Slaughter v. Friedman*, 32 Cal. 3d 149; 649 P. 2d 886 (1982).
11. *Corcoran v. United Healthcare, Inc.*, 965 F. 2d 1321 (5th Cir. Ct. 1991).

2 2

Biopsychosocial Assessment and Management of Violence in the Clinical Setting

GEORGE S. SIGEL, M.D.

Editor's Note

Avoiding the risk of malpractice involves abiding by ordinary standards of medical care. Of course, this includes the effective management of violent patients. In this lesson, the author emphasizes the importance of taking an integrated approach to such patients, using biological, psychological, and social modalities. We are reminded that mentally ill persons are not necessarily more violent than those who do not suffer with mental illness. Those patients who are given to violence usually are unhappy about their behavior and welcome efforts to help them regain control of themselves. The decision to hospitalize a potentially dangerous patient often provides relief as well as an opportunity to build a therapeutic relationship.

There is a tendency to underdiagnose psychosis in the assessment of violence. In psychotic patients, antipsychotic drugs are obviously quite useful. Anxiolytics may also be of value if agitation is present. Special care must be exerted in patients with alcohol or drug abuse. Lithium may be helpful, even in subclinical doses and in patients without a bipolar diagnosis. Carbamazepine and valproic acid can be useful as well.

CME questions for this chapter begin on page 371.

In administering medications, it is vital to foster patient compliance. Violent patients are often sensitive to and resentful of authoritarian approaches; a collaborative style is often more effective. One should derive a dynamic understanding of the underpinnings of a patient's violence and strive to help him or her learn better ways to handle anger and depression. For hospitalized patients, the environment requires careful attention to minimize triggers for violence, such as overcrowding, inactivity, and humiliation.

Introduction

Understanding the underlying processes of violence and the interventions that can be undertaken to manage it can do a great deal to help potentially violent patients regain or maintain control. Chronically mentally ill persons are not necessarily more violent than persons who are not mentally ill, but when they are violent, their assessment is especially important if therapeutic interventions are to be developed.

Several assumptions underlie this analysis. First, it is my observation that most patients who may at times be violent *do not want to be violent*; following outbursts, they become dysphoric and/or disappointed in themselves. For this reason, it is further assumed that they usually welcome the clinician's interest in helping them regain control. This is often the case even when the patient may be manifestly negative, hostile, or threatening. Most patients benefit from knowing that the psychiatrist will do whatever is necessary to keep them safe and/or others safe from them. I believe they expect this, even if seclusion and forced medication are considered necessary to stop the violence.

In the emergency-room setting, a decision to hospitalize a patient when violence and dangerousness are serious concerns may enable him or her to relax and feel more in control. Psychiatrists must take charge, but at the same time, promote opportunities for collaboration and relationship building with patients. For example, before administering intramuscular (IM) medication on an involuntary basis to contain an emergency presented by a patient's violent behavior, psychiatrists should give him or her several chances to agree to take the medication orally if appropriate. The final assumption is that patients want to regain control and that, for many, there are helpful biopsychosocial interventions. In the clinical setting, violence is rarely random or suggestive of evil and misdirected meanness.

Pharmacologic Interventions

Psychiatrists have a tendency to underdiagnose psychosis in the assessment of violence. Subtle references to problems regarding ideas of reference or conflicts with authority figures often may suggest low-grade reality distortions that predispose to violence. Today, clinicians sometimes prefer to make a diagnosis of affective disorder without psychotic features, possibly because such a diagnosis suggests a more favorable prognosis.

Antipsychotic and Anxiolytic Medications:

Antipsychotic agents are very useful in helping patients regain control, especially if reality distortions underlie the violence. If a patient has taken medication previously, the same one(s) should be used unless the experience was altogether negative. Low-dose, high-potency antipsychotic agents are used most frequently, but are not necessarily more effective. Sometimes, the sedation from chlorpromazine (Thorazine) or thioridazine (Mellaril) is more desirable. It is helpful to choose a medication that is available in both pill and injectable forms so that when different routes of administration are indicated, the same medication can be used.

Violence in the presence of psychosis is often accompanied by a degree of agitation; therefore, low doses of anxiolytic agents may be useful, especially during an emergency. Although oral medications are preferred, a combination of IM trifluoperazine (Stelazine), benztropine (Cogentin), and lorazepam (Ativan) will almost always calm down even a strong patient who is totally out of control. It is not suggested that anxiolytic medications be used on a regular basis, especially because many patients probably have a history of drug and alcohol abuse. A colleague has observed that when these agents are used appropriately as an adjunct to antipsychotic medication, patients do better on lower doses of an antipsychotic agent and do not repeatedly request higher doses. Lorazepam provides a useful example, in part because of its short half-life. However, these medications may at times initiate a paradoxical response, resulting in disinhibition.

In the subacute situation, or in between episodes when a patient is not violent, it may be very helpful to consider a trial on a mood stabilizer. Temporal-lobe epilepsy may be a consideration and clearly needs to be diagnosed carefully for clinical and forensic reasons. If this condition exists, anticonvulsant medications such as carbamazepine (Tegretol) and valproic acid (Depakene) are then used and are not considered mood stabilizers; lithium carbonate (Eskalith, Lithane) may also be used. A therapeutic relationship with the clinician must be evolving because these medications cannot be forced and usually require titration to an appropriate blood level with monitoring of liver and kidney function. Therefore, practically speaking, their use is impossible in a noncooperative patient (and then obligates the clinician to consider obtaining a court order if the need is pressing).

Lithium:

Lithium carbonate can be quite helpful, especially if the patient describes himself or herself as moody, with mood swings and episodic outbursts of violence. For example, men who hit walls often benefit from lithium. (Psychiatrists may find this behavior to be quite common if they specifically inquire about it in the initial interview.) For controlling violence, lithium doses do not necessarily have to be in the therapeutic range (as when it is used for the treatment of manic-depressive disorder). Thyroid-function tests and an electrocardiogram should be obtained; in younger patients with a history of good health, these tests can be obtained soon after the medication has been started. This medication usually is well tolerated but not always helpful. Obviously, a blood level of 1.5 mEq/L should never be exceeded. A response may take 4—7 days.

Anticonvulsants:

Carbamazepine is the next medication often considered. Although many patients who take this drug complain of nausea and sedation, it is well tolerated by most patients. A useful starting dose is 200 mg twice a day. It is often enough to provide some patients with a sense of being in better control while avoiding side effects. Higher doses can be used, but blood-level monitoring is imperative. For elderly patients who are experiencing disinhibition manifested with assaultiveness, 100 mg twice daily is suggested after liver-function tests and white blood cell counts are obtained. Carbamazepine may alter the doses of other medications given for other conditions, and this interaction must be considered.

Valproic acid is traditionally the last agent to be considered for the containment of violence. Surprisingly, however, it is more easily tolerated in some patients, with fewer gastrointestinal complaints. A starting dose of 250 mg two or three times daily is suggested, with monitoring of liver-function tests and regular white blood cell counts suggested. A blood level may be indicated if doses begin to exceed 1000 mg daily and should probably not exceed the levels considered therapeutic for the control of seizure disorders.

Propranolol:

Propranolol (Inderal) is occasionally a useful antiviolence medication. It provides some degree of tranquilization and is actually sometimes used for persons with performance anxiety. The violent patient will feel little effect from the medication, but the violence often will become less severe. One seriously violent patient always felt a "cold feeling inside" and reported that propranolol made him feel "warm inside," and this warmth coincided with his being in much better control of his violence. Blood pressure is usually not a problem with this agent, especially in younger, healthier patients, but it should be monitored. The same is true for the other ß-blockers. Some clinicians occasionally have experienced positive results with propranolol doses greater than 1000 mg daily, but I do not encourage such high doses.

Compliance:

Although polypharmacy is not encouraged, it is occasionally helpful to administer two mood stabilizers when the violence is not well controlled by either one. A mood stabilizer and a tranquilizer may be considered first before any decision to try two mood stabilizers. The use of an antipsychotic agent in conjunction with a mood stabilizer may be helpful in situations where the reaction is swift and suggestive of paranoid distortion.

Medication compliance must be a concern. Violent patients are often sensitive to issues regarding control, and they easily resent an authoritarian style. They appreciate counsel and advice, and are generally more open to using medications when they make the decision themselves. Avoid struggles, and, when the situation permits, begin to consider the psychiatric issues that often function as precursors of violence. In my experience, when these issues (to be outlined below) are defined and acknowledged, patients become more willing to consider your suggestions.

Psychiatric Interventions

Violence may be a form of social contact for some patients. When this is understood, a range of interventions becomes possible, often resulting in a marked diminution in dangerousness. When patients begin to understand the role of violence in their lives, they can substitute other behaviors for the violence and achieve a more successful adaptation through nonviolent verbal and behavioral means of problem solving.[5,6] Let us consider the numerous patterns of violence and personality sketches described below.

Violence can be a defense against sadness and depression:

"Why stay out of trouble? It enriches me," says one violent young man. His life is one long tale of impoverishment. Another person suggests that without his reputation for violence, he has little else. Through his violence, he can avoid dealing with his feelings of how little he has had throughout his life, which now can be blamed upon the violence for which he is responsible. Depression is avoided as he experiences his isolation as the direct outgrowth of his own actions—and not as a result of his past. Another person lives his life in a rage at teachers and health care providers and is at times very assaultive. In so doing, he completely avoids coming to the realization that it was his parents who sent him away at age 9 rather than the school officials. His violence enables him to avoid his depression. Through psychotic denial, for example, a patient defends against his own ambivalence by maintaining that the woman he killed was an imposter, not his mother. One patient summarized this dynamic very well when he commented, "We don't feel grief, we give it."

Violence can be used in the service of mastery and omnipotence:

"I can do what I want because I am a criminal." These words often are spoken by patients who have experienced considerable shame and humiliation. Now because they are "criminals," they have permission to act out their revenge through violence. Unfortunately, their targets are usually the wrong ones, and the good feeling generated by action after years of passivity and/or helplessness is short lived, often accompanied by further shame and humiliation. When feelings of shame and humiliation are aroused, any behavior is acceptable. One patient considered himself justified in assaulting an officer because he thought he had been humiliated through an insult. (Such patients are extremely sensitive to being insulted.) As children, many patients have felt totally helpless in the face of overwhelming abuse, neglect, and shame. As criminals, they become active in the service of acting-out their self-contempt and their conscious and unconscious wishes for revenge.

Violence can be used in the service of achieving identification/persona:

One psychotic, violent young man boasts that "they naturally know me." Another patient wavers between depression and feelings of worthlessness and omnipotent feelings of "being a legend in his time" through the reputation he has achieved by his violence. Through violence, he was a somebody, and feared he was "a nobody" without it. Yet another patient reports about an acquaintance that "he is someone here because he gets a lot of attention, and he will lose this if and when he is transferred." This statement suggests that violence may be a difficult behavior to stop due to fear that status and need gratification will be lost. For different reasons, issues of persona can become "macho" confrontations that cause situations to escalate into violent struggles.

Violence can be a way to establish a sense of self/boundaries:

One patient was clearly in the midst of a profound psychotic regression and was obviously very stressed. He appeared to be losing his sense of self as he became more psychotic and panicky. He complained that he was not sure where he stopped and others began. He intruded several times into the staff meeting room and was abruptly told to wait. He could and should have been invited to sit down in acknowledgment of the terror he was manifesting. When he was told to leave in a very confrontative style by a staff member who was clearly provoked by his intrusiveness, he became assaultive; a very violent encounter ensued. This violence paradoxically enabled him to calm down, as if it helped him establish boundaries as limits were set. This event marked the end of his regression and the beginning of his recovery.

Another patient was confronted with the observation that his fingernails were too long (and dangerous) and that they had to be cut. The symbolism of his body parts, especially in an obviously psychotic and violent young man, was overlooked; and through the confrontation, a violent struggle resulted. When his fingernails were later discussed, and his psychotic delusions about them were defined, he agreed to have them cut. An assault upon his fingernails seemed to threaten him with personality deterioration; thus, he had to fight back.

Violence can be a defense against boredom:

When institutionalized, patients are often crowded into limited space with limited activities. Boredom, even within better facilities, is a problem and can at times foster violence. Boredom also can foster regression and cause the emergence of more primitive thought patterns, which result in reality distortion, paranoid feelings, and an accompanying need for self-defense. These primitive thought patterns especially surface when patients lose their sense of identity and self-worth. For example, Richard is lucid and goal directed during a table-tennis game or when asked to do a work detail on the unit. At other times, he is aimless, very agitated, grossly delusional, and often very assaultive. When activities must be canceled because of staff shortages and especially during bad weather (when patients are confined to the unit), the level of tension and violence increases dramatically. Many patients, especially those with an Axis II diagnosis, use character defenses to deal with strongly ambivalent feelings. The principal defense for many patients is acting-out, and when meaningful outlets are thwarted, the level of violence increases.

Violence can be used to discharge sexual tension and counterdependency:

Many assaults within an institutional setting occur when a male patient believes his manhood is being challenged. Many men react with violence when they feel disrespected, but rarely do they understand what that experience is all about. An all-male environment, especially when activities are limited and space is confining, can be a stimulus to dependency longings. After years of childhood abuse and/or neglect, many patients are counterdependent in their lifestyles. When forced to be dependent, they can become extremely anxious, especially as dependency yearnings are stimulated. Homosexual advances may stimulate conflict and, because of ambivalence, often result in a display of violence. Sexual tension seems to have both pre-oedipal and oedipal derivatives. The pre-oedipal factors are linked more with dependency—wishes that are unconscious and far too painful (because of earlier frustrations secondary to abuse). Therefore, they have to be defended against, usually at all costs; violence may be the response and the defense.

Sexual feelings also may contribute to tension within a milieu and may be the reason some heterosexual men approach others for sex in settings (such as institutions) that preclude heterosexual relief. Privacy, opportunities for discharge through activities and especially competitive interactions, and milieu group meetings that permit some of these issues to be defined and discussed, can help minimize this sexual tension. Certainly, it is very important to give patients the opportunity to talk about the many ways they disrespect themselves and to explore the historic antecedents for their low self-respect and self-esteem. Their vulnerability to feeling disrespected is often central to understanding their violence, and most patients can and do want to learn about this. Psychosocial rehabilitation programs are especially important in helping patients diminish their need to act-out violent impulses. It is also important to include opportunities for enhancing self-awareness so that patients can learn about the connection between low self-esteem and violent outbursts.

Social/Contextual Issues Related to Violence

The biopsychosocial issues reviewed herein must be placed in a social context. Clearly, violence is especially likely to occur when someone's self-esteem is assaulted or threatened. Someone with marginal self-esteem is more likely to be violent if he or she loses a job and becomes more defeated and frustrated. A spouse's decision to seek a divorce can be experienced as a narcissistic assault in a vulnerable person. The loss through death or a geographical move by support persons can cause intolerable affects, and may result in episodic violence, especially if the person is prone to alcohol or drug abuse.

With the recent epidemic of domestic violence, it is important to understand the role of children in a parent's overall adjustment. In vulnerable persons, particularly those with a very narcissistic investment in their children, threats that they might be "taken away" can result in the mobilization of incredible rage and violence. The threatened loss of a spouse can affect self-esteem in ways that mobilize intense, perhaps intolerable, feelings. Violence may be the result.

For adolescents, humiliation in school may recapitulate experiences of shame and humiliation at home, perhaps leading to violence. Girlfriends or boyfriends may become important esteem aides, so their threatened loss may ignite intense feelings of rage. Gang formation is often an esteem-enhancing means of channeling aggression with substantial peer support. Psychiatrists should be aware of the desperate need for peer support that younger persons require in order to feel good about themselves.

Treatment is best considered in a social context. The patient obviously will be sizing up the therapist and may be sensitive to rejection and subtle cues of approval and disapproval. The patient will resent being told what to do and, for transference reasons, will expect disapproval and disrespect. If treated kindly and thoughtfully, patients may be willing to think about formulations and treatments that are suggested by a friendly consultant. Treatment is more likely to be tried and continued if the patient feels he or she is collaborating with a treatment team or provider who is sincerely trying to be helpful. Helping patients learn about stressors and their responses to stress is the next level of intervention to maintain or regain control.

Eventually, patients need to have a range of *corrective emotional experiences*. Such experiences may help them feel better about themselves to a degree that they want to alter their more destructive behaviors in the direction of developing new behaviors, which give them an opportunity to experience new roles and dimensions. Jobs are very important. Support groups in hospitals or within the community are essential in sustaining self-esteem. Alcoholics Anonymous and Narcotics Anonymous are very important as well, especially when substance abuse has been evident.

Conclusion

Patients can learn about their violence, and medication can help them regain or maintain control when experiencing stress. A range of corrective experiences must evolve to help them test newer ways of coping with frustration as they begin to become immersed in activities that enhance self-esteem, thereby enabling them to avoid violence. Only an integrated biopsychosocial approach will yield such results.

References

1. Corrigan P, Yudofsky S, Silver J. Pharmacologic and behavioral treatments for aggressive psychiatric inpatients. *Hosp Community Psychiatry.* 1993;44(2):125.
2. Eichelman B. Toward a rational pharmacotherapy for aggressive and violent behavior. *Hosp Community Psychiatry.* 1988;39(1):31.
3. Sheard M. Clinical pharmacology of aggressive behavior. *Clin Neuropharmacol.* 1984;7(3):173—183.
4. Schatzberg A, Cole J. *Manual of Clinical Psycho-pharmacology.* Washington, DC: American Psychiatric Press Inc; 1986:127.
5. Tardiff K. The current state of psychiatry in the treatment of violent patients. *Arch Gen Psychiatry.* 1992;49:493.
6. Sigel G. Violence as a form of social contact. Unpublished manuscript.
7. Kaplan H, Sadock B. *Pocket Handbook of Clinical Psychiatry.* Baltimore, Md: Williams & Wilkins; 1990.
8. Tardiff K. How to recognize a potentially violent patient. *Psychiatr Times.* 1993;March:13.

23

The Assessment of Violence
in the Workplace and
Its Legal Ramifications

**OTTO KAUSCH, M.D., AND
PHILIP J. RESNICK, M.D.**

Editors' Notes

*In September 1992, the Centers for Disease Control declared violence
in the workplace a national epidemic. Five categories of workplace-re-
lated violence include (1) criminal acts committed in the workplace as
a target of opportunity; (2) terrorism and hate crimes; (3) impulsive,
relatively minor violent acts resulting from interactions among employees (e.g., fights); (4) revenge homicide committed by a disgruntled employee or customer; (5) and violent acts committed by a stalker who
seeks to harm an estranged partner.*

*The typical perpetrator of nonlethal violence often has the same
risk factors associated with violent behavior, namely a male under age
30 with a prior history of violence and drug or alcohol abuse. In contrast, perpetrators of lethal violence are often older than 30 years of age
with no prior history of violence or substance abuse. The typical dis-*

CME questions for this chapter begin on page 373.

gruntled killer is a man in his 30s or 40s who has been, or believes he is about to be, fired or laid off. He often perceives that he has been treated without due respect, identifies strongly with his job, and tends to be a loner. Moreover, the disgruntled killer often is obsessed with weapons and commonly uses guns to complete his act(s) of violence. A high level of stress at work or in his personal life often triggers the violent act.

When assessing an employee's potential for violence, gather as much collateral information as possible. An employee's inability to identify thoughts and feelings represents a particularly poor prognostic sign. The use of drugs such as amphetamines, cocaine, alcohol, or phencyclidine (more commonly known as PCP) must be considered. In carrying out a full mental status exam, be alert to symptoms of paranoia. In the case of stalking, be sure to interview the potential victim.

A psychiatrist who takes no action in treating an employee who communicates a plan to kill a supervisor or coworker is at risk for malpractice. The psychiatrist's duty is not just to warn but also to protect the intended victim. Keep in mind that if a psychiatrist supervises a mental health professional working in an employee assistance program, the legal doctrine of respondeat superior applies: supervisors may bear responsibility for the actions of the professionals working under their management.

Introduction

Scientific studies have found an association among certain risk factors and violent behavior. Some factors, such as age and gender, are static (i.e., not amenable to intervention); other factors, such as active psychosis and alcohol dependence, are dynamic (i.e., amenable to treatment or intervention). In general, the more dynamic the risk factors, the greater the risk of future violent behavior. Risk factors such as antisocial personality disorder are particularly ominous.

When evaluating a patient's potential for violence, the psychiatrist should determine which risk factors are static and which are dynamic. Using this information, the mental health professional can develop a plan to reduce the risk of violence by identifying treatment strategies for the dynamic factors.

Risk Factors for Violence

Risk factors for violence include a past history of violence, young age (early 20s), gender (male), lower social class, low intelligence quotient (IQ), major mental illness (Table 1), organic brain disorder, a history of violent suicide attempts, a history of prior criminal acts, access to lethal weapons, and use of drugs and alcohol.

Past Violence:

The best predictor of future violence in a patient is a history of past violence.[1] The probability of further assault increases with each additional prior act.[2] Understanding the forces that led to past violent acts improves the clinician's ability to evaluate the current risk of violence. Thus, it is important to learn as much as possible about past violent acts.

Demographic Factors:

Several demographic factors are associated with an increased risk of violence. Violence peaks in the late teens and early twenties.[3] Men are 10 times more violent than are women.[4] Of persons arrested for homicide, 90% are male and 50% are younger than 25 years of age.[5]

Persons with low IQs are more likely to be violent than persons with average or high IQs.[6] Hodgins[7] found that intellectually handicapped men were five times more likely to commit violent offenses than were men without an intellectual handicap; intellectually handicapped women, as compared with women without an intellectual handicap, were 25 times more likely to commit violent offenses. The relationship between low IQ and violence persists down to the level of mild mental retardation. Persons with high IQs are able to deal with stress and disappointment in a variety of ways. They may talk to friends for support, respond verbally, or use other coping mechanisms. Intellectually limited persons are more likely to revert to primitive physical responses.

Psychiatric Factors:

Studies performed in the first half of this century suggested that mentally ill persons were no more violent than other citizens in the community.[8] However, despite such studies, the public continued to perceive mentally ill persons as dangerous.[9] In more recent years, studies have confirmed public fears that mentally ill persons are more dangerous than others in society. After reviewing these studies, Monahan[10] wrote, "The data that have recently become available, fairly read, suggest . . . a relationship between mental disorder and violent behavior."

Swanson, and associates[11] studied self-reports of violent behavior in an epidemiologic survey of more than 10,000 persons in the community. The higher the number of psychiatric diagnoses, the greater the likelihood of violence. The combination of substance abuse with other major psychopathology was more volatile than either alone.

In a Swedish birth cohort study followed through age 30, Hodgins[7] found that men with major mental disorders were four times more likely to commit violent offenses than were men who did not carry a psychiatric diagnosis; women with major mental disorders were 27 times more likely to commit violent offenses as compared with women who did not suffer from major mental disorders.

Klassen and O'Connor[12] reported that 25%–30% of male psychiatric patients with a history of violent behavior became violent again within 1 year of discharge. Wessely and colleagues[13] found that mentally ill patients with schizophrenia were more violent than patients with other psychiatric diagnoses.

Persecutory delusions are more likely to be acted on than other types of delusions.[14] In paranoid patients with delusions, violence is often well planned and in line with the delusion. The violence usually is directed at a specific person who is perceived as persecuting the patient. Victims are often relatives or friends. Patients with paranoid schizophrenia often commit the most serious crimes because of their ability to plan and their retention of some reality testing.

Psychotic patients with command hallucinations are at increased risk for violence.[15,16] The rate of compliance with command hallucinations is up to 40%. The likelihood of obeying commands is increased if the voice is familiar and if there is a hallucination-related delusion.[15] For example, a man who hears a voice telling him to kill his mother is more likely to act on it if he has a delusional belief that his mother is a witch.

Personality traits associated with violence include impulsive tendencies, and an inability to tolerate criticism and frustration. Such persons are often self-centered, drive automobiles recklessly, and tend to dehumanize others.[17] In addition, persons with borderline and antisocial personality disorders are more likely to be violent.[18]

Organic brain dysfunction predisposes to violence. Bryant and colleagues[19] found that prison inmates with neuropsychological deficits had significantly higher rates of violent criminal activity than inmates who were not brain damaged. Patients may become subject to explosive rages after a brain insult.[20] Diseases of the brain associated with violence include head trauma, normal-pressure hydrocephalus, cerebrovascular disease, tumors, multiple sclerosis, multi-infarct dementia, Alzheimer's disease, and Parkinson's disease.[21]

Violence in the Workplace

In September 1992, the Centers for Disease Control declared violence in the workplace a national epidemic.[22] Approximately 1 million workers are victims of violent crimes each year in the United States.[23] According to a Time and CNN poll,[24] approximately 18% of Americans have witnessed assaults at work; another 18% worry about becoming victims. According to the U.S. Labor Department, there were 1004 workplace homicides in 1992. In a study of workplace homicide between 1980 and 1988, 75% of murders in the workplace were committed with guns; cutting and piercing instruments accounted for another 14%.[25]

Although much of the research studies regarding violence in the workplace are not scientifically controlled, some efforts are in progress.[26] For now, we must rely on the patterns of violence in the workplace observed by those with practical experience.

Workplace related violence can be divided into five categories: (1) violence associated with the acts of criminals who find the workplace a target of opportunity; (2) terrorism and hate crimes, such as the bombings of the Alfred Murrah Federal Office Building in Oklahoma City and New York City's World Trade Center; (3) impulsive, relatively minor violence resulting from interactions among employees (e.g., fights); (4) revenge murder committed by a disgruntled employee or customer; and (5) violent acts committed by a stalker who seeks to harm an estranged partner.

The typical perpetrator of nonlethal violence in the workplace often has the same risk factors associated with violent behavior: male, younger than 30 years of age, and a prior history of violence and drug or alcohol abuse. In contrast, perpetrators of lethal violence in the workplace often are older than 30 years of age with no prior history of violence or substance abuse.[27]

Profile of the Disgruntled Employee Who Kills:

The typical disgruntled workplace killer is a man in his 30s or 40s.[28] He has been (or believes he is about to be) fired or laid off. Whereas a 20-year-old man can move on to another entry-level job if he is let go, a 45-year-old man may find himself out of work at a time he is expected to be at the peak of his career.

Workplace killers often perceive that they have been treated without the respect they deserve. Many workers who committed violence reported that what affected them more than being fired or demoted was the dehumanizing way in which the action was carried out.[28]

Job layoffs are known to precipitate both psychiatric disorders and alcohol abuse; each is an independent risk factor for violence. In addition, Catalano and coworkers[29] found that the incidence of violent behavior among persons who were laid off was nearly six times greater than that of their employed peers; this effect could not be attributed to psychiatric disorders or alcohol abuse.

The workplace killer usually identifies strongly with his job.[28] He may be a loner with few outside interests who isolates himself from coworkers and lacks supportive family or friends. His job may be his only source of self-esteem and stability. The workplace killer often is obsessed with weapons and uses a gun to kill. He may avidly read gun magazines and enjoy talking about weapons. Some workplace killers have an interest in survivalism.

Disgruntled workplace killers often carry a grudge. They frequently file grievances and are chronic complainers. They are likely to have difficulty accepting authority and may threaten violence directly or indirectly.

The workplace killer is sometimes undergoing a personal stress in his life. The additional burden of facing a layoff or being fired can be the "straw that broke the camel's back." Job loss following divorce or foreclosure on a home is particularly a high-risk factor.

Workplace homicide committed by disgruntled employees often involves multiple victims. Approximately one fourth of these killers then commit suicide: Burgess and colleagues[30] studied 12 men who committed revenge homicides in which 42 people were killed and 22 wounded; three of the killers committed suicide.

Joseph Wesbecker displayed many typical characteristics of the disgruntled workplace killer.[31] On September 14, 1989, he entered the printing plant where he had worked in downtown Louisville. He killed 8 coworkers and injured 12 others with a semiautomatic assault rifle; he then killed himself with a pistol. He had been described by coworkers as a "disgruntled" employee who believed that management had "done him dirty." He claimed that he had been injured by the chemicals he breathed at work. He filed a grievance and, later, a discrimination complaint against the company. He had threatened violence against his company for several months prior to the shootings, which was common knowledge among some of his coworkers and supervisors. After the shooting, one employee said, "You just hear a lot of idle threats . . . and, really, you just think the guy's blowing off steam."[18]

Stalkers Who Kill:

A number of incidents of serious workplace violence have involved stalkers of employees. Stalking is a behavior rather than a psychiatric diagnosis. Persons who stalk other persons have a wide range of psychiatric disorders. Some stalkers are victims of unrequited love.[32] Most often, they seek revenge or rapprochement after a love relationship has ended. Some stalkers suffer from erotomania (a form of delusional disorder);[33] however, most people with erotomania do not engage in stalking behavior. Employers need to worry both about employees who pose a risk of violence from within the company and angry partners of employees who may bring their violence into the workplace. In addition to killing their partners, such stalkers sometimes kill other employees during their angry rampages.

Stress as a Risk Factor:

Some employees commit violent acts when they are unable to cope with high stress in the workplace, such as chronic labor and management disputes; frequent grievances filed by employees; a large number of injury claims, especially for psychic damages; understaffing; and excess overtime. An authoritarian management style increases stress on workers as well.[34] In addition, certain individualized perceptions of employees may increase their stress levels (e.g., a sense that their workload is too demanding).[35] Some employees have conflicts with coworkers or supervisors that make them feel like they just "can't take it any more."

Psychiatric Assessment of Violence Potential

An employer or an Employee Assistance Program (EAP) representative can initiate psychiatric evaluations of potentially violent employees. The referral question to the psychiatric consultant may be vague or specific. The consultant always should have a clear understanding of why a consultation is being requested and the role the he or she will be expected to play. In the absence of valid contraindications, the consultant should expect to interview the employee. It is critical to gather as much collateral information as possible when assessing an employee for violence. Sources may include personnel files; police reports; military records; and interviews with fellow employees, supervisors, and family members.

Clinicians should perform a careful assessment of the employee's past use of violence, beginning with the person's detailed account of the nature and frequency of his or her past violent acts. The mental health professional should ask the employee to describe his or her thoughts and feelings before, during, and after previous violent acts. An inability on the part of the employee to identify thoughts and feelings is a poor prognostic sign.[36] It is useful to gather as much information as possible about events leading up to each violent act. Who said what? To what extent was the act impulsive or planned? What was the degree of injury?

In reviewing an employee's history of violence (Table 2),[37] the mental health professional should look for patterns. For example, was the violent act instigated by an insult that caused the employee to feel disrespected? Has violence occurred only in the presence of psychotic symptoms, such as paranoid delusions?

A detailed history of alcohol and drug use is critical in evaluating an employee's potential for violence. PCP is the hallucinogen most associated with violence.[38] Stimulants, such as amphetamines and cocaine, increase the risk of violence because of disinhibition, grandiosity, and a tendency toward paranoia.[39] The majority of violent employees are intoxicated at the time of their arrest.

An assessment of a history of a use of weapons may provide important information about the employee. According to Federal Bureau of Investigation statistics, firearms are used in two thirds of homicides.[5] The employee should be asked if he or she has ever owned a gun. If so, what particular weapon? Did the employee ever threaten or injure a person with a weapon? How recently did he or she acquire it? Does he or she keep a loaded gun? If an employee recently has moved a weapon, it may be an ominous sign. For example, a paranoid person who recently has moved a handgun from a closet shelf to under his or her bed is at greater risk of killing someone in misperceived self-protection.

The clinician should obtain a careful psychiatric history, noting any episodes of violence that may have precipitated psychiatric admissions. The examiner should attempt to determine patterns of symptoms the employee usually develops when becoming mentally ill. Has the employee ever had command hallucinations? If so, did he or she act on them? The psychiatrist should ask about all current medications and assess past compliance with psychotropic medications.

The examiner should perform a full examination of the employee's mental status. Special attention should be paid to symptoms of paranoia, which may result from a personality pattern or from serious mental illnesses, such as paranoid schizophrenia or delusional disorder.[40] In assessing the potential risk of violence in a paranoid employee, it is critical to ask what the employee would do if confronted by a perceived persecutor. If the clinician simply asks whether the person is homicidal, the employee may honestly answer, "No." However, many persons would strike out if they believed their lives were in danger. Ask if the employee perceives himself or herself to be singled out or mistreated at work. Does the employee carry a grudge against anyone at work or have any revenge fantasies?

The examiner should inquire about the number and severity of personal stressors in the employee's life. It is helpful to know how the employee has coped with stressful events in the past. Does the employee have support to help him or her cope with stress? Does the employee act impulsively? Does the employee talk out his problems or hold them inside, building up resentment?

In cases of stalking, the examiner should interview the potential victim. The mental health professional should inquire about threats and past acts of domestic violence committed by the stalker and attempt to determine if the stalker has pursued other victims. The examiner should look for evidence of mental illness in the stalker; it may be possible to involuntarily hospitalize the stalker if sufficient evidence of mental illness exists. The mental health professional should consult with legal counsel to determine if the stalker can be charged with a criminal offense. If so, it then may be possible to examine the stalker through a court order.

Malpractice Liability for Violent Conduct

Psychiatrists are potentially vulnerable to malpractice litigation after a patient or employee commits a violent act. In a malpractice lawsuit, a plaintiff attempts to recover monetary damages by proving in a court of law that the psychiatrist was negligent.[41] Ordinarily, a successful malpractice suit requires a psychiatric expert opinion that the defendant psychiatrist practiced below the standard of care. The only exception is in cases of res ipsa loquitur (the thing speaks for itself), where the clinician's behavior is so obviously wrong that any lay person can see that the care was inadequate.

Four elements, known as the "Four Ds," are required to prove negligence: duty, dereliction of duty, direct causation, and damages. The plaintiff must first establish that the psychiatrist had a duty to a patient or a foreseeable victim of violence. A psychiatrist is required to exercise, in both diagnosis and treatment, a reasonable degree of knowledge and skill that is ordinarily possessed and exercised by other members of his or her profession in similar circumstances.

The second element of negligence is dereliction of duty. Psychiatrists are not required to practice without error; however, they are required to exercise reasonable care. Courts make a distinction between errors of fact and errors of judgment and look less favorably upon clinicians who commit errors of fact than those who commit errors of judgment. Failure to review prior records or otherwise properly evaluate collateral sources could constitute an error of fact. For example, if one failed to review available records that documented violence in an employee who was making threats, a successful malpractice suit would likely result. Furthermore, if the evaluator failed to interview the employee and based his or her opinion solely on the report of an employer, the clinician could be sued by the employee who unjustly lost his or her job. Therefore, in performing an evaluation of a possibly violent worker, it is imperative that the clinician gather sufficient data before offering an opinion.

Errors of judgment will not result in a successful suit if the clinician acted in good faith and exercised the requisite care in obtaining necessary information, in formulating a diagnosis, and in treating the patient's condition. A psychiatrist who takes no action in treating an employee who communicated a plan to kill his supervisor is at risk for a malpractice suit. However, if the psychiatrist took some reasonable steps to protect the victim, the psychiatrist is unlikely to be sued successfully even if there is a bad outcome because he or she made an error of judgment.

The third element of negligence is proof of direct causation between the dereliction of duty and the resulting harm; the legal term for this is proximate cause. The final element is actual damages, which may include the costs associated with injury to others, suicide, or loss of employment.

Psychiatrists must be mindful of the Tarasoff doctrine when dealing with potentially dangerous employees. In the landmark Tarasoff decision,[42] the California Supreme Court stated:

When a therapist determines, or according to the standard of his profession should determine, that his patient presents a serious danger of violence to another, he incurs an obligation to use reasonable care to protect the intended victim from danger. The discharge of such duty, depending on the nature of the case, may call for the therapist to warn the intended victim or others likely to apprise the victim of danger, to notify the police, or take whatever other steps are reasonable under the circumstances.

Although an earlier Tarasoff decision in 1974 specified a duty to warn,[43] the superseding 1976 Tarasoff case clearly enunciated that the duty was to protect the potential victim from danger. Because of the publicity in the first Tarasoff case, clinicians commonly make the error of thinking that their duty is to warn, rather than to protect, the intended victim.

In cases of potentially violent employees, protective steps may include warning an employer or coworkers, notifying the police, hospitalizing the employee, placing the employee in a drug rehabilitation program, or other reasonable interventions. If there is a violent outcome, the court will judge in retrospect whether the psychiatrist took reasonable steps to prevent foreseeable violence.

Some state courts have applied the Tarasoff doctrine only to identifiable victims; other courts have included broader categories of potential victims.[44] By 1989, 12 states had adopted some form of a Tarasoff limiting statute.[45] Needless to say, psychiatrists should be aware of the Tarasoff requirements in their particular states.

When psychiatrists are acting as supervisors for an EAP program, they should be aware that they may bear responsibility for the actions of those they supervise under the legal doctrine of respondeat superior. The supervisor should monitor closely cases of potential workplace violence and be readily available for consultation.

Psychiatrists should be familiar with their organization's policies and procedure manuals because they may be held liable for failing to adhere to them. For example, if an examiner worked as a consultant to an EAP program that required that a risk-assessment form be completed on all employees who made threats, the examiner is more likely to be held liable in a suit if he or she did not fulfill this requirement. It is better for an organization to have no policy than to have one that sets unrealistically high standards.

Strategies for Reducing Malpractice Risk

Psychiatrists who assess potential violence in the workplace can reduce their risk of being sued for malpractice by keeping in mind the following recommendations:

- Stay abreast of the literature regarding the assessment of the risk of violence in general and in the workplace in particular.
- Obtain all relevant data, including past records, before assessing an employee. Be sure to obtain a signed release of information from the employee.
- Carefully document your reasoning for recommending a particular course of ac-tion in cases of potentially violent em-ployees. Provide a detailed risk-benefit analysis for the decision that you reach.
- Be aware of the specific Tarasoff doctrine and relevant case law in your state regarding protection of potential victims.
- Obtain consultation in complex cases. It is much more difficult for

a plaintiff to prove that no prudent clinician would make the decision you made if a consultant contemporaneously agreed with you. You also might consider seeking legal advice in complex cases.

- If you are being employed as a consultant, be clear about the referral questions and the role you will be expected to play in any subsequent proceedings.
- Before an employee evaluation, clearly inform the employee of the limits of confidentiality. If an employee mistakenly thinks you are mistreating him or her, that person could bring a suit against you for breach of confidentiality.
- If you are working for an organization or agency, be sure to follow its policies and procedures. If some policies are difficult to implement, help the organization de-velop more realistic policies.
- Do not offer an opinion when an em-ployer provides background data and you are not allowed to interview the employee.
- Closely monitor the work of supervisees who evaluate or treat potentially violent employees.

Conclusion

Assessing dangerous patients is both challenging and intellectually stimulating. Unfortunately, a wrong decision can have devastating consequences. In the event of a bad outcome, the consultant's evaluation will be scrutinized. The consultant can best protect himself or herself by being knowledgeable about risk assessments, performing thorough evaluations, documenting reasons for decisions, and obtaining consultation in difficult cases.

References

1. Klassen D, O'Connor WA. A prospective study of predictors of violence in adult male mental health admissions. Law Hum Behav. 1988;12:143_158.
2. Shah SA. Dangerousness: a paradigm for exploring some issues in law and psychology. Am Psychol. 1978;33:224–238.
3. Monahan J. The Clinical Prediction of Violent Behavior. Washington, DC: Government Printing Office; 1981. DHHS Publication No. ADM81-921.
4. Tardiff K, Sweillam A. Assault, suicide, and mental illness. Arch Gen Psychiatry. 1980;37:164–169.
5. Federal Bureau of Investigation. Crime in the United States. Washington, DC: U.S. Department of Justice; 1992.

6. Quinsey V, MacGuire A. Maximum security psychiatric patients: actuarial and clinical prediction of dangerousness. J Interpers Violence. 1986;1:143–171.

7. Hodgins S. Mental disorder, intellectual deficiency, and crime: evidence from a birth cohort. Arch Gen Psychiatry. 1992;49:476–483.

8. Brown P. The Transfer of Care: Psychiatric Deinstitutionalization and Its Aftermath. London: Routledge & Kegan Paul; 1985.

9. Link BG, Cullen FT, Frank J, et al. The social rejection of former mental patients: understanding why labels matter. Am J Sociol. 1987;92:1461–1500.

10. Monahan J. Mental disorder and violent behavior. Am Psychol. 1992;47:511–521.

11. Swanson JW, Holzer CE, Ganju VK, et al. Violence and psychiatric disorder in the community: evidence from the Epidemiologic Catchment Area surveys. Hosp Community Psychiatry. 1990;41:761–770.

12. Klassen D, O'Connor WA. Assessing the risk of violence in released mental patients: a cross-validation study. J Consult Clin Psychol. 1990;1:75–81.

13. Wessely SC, Castle D, Douglas AJ, et al. The criminal careers of incident cases of schizophrenia. Psychol Med. 1994;24:483–502.

14. Wessely SC, Buchanan A, Reed A, et al. Acting on delusions, I: prevalence. Br J Psychiatry. 1993;163:69–76.

15. Junginger J. Predicting compliance with command hallucinations. Am J Psychiatry. 1990;147:245–247.

16. Junginger J. Command hallucinations and the prediction of dangerousness. Psychiatr Services. 1995;46: 911–914.

17. Reid WH, Balis GU. Evaluation of the violent patient. Am Psychiatr Assoc Annu Rev. 1987;6:491–509.

18. Tardiff K. Violence: causes and nonpsychopharmacologic treatment. In: Rosner R, ed. Principles and Practice of Forensic Psychiatry. New York: Chapman & Hall; 1994.

19. Bryant ET, Scott ML, Golden CJ, et al. Neuropsychological deficits, learning disability, and violent behavior. J Consult Clin Psychol. 1984;52:323–324.

20. Krakowski M, Convit A, Jaeger J, et al. Neurologic impairment in violent schizophrenic patients. Am J Psychiatry. 1989;146:849–853.

21. Tardiff K. The current state of psychiatry in the treatment of violent patients. Arch Gen Psychiatry. 1992; 49:493–499.

22. Centers for Disease Control. Homicide in the U.S. Workplace: A Strategy for Prevention and Research. Atlanta: Centers for Disease Control; 1992. NIOSH Publication #92-103.

23. Bachman R. National Crime Victimization Survey: Violence and Theft in the Workplace. Washington, DC: U.S. Department of Justice; 1994. NCJ–148199.

24. Toufexis A. Workers who fight firing with fire. Time. 1994;143:36.

25. Jenkins EL, Layne LA, Kisner SM. Homicide in the workplace: the U.S. experience. AAOHN J. 1992; 40:215–218.

26. Johnson PW, Meyer RG, Feldmann TB. Violence in the workplace: new empirical data. Bull Am Acad Foren Psychol. 1995;August:3–5.

27. Filipczak B. Armed and dangerous at work. Training. 1993;30:40.

28. Bensimon HF. Violence in the workplace. Training and Development. 1994;48:27–32.

29. Catalano R, Dooley D, Novaco R, et al. Using ECA survey data to examine the effects of job layoffs on violent behavior. Hosp Community Psychiatry. 1993; 44:874–879.

30. Burgess AW, Burgess AG, Douglas JE. Examining violence in the workplace. J Psychosoc Nurs. 1994; 32:14.

31. Kuzmits FE. When employees kill other employees: the case of Joseph T. Wesbecker. J Occup Med. 1990;32:1014–1020.

32. Zona MA, Sharma KK, Lane J. A comparative study of erotomanic and obsessional subjects in a forensic sample. J Forensic Sci. 1993;38:894–903.

33. Diagnostic and Statistical Manual of Mental Disorders. 4th ed. Washington, DC: American Psychiatric Association; 1994.

34. Kinney J, Johnson DL. Breaking Point: The Workplace Violence Epidemic and What to Do About It. Washington, DC: U.S. Department of Health and Human Services; 1993.

35. Sauter SL, Murphy LR, Hurrell JJ. Prevention of work-related psychological disorders. Am Psychol. 1990;45:1146–1158.

36. Ball EM, Dotson LA, Brothers LT, et al. Prediction of dangerous behavior. Presented at the 23rd Annual Meeting of American Academy of Psychiatry and the Law, Boston; October 1992.

37. Wack RC. The ongoing risk assessment in the treatment of forensic patients on conditional release status. Psychiatr Q. 1993;64:275–293.

38. Budd RD, Lindstrom DM. Characteristics of victims of PCP-related deaths in Los Angeles county. J Toxicol Clin Toxicol. 1982;19:997–1004.

39. Honer WE, Gewirtz E, Turey M. Psychosis and violence in cocaine smokers. Lancet. 1987;i:451.

40. Boxer PA. Assessment of potential violence in the paranoid worker. J Occup Med. 1993;35:127–131.

41. Simon RL, Sadoff RL. Psychiatric Malpractice. Washington, DC: American Psychiatric Press; 1992.

42. Tarasoff v Regents of the University of California, 17 Cal 3d 425, 131 Cal Rptr 14, 551 P 2d 334 (1976).

43. Tarasoff v Regents of the University of California, 118 Cal Rptr 129, 529 P 2d 553 (1974).

44. Felthous AR. The duty to protect. In: Rosner R, ed. Principles and Practice of Forensic Psychiatry. New York: Chapman & Hall; 1994.

45. Appelbaum PS, Zonana H, Bonnie R, et al. Statutory approaches to limiting psychiatrists' liability for their patients' violent acts. Am J Psychiatry. 1989;146:821–828.

QUESTIONS

How to earn CME using this section

*T*he dual mission of a Hatherleigh CME Book is to provide medical professionals with a review of authoritative, practical information that illuminates the common and challenging clinical issues they encounter in their daily work, and to include with that information an exam that enables them to earn Category I credit toward the recertification of their license.

The chapters in this book were originally published Hatherleigh's our peer reviewed *Psychiatric Malpractice Risk Management* continuing medical education program. They were selected for inclusion on the basis of their fundamental importance to this topic area. The material should provide the practicing psychiatrist with detailed knowledge about the various professional standards he or she must uphold to practice medicine effectively and prudently.

Nineteen of the chapters in this book can be used to earn continuing medical education credits via the CME Appendix. The editor's notes at the beginning of each chapter highlight the learning points. To earn CME credits using this book, simply call Hatherleigh to order a quiz response form using the toll-free number, 1-800-367-2550. Hatherleigh representatives will inform you of the options available to you as a participant in one of our CME programs.

The Hatherleigh Company, Ltd., is accredited by the Accreditation Council for Continuing Medical Education (ACCME) to sponsor continuing medical education for physicians. The Hatherleigh Company, Ltd. designates *Psychiatric Malpractice Risk Management: A Comprehensive Guide* for no more than 2 credit hours per chapter in Category 1 of the Physician's Recognition Award of the American Medical Association. This CME Activity was planned and produced in accordance with the ACCME Essentials.

CHAPTER 4

Reducing the Risk of Malpractice

page 48

1. **Specific accepted standards of care:**
    A. Include the application of knowledge from the cutting edge of research.
    B. Involve a reasonableness of practice following guidelines observed by most practitioners.
    C. Preclude the use of any and all nonestablished approaches to therapy, even when these are noninvasive, carry no significant sequellae, and may be used in conjunction with specific accepted standards of care.
    D. Include always making the right diagnosis, regardless of how the diagnosis may have been made.

2. **Which of the following procedures may raise the question of not following accepted standards of care and thus threatening the patient's welfare?**
    A. Excessive monitoring of medications
    B. Using neuropsychological testing to clarify diagnosis when the clinical evidence is insufficient
    C. Failing to provide the patient's family with information they may require to assure that the patient has a better chance of staying well and not reverting to self-destructive behavior when the patient is expected to be living home
    D. Refusing to see a new patient referred by a colleague, and instead referring him or her to an outpatient clinic

3. **Which of the following statements is correct?**
    A. If a patient succeeds in committing suicide in a hospital, negligence can always be assumed.
    B. If a psychiatrist is not certain of a patient's potential for violence or self-destructive behavior at the time of discharge from hospital, he can request the decision be made by a court.
    C. In prescribing a biological treatment, it is not necessary to explain to a patient or his family what might happen if the treat-

ment is withheld or inform them about alternate methods of care.

D. Sexual activities between a therapist and patient are not considered unethical if they have fallen in love with each other.

4. **In which of the following situations is the psychiatrist least likely to be confronted with malpractice charges?**

   A. A patient gives a history of exhaustion, weight gain, cloudy thinking, dry skin, and sensitivity to cold. Her referring physician attests to the fact that her blood thyroid levels are normal. The psychiatrist prescribes antidepressants, but the patient only becomes worse. The patient independently seeks advice from another physician who diagnoses hypothyroidism and treats the patient with thyroid hormone resulting in dramatic clinical improvement within a month.

   B. Although a patient manifests clear-cut symptoms of depression, the therapist chooses to continue individual psychotherapy and conjoint marital therapy for months while refraining from using antidepressants. The patient's depression deepens, and in a panic state he attempts suicide and is hospitalized. Although he then recovers with six weeks of antidepressant treatment, he loses his employment as a consequence of the hospitalization.

   C. A psychiatrist recommends clozapine for a chronically ill schizophrenic patient. He does not think it necessary to offer any other options, such as electric convulsive treatments or psychiatric rehabilitation, neither of which has ever been previously afforded the patient. He warns the patient and the family about the potential side effects of the drug and obtains signed consent to proceed. He uses active monitoring. Nonetheless, the patient develops a serious blood dyscrasia and dies.

   D. A patient, in a state of agitation because he has discovered his wife is having an affair, consults a psychiatrist. After seeing the patient once, the psychiatrist tells him that he is not suffering with mental illness and does not need any professional care. Two days later, the patient brutally beats his wife and then attempts suicide.

CHAPTER 5

Vulnerability of Psychiatrists in Assessment of Risk for Malpractice

page 59

5. In considering committment:
   A. The concept of dangerousness is clear and easily defined by psychiatrists.
   B. Dangerousness may better be redefined in clinical terms, such as potential violence to self or others under various clinical conditions.
   C. If the doctor is uncertain, the safest course is always to contact the legal system and do whatever their representative decides.
   D. Always try to get the patient to enter the hospital voluntarily, no matter how psychotic he or she may be.

6. Which of the following statements is correct?
   A. Merely having a side effect from a medication is a common ground for a major malpractice suit.
   B. The doctor must be aware of the risk of lawsuits caused by unexpected side effects from *combinations* of medications that may damage patients.
   C. Courts have ruled that competent patients who are not emergencies have the right to refuse only antidepressant medications.
   D. In following the rule of informed consent, it is usually not necessary to offer patients information about alternative treatment modalities when a choice exists.

7. Which of the following statements is correct?
   A. When releasing a patient to the community, economic issues should be given as much importance in the decisions as clinical findings.
   B. If, at the time of considering hospital discharge, the treating psychiatrist is uncertain about the possibility of self-destructive or violent behavior following release, consult the court and follow the judge's decision.
   C. The *Tarasoff* duty to protect requires therapists to personally

warn prospective victims and provides no other avenues for carrying out the professional mandate.

D. The rule of confidentiality should never be broken, even when it comes to informing families about the care of patients after discharge or responding to court demands for such information.

8. Which of the following statements is correct?

A. It is not necessary to demonstrate related damage in order to win a malpractice suit against a physician.

B. Incompetent patients can legally sign themselves into the hospital.

C. There is no way to hospitalize incompetent patients against their will.

D. Psychiatrists have been sued for improper commitment because they found evidence of "dangerousness," but no evidence for a bona fide mental illness linked to it.

CHAPTER 6

Practical Legal Consideration for the Psychiatrists Being Sued for Malpractice

page 71

9. When threatened by a malpractice lawsuit:

A. It's best to be your own attorney.

B. Don't take things seriously until you actually receive a subpoena.

C. Report any indications of a threatening claim to your insurance company at once.

D. Be careful about what you reveal to the attorney assigned to you, and only give him records he specifically requests.

10. Which of the following statements is correct?

A. If the attorney for a patient calls informally and says he's just gathering some information about your treatment with the patient, tell him anything he wants to know.

B. It's best to be belligerent toward any and all individuals connected with a malpractice claim brought against you, including your own insurance carrier.

C. If you receive a summons or complaint about a malpractice suit against you, don't feel you have to respond within any specific time period.

D. If you receive a summons or complaint, be sure to note every detail about how it was delivered because, the way the law works, improper delivery of a summons can force dismissal of the whole case against you.

11. A deposition is:

A. An informal, inconsequential discussion between lawyers in search of compromises, with clients present.

B. A serious meeting between the sides for which you should be well prepared by your attorney because the information brought out can be used later in a court hearing.

C. The official document delivered by the sheriff informing you that you are being sued for negligence.

D. Another term for settlement, in which an agreement to drop the suit is made in return for financial compensation.

12. If you are involved in a malpractice suit:

A. Never settle.

B. Never participate with your lawyer in the selection of a jury.

C. Realize that any hearing is a civil hearing and not a criminal one, and can only lead to a verdict of negligence, not one of guilt.

D. Always enter into a countersuit for damages if you are found not negligent, even if it takes another five years to trek through the legal mazes.

CHAPTER 8

Recent Developments in Clinical Psychiatry and the Law

page 96

13. **Which of the following statements is correct?**
    A. Involuntary commitment regulations that impose a standard of "clear and present danger" because of a dangerous patient's mental illness exist in only 30 states.
    B. If a therapist discharges a "dangerous" patient under the administrative mandate of a managed care company and the patient commits suicide or kills someone, it is the psychiatrist who faces liability in malpractice charges.
    C. Thus far, courts have unanimously agreed that managed care companies are liable for decisions related to patient discharge; treating psychiatrists operating under the company's directive cannot be held accountable in this regard.
    D. All of the above statements are correct.

14. **If a psychiatrist cannot obtain an extension for hospitalization from the patient's managed care company and absolutely believes that a patient will be harmed or others will be harmed if the patient is released from the hospital, the psychiatrist should:**
    A. Proceed with the mandated discharge, but make a clear note in the chart that he or she disagrees with the decision.
    B. Increase the patient's medication to decrease the likelihood of impulsive violent behavior.
    C. Demand to speak to and review the case with the medical director of the managed care company.
    D. Obey the mandate, but insulate himself or herself from future liability by writing a letter about the case to the local newspaper.

15. **Which of the following statements is correct?**
    A. A patient's right to confidentiality cannot be breached, even when he or she threatens to commit suicide.
    B. Boundary violations occur most frequently in the treatment of patients with obsessive-compulsive disorder.

    C. The term boundary crossing applies only to sexual behavior between therapist and patient.

    D. Most of the false accusations regarding boundary violations against psychiatrists come from patients with borderline personality disorder.

16. **When a patient allegedly has no memory of early childhood sexual abuse before entering therapy and, during the course of therapy, begins to remember such episodes, the therapist should:**

    A. Understand that courts will not support such memories as facts without corroborating evidence.

    B. Routinely encourage the patient to confront those responsible for the abuse and take legal action to obtain retribution.

    C. Recommend group attendance with verified incest survivors even if the patient's own recollections cannot be verified.

    D. Reject the memories as false, inasmuch as the patient was unaware of them prior to treatment.

CHAPTER 9

Malpractice Liability Prevention in Hospital Psychiatry

page 109

17. **Which of the following statements is correct?**

    A. Psychiatrists cannot be sued by patients for false imprisonment.

    B. During an intake evaluation, it is not necessary to write anything about a patient's preliminary assessment and treatment plan if extensive data obtained during the interview with the patient have been recorded.

    C. An intake report must reflect that the psychiatrist has taken into account relevant sources of information in addition to his or her own interview of the patient.

    D. All of the above statements are correct.

18. **The doctrines of vicarious liability, such as** *respondeat superior:*
   A. Require psychiatrists to make a reasonable attempt to contact third parties expected to be of potential relevance to their evaluation of a patient.
   B. Impose potential liability upon psychiatrists for negligent acts committed by other members of the treatment team who are under their supervision or control.
   C. Excuse psychiatrists from the necessity of noting and responding to observations or opinions expressed in a patient's chart by other members of the treatment team.
   D. Releases the treating psychiatrist of the duty to procure a signed release of information from the patient when information must be obtained from another professional who has worked with the patient.

19. **The psychiatrist who is in charge of a hospitalized patient's care:**
   A. Is only responsible for the treatment of the patient's mental disorder and need not be concerned with the patient's physical health.
   B. Is only required, under most circumstances, to read a patient's prior hospital discharge summaries, not the other details of the record.
   C. Is legally expected to predict suicide when conducting an assessment of suicidality.
   D. Cannot be held liable if a suicidal patient commits suicide after discharge from the hospital.

20. **Which of the following can serve as the basis of a liability action arising from the use of psychopharmacologic agents?**
   A. Instituting pharmacotherapy without baseline medical clearance
   B. Prescribing psychotropic medication during pregnancy
   C. Long-term use of benzodiazepines
   D. All of the above

CHAPTER 10

The Risk of Misdiagnosing Physical Illness as Depression

page 131

21. Which of the following statements is correct?

A. If a patient has had a recent physical examination, the psychiatrist can rest assured no physical illness is present.

B. In Hall's study of psychiatric outpatients, not one revealed a physical disorder producing psychopathologic symptoms.

C. In Hall's study of state hospital patients, 46% had previously unrecognized, undiagnosed physical illnesses specifically related to their psychiatric symptoms.

D. Failure to detect a physical disorder presenting as a psychiatric disorder is exclusively the problem of psychiatrists.

22. In Koranyi's study, what percentage of nonpsychiatric physicians failed to diagnose physical illness in patients they referred to psychiatrists?

A. 10%

B. 20%

C. 32%

D. 48%

23. Which of the following statements is correct?

A. In Hall's study of state hospital patients, over half the patients with physical disease improved dramatically with regard to psychiatric symptoms once the physical disorder was adequately treated.

B. In Koranyi's study, 83% of all patients referred for psychiatric care by social agencies or who were self-referred had undetected physical illness.

C. No matter how closely the first presentation of a patient conforms to classical DSM-III descriptive criteria, it does not guarantee that he or she suffers only or primarily from a psychiatric illness.

D. All of the above

24. Which of the following statements is correct?

A. Malignant tumors may present to the psychiatrist as depressive symptomatology months before any physical signs or symptoms appear.

B. Increased urinary excretion of 5-hydroxyindolacetic acid confirms a diagnosis of diabetes mellitus.

C. Sexual dysfunction, marital problems, and depression are rarely, if ever, seen in patients with diabetes mellitus.

D. Cushing's syndrome never presents as an affective illness.

CHAPTER 11

The Suicidal Patient

page 148

25. In the management of suicidal patients:

A. The physician need not be concerned about malpractice complaints, since it is the patient who takes his own life.

B. In asessing physician culpability in the case of a suicide, the usual procedure of comparing a physician's actions against other practitioners as to whether they would have been able to predict the risk and what steps they might have taken to prevent it is not employed.

C. Physicians and psychotherapists are obligated to carefully and systematically assess the level of suicidal risk in all patients.

D. When a seriously suicidal patient refuses to cooperate with a recommendation of hospitalization in a protective setting, there is nothing a psychiatrist can do since the patient's right to refuse treatment takes precedence over all other considerations.

26. In representative cases involving suicide, liability ws found when:

A. The treating physician had failed to obtain a patient's relevant prior records.

B. There was evidence that a patient who had walked away from a hospital and killed hjimself by jumping in front of a truck could not have been located even if appropriate search procedures had been carried out.

C. A patient had not previously exhibited any suicidal risk.

D. A psychiatrist had never been informed about a specific delusion that a patient believed he could breathe under water.

27. **In assessing a patient with regard to suicide risk, which of the following areas for investigation seems least relevant?**

A. The patient's familiarity with stories of famous people who have attempted suicide

B. Previous suicidal attempts

C. Specific means by which the patient proposes to kill himself and whether he posesses the means

D. Depth of hopelessness and depression

28. **In order to protect patients from self-injury, courts have established that:**

A. Open door policies are no longer tenable.

B. Hospitals and health care professionals are responsible regardless of what measures have been taken to protect the patient, if a significant injury has been sustained.

C. A reasonable balance between protecting the patient and taking intelligent risks to promote treatment and recovery is acceptable.

D. Nursing homes are exempt from malpractice claims.

CHAPTER 12

Management of Suicidal Patients

page 159

29. **The most apparent common denominator of all factors conducive to suicide is:**

A. Age level

B. Family circumstances

C. The level of psychological pain and the patient's ability to tolerate it

D. A recent experience of loss

30. **In the management of the suicidal patient, the therapist should:**
   A. Be active in developing a relationship with the patient.
   B. Assume a more passive and reflective approach to treatment.
   C. Delay the relief of symptoms as a motive for treatment.
   D. Minimize, or avoid contact with, the patient's family.

31. **A high suicide risk patient should usually be hospitalized:**
   A. When he or she has made a recent suicide attempt.
   B. When it is difficult to establish rapport with the patient.
   C. If organic or toxic brain syndrome are present.
   D. All of the above.

32. **If seems preferable to avoid hospitalization for the patient with suicidal ideas who denies intent:**
   A. When the family and patient firmly request hospitalization but are considered manipulative
   B. When the patient assures everyone that a recent suicide attempt was only a "gesture" for attention
   C. When a good relationship exists with the patient and responsible, caring persons are available in his or her environment
   D. When the suicide impulses are part of a bipolar depression reaction

---

CHAPTER 13

Liability Potential for Psychiatrists Who Supervise the Care Given by Other Mental Health Professionals

page 177

33. **You are asked to see a patient receiving counseling from a social worker to evaluate and possibly prescribe antidepressants. Once you take on this responsibility:**
   A. Your relationship to the social worker becomes supervisory and you are ultimately responsible for everything he/she does with the patient.

B. You are essentially a consultant, and your legal liability stops after you make your recommendations, whether or not you prescribe medication.

C. You should spell out for the patient where your responsibilities begin and end—with the initiation and monitoring of medication—and arrange ground rules for ongoing communication with the patient's therapist.

D. You should insist that the patient terminate treatment with the social worker and see you for both psychotherapy and pharmacotherapy.

34. **In the case vignette, Dr. A provides medical backup for patients of a social worker she's never met. One of these patients is distressed and asks to see her because the social worker is away, an exigency not discussed between the professionals beforehand. According to the authors, Dr. A:**

A. Is at risk for a lawsuit based on confused communication in spite of the fact that the patient experiences no damage from this situation.

B. Can fully evaluate the patient and handle the emergency.

C. Should, because of the poor communications, refuse to collaborate on any new patients with the social worker.

D. Should abruptly refuse to continue treating any patients now shared with this social worker and make no provisions for referral to another psychiatrist for drug therapy and monitoring.

35. **Which of the following statements is correct?**

A. Consultation transfers responsibility for a patient to the consultant.

B. A patient can never object to anything that one professional relates to another about him/her if the two are working collaboratively.

C. The signature of a physician places the physician in a legally and ethically responsible status for the action or consequences of the signed document.

D. An academic or hospital staff psychiatrist supervising staff who treat patients cannot be held liable for damages to patients re-

sulting from poor treatment if the staff in question are trainees
or nonmedical professionals.

36. **Which of the following suggestions is not cited by the authors as a way to minimize medicolegal risk in interactions with other mental health professionals?**
    A. Make an effort to do a better job than the other professional(s)
       and hope the patient appreciates it
    B. Choose collaborating clinicians very carefully
    C. Clearly define the roles to be assumed by each party
    D. Assess differing personality styles and perspectives on therapy

CHAPTER 14

Liability Prevention in Psychopharmacology
page 188

37. **Which of the following statements is correct?**
    A. Courts are only concerned with what treatment a doctor ordered, not with the reasons for its choice.
    B. There is no reason for psychiatrists to be up to date in psychopharmacology (or any other treatment modality for that matter) as long as they are skilled in the particular type of therapy that they provide.
    C. The only malpractice claims that have been brought against psychiatrists involve tardive dyskinesia induced by neuroleptics.
    D. Psychiatrists are required to inform patients of all material risks of taking a medication, but not of every conceivable risk.

38. **Which of the following procedures is not always required prior to starting a patient on a psychopharmacologic agent?**
    A. Complete clinical history, with diagnostic and psychopathologic assessment
    B. Complete documentation of treatment decisions
    C. Signed permission from the patient's family
    D. A complete physical examination and appropriate laboratory tests within a reasonable time prior to treatment

39. **Which of the following areas is not cited as a common cause of liability for drug treatment?**
  A. Lack of informed consent
  B. Lack of concomitant psychotherapy
  C. Failure to monitor response to medication properly
  D. Excessive dosages of medication

40. **Which type of information is the psychiatrist not required to point out to a patient who is about to be administered medication?**
  A. The names of all similar drugs, explaining in detail each difference among them
  B. Whether the action of the drug is to treat the disease or to relieve symptoms
  C. Alternative approaches to treatment, if any
  D. An explanation of possible effects on driving and working around machinery

CHAPTER 15

Malpractice in Child and Adolescent Psychiatry
page 206

41. **In the case examples, the events that triggered lawsuits against treating psychiatrists included all but which of the following?**
  A. Assault by another hospitalized patient
  B. Agranulocytosis during the use of barbiturates without sufficient pretreatment warning
  C. Sexual encounter with a seductive patient
  D. Arranging to treat a child without the knowledge of the custodial parent

42. **According to the author, the most frequent medication-related allegations in psychiatric practice involve all of the following except:**
  A. Failure to monitor potential side effects
  B. A psychotic patient discontinuing medications and committing suicide or homicide

C. Side effects arising from combining psychopharmacologic agents

D. Lack of informed consent

43. Which of the following statements is correct?

A. The rule that "the release of information regarding a minor, unemancipated child, or adolescent to persons outside the family requires the agreement of parents or guardians" *does not apply* to giving information to noncustodial parents or managed care companies.

B. The patient's knowledge or permission (depending on age and circumstances) is required before advising the custodial family of such matters as diagnosis, treatment, prognosis, and the like.

C. For young minors, request for information from a third party must be agreed to in writing by both child and parent.

D. As long as the patient is under 18 years of age, there is no need for psychiatrists intending to give medication to obtain his or her informed consent if the parents have already given theirs.

44. Which of the following is not cited as a possible exception to confidentiality:

A. Child abuse

B. Gunshot wounds

C. Court-ordered examinations

D. Severe insomnia

CHAPTER 16

Protecting Others from Violence

page 218

45. The California court decision, which established the responsibility of professionals to act to protect potential victims of viokence, is known as the:

A. Poddar Case

B. Tarasoff Case

C. Powelson Case

D. Tatian Case

46. In the evaluation and management of violent or potentially violent patients:

A. The need for strict confidentiality always prevents the physican from informing anyone of such a risk.

B. A careful assessment of the threat of violence must be carried out before discharge form hospital, and such an evaluation must be diligently recorded.

C. Nonmedical therapists cannot be held liable in the event of violence.

D. The rights of patients to refuse treatment has eliminated all possibility of committing even the most potentially violent patients today.

47. In assessing cases having to do with portection of others, which of the following dimensions will be considered?

A. The existence of a special relationship, such as that between doctor and patient, between the defendant and the dangerous person?

B. An identifiable victim

C. Whether the therapist's evaluation that confidentiality took precedence over the duty to warn was indeed based on reasonable criteria.

D. All of the above

48. Which of the following statements is not correct?

A. A well-trained psychiatrist should be capable of predicting dangerousness per se.

B. Ptaients who are both mentally ill and reveal a clear and present danger of harm to themselves or others are committable.

C. If a formerly hospitalized patient witha history of violence is not compliant with a treatment regimen, the extent to which the psychiatrist must reach out to locate and amange such a case is currently disputable.

D. Before releasing any patient from the hospital with a history of violence, a careful evaluation of the risk should be done and duly recorded.

CHAPTER 17

Tarasoff v. Regents *and the Duty to Protect*

page 243

49. In the *Tarasoff* case, the psychiatrist who was sued:
A. Failed to inform anyone of the patient's dangerousness.
B. Refused to reveal confidential information about the patient during the patient's murder trial.
C. Informed the campus police but failed to inform the victim or the victim's family.
D. Did not even consider the possibility of the patient being dangerous.

50. Which of the following statements is correct about decisions following the *Tarasoff* case?
A. Foreseeable violence might involve a "class of persons at risk."
B. They have been solidly unanimous in their interpretation of that decision.
C. They have made it clear that only psychiatrists can be held responsible in such a situation.
D. They have exempted all cases in which injury or death has resulted from patients driving automobiles while on medication causing side effects.

51. When a therapist encounters a patient who harbors homicidal intent toward a particular person, he or she should:
A. Refer the case to a colleague.
B. Consult a colleague immediately and proceed on a plan to warn the potential victim.
C. Refrain from writing this information down in the record.
D. Notify the American Psychiatric Association Task Force on Violence.

52. Which of the following statements about the Tarasoff ruling is correct?
A. It has been applied only to threats against people, not property.
B. It is unconstitutional because it violates the principle of confidentiality.

C. It creates a climate in which therapists will always react impulsively and warn anyone and everyone should a patient express intense hostility toward a particular person.

D. It creates a climate in which warnings may actually strengthen the therapeutic alliance and be of help to the patient.

CHAPTER 18

Boundary Issues in Psychiatric Treatment

page 261

53. According to the author, the most serious boundary violation in therapy consists of:

A. Using information given by a patient for personal gain.

B. Talking to a patient whom the therapist encounters in a social situation.

C. Sexual involvement.

D. Revealing personal information about oneself to patients.

54. In order to preserve the integrity of the doctor-patient relationship:

A. Boundaries should be crossed only when it will help reassure a patient of the therapist's love and affection.

B. One should be especially alert for patients with a history of childhood abuse or seductive qualities that might threaten to compromise boundaries.

C. One need not be concerned about setting special fees, giving extra time, or being available to patients any time they wish, unless erotic elements are obvious in the transference.

D. Do not turn to patients for help in dealing with one's own problems, unless there is no one else to turn to.

55. Which of the following statements is correct?

A. There have never been reports of sociopathic psychiatrists taking vicious advantage of their patients sexually and otherwise.

B. Most psychiatrists who become involved in serious boundary violations with patients are sociopathic.

C. It's fine for therapists to employ patients (as baby sitters or maids, for example) as long as they pay the minimum wage and social security.

D. Avoiding minor infractions of boundaries on a routine basis will help most therapists to reduce their risk of getting involved in major boundary violations.

56. Which of the following statements is correct?

A. If a psychiatrist begins to have strong and persistent feelings of love for a patient which he/she cannot handle, these should be discussed with an appropriate colleague and referral to another therapist should always be considered.

B. It is unethical for therapists to let patients know anything at all about their personal lives.

C. Psychiatrists should never treat as patients anyone with whom they have any outside contact whatsoever.

D. If a relative of a psychiatrist's friend wishes to see the psychiatrist for treatment, the doctor must refuse or must end his or her friendship.

CHAPTER 19

Sexual Boundary Violations

page 277

57. Which of the following is *not* cited as a result or consequence of sexual intimacies between therapists and clients?

A. Distrust of the opposite sex

B. Serious interference with and possibly outright rejection of further treatment with anyone

C. Much-improved sexual relations

D. Suicidal ideation, guilt, depression, and shame

58. Which of the following statements is correct?

A. Sexual relations between therapist and client are unequivocally permitted long after treatment has ended.

B. Unexpectedly, surveys have shown that wheras 2.5% of men therapists report having had sexual intimacies with one or more clients, the rate is 9.4% for women therapists.

C. Men patients appear to be more likely to combine dependency needs with erotic desires in their relationship with their therapists.

D. Women clients are more likely to eroticize dependency and emotional intimacy needs in therapy than men clients.

59. **Which of the following features is cited as part of the make-up of the "lovesick" therapist?**

A. Strong independence and a tendency to exploit others

B. An altered state of consciousness impairing judgment in the presence of the loved one

C. A lack of feeling and overall numbness

D. Successful social and professional interactions with others

60. **Which type of therapist personality is described as knowing professional standards, suffering from personal distress, showing remorse for unethical behavior, stopping such behavior on his or her own, and commonly seeking consultation from colleagues?**

A. Mildly neurotic

B. Severely neurotic and socially isolated

C. Impulsive character disorder

D. Narcissistic character disorder

CHAPTER 20

Are You liable for Your Patients' Sexual Behavior?

page 289

61. **With Youngberg v. Romero, the U.S. Supreme Court decided that:**

A. The only legal means to seek compensation from professional wrongdoing is by instituting a malpractice suit.

B. A professional can be held liable only when damages stem from a decision that was a substantial departure from accepted professional judgment, practice, or standards in a manner indicating that the practioner did not base his action on a professional judgment.

C. It is permissible for psychiatrists to inform third parties at risk of infection if HIV-positive patients refuse to cease risk-creating behavior or to inform their contacts about their HIV seropositivity.

D. A man who contracted hepatitis had standing to sue his sexual partner's physician, who failed to offer the partner proper advice regarding the need to refrain from intercourse for a certain period.

62. **In the management of patients with AIDS, clinicians should keep in mind that:**

A. A psychiatrist may hospitalize HIV-positive patients involuntarily if they are endangering others, irrespective of such patients' mental status.

B. State statutes do not vary greatly in delineating the circumstances requiring warnings to at-risk third parties.

C. All states require physicians to report AIDS cases to public health authorities.

D. Decisions reached after *Tarasoff* have never found physicians liable for third-party injuries when caused by transmission of an infectious disease.

63. **In the case of the analyst of the psychiatric resident who revealed that he was a pedophile:**

A. A suit was brought against the psychiatric resident's analyst by a boy and his parents who alleged that the resident had sexually assaulted the boy while hospitalized, and the court upheld that the boy had grounds for suit.

B. A suit was brought against the resident's analyst by a boy and his parents who alleged that the resident had sexually assaulted the boy while hospitalized, but the court determined that the boy had no grounds for suit.

C. The resident's analyst was under no obligation to act to prevent the resident from specializing in child psychiatry.

D. The resident's analyst successfully countersued the parents for defamation.

64. Which of the following statements is correct?

A. Administrators and professionals who care for mentally disabled patients are required by law to discuss in explicit detail the patients' sexual behavior and provide adequate guidance for patients and staff members.

B. A patient's ability to consent to sexual interaction is not relevant in determining a hospital caregiver's responsibility for a patient's sexual behavior because the mere fact that the patient is hospitalized establishes lack of ability to consent.

C. Evidence that a clinician or hospital followed a policy regarding sexual behavior among patients suggests action with forethought, which is a powerful argument against a claim of negligence.

D. All of the above

CHAPTER 21

Guidelines to Avoid Liability in Managed Care

page 309

65. The most important step to reduce a physician's risk of malpractice liability is to:

A. Always follow the instructions of a utilization review

B. Always practice according to the "standard of care" in rendering treatment to each patient

C. Never participate in managed care programs, because each doctor can be held liable for the level of practice of all the other physicians

D. All of the above

66. If a physician feels that the decision of the utilization review process is not good for a patient's well being, he or she should:

A. Follow the decision nonetheless.

B. Encourage the patient to immediately initiate a lawsuit against the physician or other professionals who have carried out the review.

C. Go to court to defend his or her treatment recommendations

D. Continue treatment even if payment will not be made and make a second request for support of continued treatment.

67. **Which of the following is not one of the authors' recommendations for the independent practicing physician?**

A. Vigorously challenge or appeal any utilization review denial that conflicts with your medical judgment

B. Document all contacts with utilization reviewers

C. Save money by terminating your own professional liability insurance, because you will inevitably be fully covered by the managed care organization with which you deal

D. Demand to know in writing the basis for any utilization review decision, especially those with which you do not agree

68. **Which of the following is not one of the authors' recommendations for the managed care physician?**

A. Be assured that you will not personally be held liable for any malpractice claims and only the managed care organization for which you work can be sued

B. Carefully review and negotiate any contract that imposes managed care techniques on patient treatment

C. Review all practice protocols and determine the degree to which they conform to the standard of care

D. Review all written materials provided to patient members to ensure no references to "guarantees" or false representation

---

CHAPTER 22

Biopsychosocial Assessment and Management of Violence in the Clinical Setting

page 321

69. **Which of the following statements is correct?**

A. Contrary to popular opinion, mentally ill women are more prone to violence than their male counterparts.

B. Violence is three times more common in chronically mentally ill persons than in those lacking such illness.

C. There is a tendency to underdiagnose psychosis in the assessment of violence, and hence a delay or failure to use antipsychotic medications appropriately.

D. In an emergency room setting, a decision to hospitalize a potentially dangerous patient inevitably intensifies the risk of violence and eliminates any possibility of a therapeutic alliance.

70. **Which of the following statements is correct?**
    A. Violence is never seen among patients with affective disorders.
    B. When lithium is used in non-bipolar patients to reduce mood swings and episodic outbursts of violence, it often need not be given in as high dosages as would be indicated for treating manic-depressive disorder.
    C. Anticonvulsants such as carbamazepine or valproic acid have no place in the management of violent patients regardless of diagnosis.
    D. Sharp rises in blood pressure frequently induced by the drug propranolol preclude its use in violent patients.

71. **Violent patients:**
    A. Seem particularly sensitive to being insulted and particularly vulnerable to feelings of shame and humiliation
    B. Respond best when managed in a strongly authoritarian way
    C. Respond best when managed in a strongly permissive way
    D. Are rarely amenable to exploring underlying issues giving rise to violence, such as the inability to handle hostile or depressive feelings

72. **Which of the following is not cited in the lesson as a potential trigger for violence in institutionalized patients?**
    A. Boredom and inactivity
    B. Individual or group therapy designed to help them learn new ways to deal with provocative situations
    C. Conflictual dependency longings, especially in an all-male environment
    D. Sexual tensions

CHAPTER 23

The Assessment of Violence in the Workplace and its Legal Ramifications

page 332

73. **Risk factors for violence include:**
    A. Age higher than 45 years
    B. Female gender
    C. High IQ
    D. Prior criminal history

74. **Which of the following statements is correct?**
    A. According to Monahan, data suggest a relationship between mental disorders and violent behavior.
    B. Persecutory delusions are less likely to be acted on violently than other types of delusions.
    C. Psychotic patients with command hallucinations are at reduced risk for violence.
    D. Organic brain dysfunction does not predispose to violence.

75. **The typical perpetrator of lethal violence in the workplace is a man who:**
    A. Is under 30 years of age.
    B. Has been or believes he is about to be fired or laid off.
    C. Perceives that he has been treated with more respect than he deserves.
    D. Has never identified much with his job.

76. **Which of the following is not listed as a recommendation to reduce the risk of malpractice in dealing with a potentially violent employee?**
    A. Keep current in your knowledge of the literature regarding assessment of the risk of violence.
    B. Before an employee evaluation, clearly inform the employee of the limits of confidentiality.
    C. Closely monitor the work of supervisees who evaluate or treat potentially violent employees.
    D. Be prepared to offer the employer an intelligent opinion about a worker's potential for violence based on information provided by the employer when an interview of the employee cannot be arranged.

INDEX